Pocket Nurse Guide to
Drugs

Pocket Nurse Guide to Drugs

Julia B. Clark, Ph.D.

Professor of Pharmacology,
Indiana University School of Medicine,
Department of Pharmacology and Toxicology
Indianapolis, Indiana

Sherry F. Queener, Ph.D.

Professor of Pharmacology,
Indiana University School of Medicine,
Department of Pharmacology and Toxicology
Indianapolis, Indiana

Virginia Burke Karb, M.S.N., R.N.

Associate Professor,
School of Nursing,
University of North Carolina at Greensboro,
Greensboro, North Carolina

Coordinating Editor
Thomas A. Lochhaas

The C. V. Mosby Company

St. Louis • Toronto • Princeton   1986

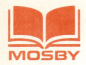

A TRADITION OF PUBLISHING EXCELLENCE

Editor Nancy L. Mullins
Assistant Editor Maureen Slaten
Designer Diane M. Beasley
Production Publication Services

Cover photograph © G. Robert Bishop 1985

Copyright © 1986 by The C.V. Mosby Company

All rights reserved. No part of this publication may be reproduced, stored in a retrieval system, or transmitted, in any form or by any means, electronic, mechanical, photocopying, recording, or otherwise, without prior written permission from the publisher.

Printed in the United States of America

The C.V. Mosby Company
11830 Westline Industrial Drive, St. Louis, Missouri 63146

Library of Congress Cataloging-in-Publication Data

Clark, Julia B.
  Pocket nurse guide to drugs.

  Includes index.
  1. Drugs—Handbooks, manuals, etc. 2. Nursing—Handbooks, manuals, etc. I. Queener, Sherry F.
II. Karb, Virginia Burke. III. Lochhaas, Thomas A.
IV. Title. [DNLM: 1. Drugs—handbooks. 2. Drugs—nurses' instruction. QV 39 C593p]
RM300.C512 1986   615'.1   85-28432
ISBN 0-8016-1013-3

TY/RRD/RRD 9 8 7 6 5 4 3 2 01/C/087

Consultant Board

Barbara Carruthers
Coordinator
First Year Nursing
Health Sciences Division
Humber College
North Campus
Ontario, Canada

Bonnie Klank, Pharm.D.
Drug Information Center
Pharmacy Department
Indiana University Hospitals
Indianapolis, Indiana

Kay See-Lasley, M.S., R.Ph.
Medical Editorial Consultant
Writer/Consultant Medicine and Christian Literature
Christian Pharmacy Fellowship International
Board Member
Chairman of Missions
Lawrence, Kansas

Katherine Stefos, Ph.D., R.Ph.
Adjunct Associate Professor
School of Nursing
University of Texas
Houston, Texas

Lynn Roger Willis, Ph.D.
Professor of Pharmacology and Medicine
Department of Pharmacology and Toxicology
Indiana University School of Medicine
Indianapolis, Indiana

Preface

The *Pocket Nurse Guide to Drugs* is intended as a ready reference in the clinical setting, offering immediate information in a concise format. Brevity is achieved by minimizing discussion or extensive explanation of individual agents. Properties of classes of drugs are presented and discussed as necessary for clarity; individual agents appear in summary tables. The *Pocket Nurse Guide to Drugs* is not intended to replace a textbook of pharmacology, where greater depth of coverage on any individual agent is available.

The guide is divided into eleven units: central nervous system drugs (nine chapters), sensory system drugs (two chapters), cardiovascular system drugs (nine chapters), gastrointestinal system drugs (six chapters), respiratory system drugs (three chapters), body defense system drugs (five chapters), endocrine system drugs (four chapters), female reproductive system drugs (five chapters), male reproductive system drugs (two chapters), antiinfective agents (four chapters), and antineoplastics (five chapters). These units conform to useful clinical groupings.

Within each chapter, a consistent format is used to make finding material quite easy. Chapters begin with an alphabetic listing of drugs included. Following the list of drugs, there are overviews of the class of drugs covered in the chapter: general actions, general side effects, and general nursing implications. After the overview, groups of drugs within the classes are summarized under the following headings: drug group (alphabetic list), actions, indications, nurse alert, administration (summarized in tabular form), side effects, and nursing implications. The section entitled "Nurse alert" contains information on contraindications of the agents; "Nursing implications" contains information on the proper nursing activities associated with the use of the agents.

Five appendixes complete the *Pocket Nurse Guide to Drugs*. These appendixes summarize reference information. They include lists of common, clinically important drug interactions; vaccines; and physical symptoms produced by common poisons; charts showing conversion of units; and tables of abbreviations.

Julia B. Clark
Sherry F. Queener
Virginia Burke Karb

Contents

Part I Central Nervous System Drugs 1

1 Sedative-hypnotics, Antianxiety Agents, and Anti-Alcohol Agents 2

Barbiturates 5
Nurse Alert for Barbiturates 5
Benzodiazepines 11
Nurse Alert for Benzodiazepines 16
Other Sedative-hypnotics and Antianxiety Drugs 17
Nurse Alert for Other Sedative-hypnotic and Antianxiety Agents 18
Antialcohol Agent 19
Nurse Alert for Disulfiram 21

2 Antipsychotic Drugs 24

Nurse Alert for Antipsychotics 25

3 Antidepressant Drugs 43

Tricyclic Antidepressants 43
Nurse Alert for Tricyclic Antidepressants 44
Second Generation Antidepressants 48
Nurse Alert for Second Generation Antidepressants 49
MAO Inhibitors 49
Nurse Alert for MAO Inhibitors 50
Lithium 51
Nurse Alert for Lithium 52

4 Central Nervous System Stimulants 54

CNS Stimulants for Narcolepsy and Hyperkinesis 56

Contents   ix

Nurse Alert for CNS Stimulants for
   Narcolepsy and Hyperkinesis 57
CNS Stimulants to Suppress Appetite 63
Nurse Alert for CNS Stimulants for Appetite
   Suppression 63
CNS Stimulants for Respiratory
   Stimulation 66
Nurse Alert for CNS Stimulants for
   Respiratory Stimulation 68

5   Narcotic Analgesics and Antagonists 71

Narcotic Analgesics 71
Nurse Alert for Narcotic Analgesics 72
Narcotic Antagonists 80
Nurse Alert for Narcotic Antagonists 82

6   General Anesthetics 83

Inhalation Anesthetics 83
Nurse Alert for Inhalation Anesthetics 84
Intravenous Anesthetics 86
Nurse Alert for Intravenous Anesthetics 87

7   Anticonvulsants 91

Nurse Alert for Anticonvulsants 91

**8   Drugs for Central Motor Control: Parkinsonism
and Spasm 108**

Drugs for Parkinsonism 108
Nurse Alert for Drugs for Parkinsonism 109
Centrally Acting Skeletal Muscle
   Relaxants 116
Nurse Alert for Centrally Acting Skeletal
   Muscle Relaxants 117

9   Neuromuscular Drugs 122

Acetylcholinesterase Inhibitors 122

x   Pocket Nurse Guide to Drugs

Nurse Alert for Acetylcholinesterase
Inhibitors 123
Neuromuscular Blocking Drugs 128
Nurse Alert for Neuromuscular Blocking
Drugs 129

Part II Sensory System Drugs 135

10   Drugs Affecting the Eye 136

Drugs for Mydriasis and Cycloplegia 136
Nurse Alert for Anticholinergic Drugs 137
Drugs Used to Treat Glaucoma 141
Nurse Alert for Drugs for Glaucoma 145

11   Local Anesthetics 148

Nurse Alert for Local Anesthetics 149

Part III Cardiovascular System Drugs 155

12   Drugs to Improve Circulation 156

Sympathomimetics for Hypotension
and Shock 156
Nurse Alert for Sympathomimetics for
Hypotension and Shock 157
Antianginal Drugs 164
Nurse Alert for Antianginal Drugs 165
Vasodilators for Peripheral Vascular
Disease 171
Nurse Alert for Vasodilators for Peripheral
Vascular Disease 172

13   Antihypertensive Drugs 176

Nurse Alert for Antihypertensive Drugs 180

14   Diuretics 203

Loop Diuretics 206
Nurse Alert for Loop Diuretics 206
Thiazide and Related Diuretics 211

Contents **xi**

Nurse Alert for Thiazide Diuretics 211
Potassium-sparing Diuretics 216
Nurse Alert for Potassium-sparing
    Diuretics 216
Carbonic Anhydrase Inhibitors 218
Nurse Alert for Carbonic Anhydrase
    Inhibitors 219
Osmotic Diuretics 222
Nurse Alert for Osmotic Diuretics 222
Organomercurials 224
Nurse Alert for Organomercurials 226

15 **Cardiotonic Drugs: Cardiac Glycosides and Drugs for Congestive Heart Failure 228**

Nurse Alert for Cardiac Glycosides 229

16 **Fluids and Electrolytes 236**

Nurse Alert for Fluid and Electrolyte
    Therapy 237

17 **Antiarrhythmic Drugs 252**

Nurse Alert for Antiarrhythmic Drugs 253

18 **Anticoagulant, Thrombolytic, and Hemostatic Drugs 270**

Anticoagulants 270
Nurse Alert for Anticoagulants 271
Thrombolytics 277
Nurse Alert for Thrombolytics 278
Hemostatic Agents 279
Nurse Alert for Hemostatic Agents 282

19 **Antilipemics 285**

Nurse Alert for Antilipemics 287

20 **Drugs to Treat Nutritional Anemias 291**

Iron Deficiency Anemia 291
Nurse Alert for Drugs for Iron
    Deficiency Anemias 294

xii Pocket Nurse Guide to Drugs

Megaloblastic Macrocytic Anemias 296
Nurse Alert for Drugs for Megaloblastic
Macrocytic Anemias 296

Part IV Gastrointestinal System Drugs 299

21 Drugs Affecting Motility and Tone 300

Nurse Alert for Drugs Affecting Motility and
Tone 301

22 Drugs to Treat Ulcers 310

Nurse Alert for Drugs to Treat Ulcers 311

23 Antiemetic Drugs 316

Nurse Alert for Antiemetic Drugs 317

24 Antidiarrheal Drugs 326

Nurse Alert for Antidiarrheal Drugs 326

25 Laxatives and Cathartics 329

Nurse Alert for Laxatives and Cathartics 330

26 Digestants 338

Nurse Alert for Digestants 338

Part V Respiratory System Drugs 341

27 Bronchodilators and Other Drugs for Asthma 342

Adrenergic Bronchodilators 342
Nurse Alert for Adrenergic
Bronchodilators 348
Xanthines 350
Nurse Alert for Xanthines 351
Other Drugs to Treat Asthma 354
Nurse Alert for Other Drugs to Treat
Asthma 356

28 Nasal Decongestants 358

Nurse Alert for Nasal Decongestants 358

Contents **xiii**

29 Drugs to Treat a Cough 362

Nurse Alert for Anticough Drugs 363

Part VI Body Defense System Drugs 369

30 Nonnarcotic Analgesic-antipyretic Drugs 370

Nurse Alert for Analgesic-antipyretic Drugs 371

31 Antihistamines for Allergic Reactions 375

Nurse Alert for Antihistamines for Allergic Reactions 376

32 Nonsteroidal Antiinflammatory Drugs 382

Nurse Alert for Nonsteroidal Antiinflammatory Drugs 383

33 Antirheumatoid Drugs 390

Nurse Alert for Antirheumatoid Drugs 390

34 Drugs for Gout 395

Nurse Alert for Drugs for Gout 395

Part VII Endocrine System Drugs 401

35 Drugs Affecting the Pituitary Gland 402

Neurohypophyseal Hormones for Diabetes Insipidus 403
Nurse Alert for Neurohypophyseal Hormones 404
Adenohypophyseal Hormones 408

36 Adrenal Steroids and Other Drugs Affecting the Adrenal Gland 412

Nurse Alert for Adrenal Steroids 416

37 Antidiabetic Agents 426

Insulin Preparations 426
Nurse Alert for Insulin Preparations 426

xiv Pocket Nurse Guide to Drugs

Oral Hypoglycemic Agents 435
Nurse Alert for Oral Hypoglycemic
Agents 435

38 Drugs Affecting the Thyroid and Parathyroid
Glands 438

Drugs for Hypothyroidism 438
Nurse Alert for Drugs for Hypothyroidism 439
Drugs for Hyperthyroidism 443
Nurse Alert for Drugs for Hyper-
thyroidism 444
Drugs to Alter Calcium Metabolism 448
Nurse Alert for Drugs Affecting Calcium
Metabolism 449

Part VIII Female Reproductive System Drugs 453

39 Estrogens 454
Nurse Alert for Estrogens 455

40 Progestins 462
Nurse Alert for Progestins 462

41 Fertility Agents 465
Nurse Alert for Fertility Agents 465

42 Oral Contraceptives 469
Nurse Alert for Oral Contraceptives 469

43 Oxytocic Drugs 478
Nurse Alert for Oxytocic Drugs 479

Part IX Male Reproductive System Drugs 483

44 Androgens 484
Nurse Alert for Androgens 484

45 Anabolic Steroids 489
Nurse Alert for Anabolic Steroids 492

Contents   xv

Part X Antiinfective Agents 495

46 Antibiotics 496

Penicillins 498
Nurse Alert for Penicillins 499
Cephalosporins 505
Nurse Alert for Cephalosporins 509
Penicillin Substitutes 511
Nurse Alert for Penicillin Substitutes 515
Tetracyclines 518
Nurse Alert for Tetracyclines 520
Chloramphenicols 521
Nurse Alert for Chloramphenicol 522
Aminoglycosides 523
Nurse Alert for Aminoglycosides 526
Polymyxins 532
Nurse Alert for Polymyxins 532
Sulfonamides 534
Other Drugs for Urinary Tract
    Infections 541
Nurse Alert for Other Drugs for Urinary Tract
    Infections 541
Antituberculosis Drugs 544
Nurse Alert for Antituberculosis Drugs 545
Antileprosy Drugs 550

47 Antifungal Agents 552

Drugs for Systemic Fungal Infections 552
Nurse Alert for Drugs for Systemic
    Fungal Infections 553
Drugs for Topical Fungal Infections 558
Nurse Alert for Drugs for Topical
    Fungal Infections 558

48 Antiviral Agents 562

Nurse Alert for Antiviral Agents 563

49 Antiparasitic Agents 569

Nurse Alert for Antiparasitic Agents 576

xvi Pocket Nurse Guide to Drugs

Part XI Antineoplastics 585

50 Anticancer Drugs: Drugs that Directly Attack DNA 586

Nurse Alert for Drugs that Directly Attack DNA 587

51 Anticancer Drugs: Drugs that Block DNA Synthesis 596

Nurse Alert for Drugs that Block DNA Synthesis 597

52 Anticancer Drugs: Drugs that Block RNA and Protein Synthesis 602

Nurse Alert for Drugs that Block RNA and Protein Synthesis 603

53 Anticancer Drugs: Drugs that Block Mitosis 607

Nurse Alert for Drugs that Block Mitosis 607

54 Drugs to Control Cancer of Specific Tissues 611

Nurse Alert for Drugs to Control Cancer of Specific Tissues 612

Appendix A Representative Common Drug Interactions 619

Appendix B Vaccines Useful in Preventing Bacterial or Rickettsial Diseases 637

Appendix C Physical Symptoms Produced by Common Poisons 640

Appendix D Common Conversions 644

Appendix E Abbreviations 646

Generic Drug Index 649

Trade Name Index 666

General Index 682

Pocket Nurse Guide to
Drugs

CENTRAL NERVOUS SYSTEM DRUGS

PART

I

Sedative-hypnotics, Antianxiety Agents, and Anti-Alcohol Agents

1

Barbiturates
  Amobarbital
  Butabarbital
  Pentobarbital
  Phenobarbital
  Secobarbital
Benzodiazepines
  Alprazolam
  Chlorazepate
  Chlordiazepoxide
  Diazepam
  Flurazepam
  Halazepam
  Lorazepam
  Oxazepam
  Prazepam
  Temazepam
  Triazolam

Other sedative-hypnotics and antianxiety drugs
  Chloral hydrate
  Triclofos sodium
  Methyprylon
  Ethchlorvynol
  Ethinamate
  Glutethimide
  Hydroxyzine hydrochloride
  Hydroxyzine pamoate
  Meprobamate
Antialcohol agent
  Disulfiram

General Actions of Sedative-hypnotics and Antianxiety Agents

All of these drugs act pharmacologically as general depressants of the central nervous system. They depress the reticular activity of the brain stem, thus decreasing the general level of arousal. The stage and degree of depression are dose dependent.

General Side Effects of Sedative-hypnotics and Antianxiety Agents

Continued administration of general CNS depressants can cause drug dependence and tolerance, including cross tolerance among different sedative-hypnotics, antianxiety agents, and alcohol. Withdrawal symptoms occur with cessation after dependence is established.

General Nursing Implications for Sedative-hypnotics and Antianxiety Agents

- Patients should be instructed to take their medications only as directed and not to increase the dose without prior physician approval.
- Caution patients to keep all health care providers informed of all medications they are taking, so that inadvertent drug interactions can be avoided.
- Caution patients to avoid the use of alcohol.
- Use with caution in patients with chronic respiratory diseases such as chronic obstructive pulmonary disease, emphysema, and chronic bronchitis.
- Urge patients to seek appropriate therapy for anxiety or insomnia and not to rely on the drugs alone.
- Any of the CNS depressants can produce drowsiness, so these drugs should not be taken prior to driving, operating machinery, or engaging in other activities requiring mental alertness unless it is known that the patient can tolerate the particular dose of medication. Individual patient assessment should be done. The elderly may not subjectively recognize sedation or decreased mental performance.
- Health care providers should be alert to patients who return for prescription refills on an increasingly frequent basis, because this may indicate improper use or abuse of the particular requested drug. Depressed patients should be evaluated carefully for possible suicidal tendencies.
- The usual dose of the medications should be reduced in the elderly, the debilitated, or those with known liver or renal disease.

Pocket Nurse Guide to Drugs

- Paradoxical restlessness, agitation, or even rage can occasionally occur with some of the drugs. If an unanticipated reaction occurs, the patient and family should be instructed to seek medical assistance.
- As with all medications, patients should be reminded not to "share" drugs with friends or family.
- Patients should be reminded to keep these and all medications out of the reach of children. Childproof caps should be used on medications.
- Instruct patients not to keep these drugs on the nightstand or any other place where the patient could accidentally repeat a dose of medication if awakened during the night.
- Hospitalized patients receiving any sleeping medication should have the siderails up during the night, and the patients should be instructed to call for assistance before getting up during the night. Keeping a night-light on in the room may be helpful to some patients. Report any symptoms of confusion or disorientation in the patient that occur during the night; these symptoms may indicate a need to change drugs or dosages.
- Being hospitalized is stressful to most individuals, and for this reason, many physicians prescribe some form of sleeping medication that the patient may take as needed, once or twice per night. The patient should not be denied needed medication, but on the other hand, patients should not automatically be given the sleeping medication without individual assessment. A back rub, a small snack, a glass of warm milk, or other aids to sleep may be more effective than medications in promoting sleep in some individuals.
- With chronic use, some of the medications may produce changes in libido or sexual activity. Careful questioning of the patient may reveal this problem; it may justify changing the patient to a different medication.
- The medications are generally not recommended for use during pregnancy or during lactation. Some women may wish to consider using birth control measures while taking these medications. If a woman suspects she may be pregnant, she should consult her physician immediately.

Barbiturates

| Amobarbital | Pentobarbital | Secobarbital |
| Butabarbital | Phenobarbital | |

Actions of Barbiturates

Barbiturates cause a spectrum of CNS depression ranging from sedation to anesthesia and are classified according to the duration of their depressant actions: ultra short-acting, short-acting, intermediate-acting, and long-acting.

Indications for Barbiturates

Amobarbital is used for daytime sedation, preanesthetic sedation, and hypnosis. *Butabarbital* is used for sedation or for insomnia when the need is to prolong sleep rather than induce sleep. *Pentobarbital* is used mainly for insomnia and preanesthetic sedation, and occasionally for daytime sedation. *Phenobarbital* is used as a sedative. See Chapter 7 for use as an anticonvulsant. *Secobarbital* is used mainly for insomnia and preanesthetic sedative.

Nurse Alert for Barbiturates

- Barbiturates are widely abused because of their euphoric effects.
- Secobarbital, pentobarbital, and amobarbital are Schedule II controlled drugs, butabarbital is a Schedule III drug, and phenobarbital and mephobarbital are Schedule IV drugs.
- Withdrawal symptoms in a dependent patient are severe and begin within 24 hours after the last dose of the barbiturate. They include grand mal seizures, delirium, fever, coma, and, rarely, death.
- Barbiturates have an additive effect with other general CNS depressants and are potentiated by antipsychotic drugs and narcotic analgesics; barbiturates administered for insomnia must be given at least 8 hours before major tranquilizers, narcotic analgesics, or general anesthetics are given to a patient undergoing surgery.

Text continued on p. 10

Table 1-1 Administration of barbiturates

Generic Name	Trade Name	Dosage and Administration	Duration
Amobarbital*	Amytal† Isobec‡	ORAL: *Adult*—as sedative 50 to 300 mg daily in divided doses; as hypnotic, 65 to 200 mg at bedtime. *Children*—as sedative, 6 mg/kg body weight in 3 divided doses.	An intermediate-acting barbiturate that acts like a short-acting barbiturate in humans.
Butabarbital	Butalan Buticaps Butisol Sodium† Day-Barb‡ Neo-Barb‡	ORAL: *Adult*—as sedative, 50 to 120 mg/day in 3 or 4 divided doses; as hypnotic, 50 to 100 mg at bedtime. *Children*—as sedative, 6 mg/kg body weight in 3 divided doses daily.	An intermediate-acting barbiturate.
Pentobarbital*	Nembutal† Novopentobarb‡ Pentogen‡	ORAL: *Adults*—as sedative, 30 mg 3 or 4 times daily or 100 mg in timed-release form in the morning; as hypnotic, 100 mg at bedtime. *Children*—as sedative, 6 mg/kg in 3 divided doses daily. RECTAL: *Adults*—120 to 200 mg for sedation or hypnosis.	A short-acting barbiturate.

		Children—as sedative, 30 to 120 mg daily. INTRAMUSCULAR: *Adults*—as hypnotic, 150 to 200 mg. INTRAVENOUS: *Adults*—as hypnotic, 100 mg. After 1 min, can administer small increments, but no more than 500 mg total. *Children*—as hypnotic, 50 mg initially. Can administer small increments after 1 min if necessary.	
Phenobarbital*	Luminal† Solfoton PBR/.2 Barbita	ORAL: *Adults*—as sedative, 30 to 120 mg daily in 2 or 3 divided doses; as hypnotic, 100 to 320 mg at bedtime. *Children*—as sedative, 6 mg/kg daily in 4 divided doses.	A long-acting barbiturate.

cont'd. next page

*Also available as the sodium salt. Only the sodium salt is suitable for administration as a solution by the rectal, intramuscular, or intravenous route.
†Available in U.S. and Canada
‡Available in Canada only

Table 1-1   Administration of barbiturtates—cont'd.

Generic Name	Trade Name	Dosage and Administration	Duration
Phenobarbital—cont'd.		INTRAMUSCULAR, INTRAVENOUS: *Adults*—as sedative, 30 to 120 mg; as hypnotic, 100 to 320 mg, with no more than 100 mg (2 ml of 5% solution) per minute IV. RECTAL: *Children*—as sedative, 6 mg/kg daily divided in 3 doses.	
Secobarbital*	Novosecobarb‡ Secogen Sodium‡ Seconal† Seconal Sodium†	ORAL: *Adults*—as sedative, 30 to 50 mg; as hypnotic, 100 to 200 mg at bedtime; for preoperative sedation, 200 to 300 mg 1 to 2 hr before surgery. *Children*—as sedative, 6 mg/kg body weight in 3 divided doses; for preoperative sedation, 50 to 100 mg 1 to 2 hrs before surgery.	A short-acting barbiturate. Not indicated for repeated use because tolerance develops, rebound insomnia becomes marked, and the addiction potential is high.

RECTAL: *Adults*—120 to 200 mg
as required for sedation or
hypnosis. *Children*—15 to 120
mg
INTRAMUSCULAR: *Adults*—as
hypnotic, 100 to 200 mg.
Children—as hypnotic, 3 to 5
mg/kg body weight, up to 100
mg.
INTRAVENOUS: *Adults*—as
hypnotic, 50 to 250 mg; inject
only 50 mg in 15 sec.

*Also available as the sodium salt. Only the sodium salt is suitable for administration as a solution by the rectal, intramuscular, or intravenous route.
†Available in U.S. and Canada
‡Available in Canada only

Side Effects of Barbiturates

Barbiturates may cause allergic reactions including rashes, skin changes, and photosensitivity. Barbiturates suppress REM sleep and are not effective as hypnotics after 3 weeks. Drowsiness generally occurs. Acute overdose causes respiratory depression, tachycardia, hypotension, and shock, potentially leading to coma and death from respiratory and cardiovascular collapse. Mild withdrawal symptoms include nightmares, daytime agitation, and a "shaky" feeling.

Nursing Implications for Barbiturates

- Individuals taking phenobarbital for its anticonvulsant activity may find the drowsiness produced to be troublesome. With continued use, tolerance to the drowsiness will usually develop.
- The barbiturates have no analgesic properties and should not be substituted for analgesics in the patient with pain. In the presence of pain the barbiturates may produce paradoxical restlessness and excitement. If used concomitantly with narcotic analgesics, the dose of barbiturate may need to be reduced because both groups of drugs cause CNS depression.
- The hangover effect seen with many barbiturates is a side effect of the medication and not an indication for increasing the dose the next night to "sleep better."
- The barbiturates increase the metabolism of the tricyclic antidepressants, corticosteroids, digitoxin, phenothiazines, quinidine, doxycycline, oral anticoagulants, and phenytoin, so the dose of any of these medications may need to be increased while the patient is taking barbiturates.
- Patients should be carefully assessed for suicide potential before barbiturates are prescribed. In addition, large quantities of the prescribed drug should not be dispensed to avoid potentially fatal overdose.
- Intravenous barbiturates: The intravenous route is used infrequently, except in surgery. Administer the prescribed drug slowly, observing the patient carefully for respiratory

Sedative-hypnotics, Antianxiety Agents, and Anti-Alcohol Agents **11**

depression, which might result in apnea, and for vasodilation, which might produce shock. Monitor the pulse and blood pressure carefully. Use only in a setting where supportive emergency care is available. For instructions regarding dilution and rate of administration, see the manufacturer's literature.

- Agranulocytosis and thrombocytopenia occur rarely. Instruct patients to report a fever, sore throat, malaise, easy bruising, or unexplained bleeding.
- Symptoms of barbiturate overdose include ataxia, decreased level of consciousness or mental dullness, nystagmus, and respiratory depression. Eventually coma will develop. Treatment should be supportive and should involve respiratory assistance as needed, intravenous fluids, appropriate drugs to correct cardiovascular difficulties, and oxygen. Dialysis may be used if necessary.

Benzodiazepines

Alprazolam	Flurazepam	Prazepam
Chlorazepate	Halazepam	Temazepam
Chlordiazepoxide	Lorazepam	Triazolam
Diazepam	Oxazepam	

Actions of Benzodiazepines

The benzodiazepines have actions similar to other general CNS depressants but with fewer problems associated with overdose or side effects.

Indications for Benzodiazepines

Alprazolam, chlorazepate, halazepam, oxazepam, and *prazepam* are used to treat anxiety. *Chlordiazepoxide* is used to treat anxiety and alcohol withdrawal. *Diazepam* is used to treat anxiety, severe muscle spasm, status epilepticus, acute alcohol withdrawal symptoms, and for sedation. *Flurazepam* and *temazepam* are used only as hypnotics. *Lorazepam* is used to treat anxiety and insomnia. *Triazolam* is used as a hypnotic, antianxiety agent, and anticonvulsant.

Text continued on p. 16

Table 1-2 Administration of benzodiazepines

Generic Name	Trade Name	Dosage and Administration	Duration
Alprazolam	Xanax*	ORAL: *Adults*—0.25 to 0.5 mg 3 times daily; Maximum daily dose: 4 mg. *Elderly*—0.25 mg 2 or 3 times daily.	Metabolites are only weakly active.
Chlorazepate	Tranxene* Azene*	ORAL: *Adults*—13 to 60 mg divided into 2 to 4 doses or at bedtime. *Elderly*—6.5 to 15 mg daily.	Half-life is 30 to 200 hr. Metabolites are active.
Chlordiazepoxide	A-Poxide Apo-Chlordiaz-epoxide† Libritabs Librium* Medilium† Relaxil† Trilium† SK-Lygen Murcil Sereen Reposams .10	ORAL: *Adults*—for anxiety, 15 to 100 mg divided in 3 to 4 doses or in 1 dose at bedtime. *Elderly*—5 mg 2 to 4 times daily. *Children*—0.5 mg/kg body weight daily in 3 to 4 doses. May be given IM. INTRAVENOUS: *Adults*—for alcohol withdrawal, 50 to 100 mg slowly over at least 1 min, then 25 to 50 mg every 6 to 8 hr, with the total dose not more than 300 mg.	Half-life is 24 to 48 hr. Metabolites are active. The hydrochloride salt is used for injection.

| Diazepam | Apo-Diazepam†
 E-Pam†
 Meval†
 Novodipam†
 Valium*
 Valrelease | ORAL: *Adults*—4 to 40 mg divided into 2 to 4 doses or a single dose of 2.5 to 10 mg at bedtime. *Elderly*—2 to 2.5 mg once or twice daily. *Children*—0.12 to 0.8 mg/kg daily in 3 to 4 doses.
 INTRAVENOUS: administer no more than 5 mg/min. For severe anxiety, severe muscle spasm, status epilepticus, or recurrent seizures: *Adults*—5 to 10 mg initially, repeated in 3 to 4 hr if needed. *Children*—0.04 to 0.2 mg/kg initially; repeat in 3 to 4 hr if necessary. Sedation for cardioversion or endoscopic procedures: *Adults*—10 to 20 mg as required. For acute alcohol withdrawal symptoms: *Adults*—5 to 20 mg in 3 to 4 hr if necessary. | Half-life is 48 to 200 hr. Metabolites are active. |

cont'd. next page

*Available in U.S. and Canada
†Available in Canada only

Table 1-2 Administration of benzodiazepines—cont'd.

Generic Name	Trade Name	Dosage and Administration	Duration
Flurazepam	Apo-Flurazepam† Dalmane* Novoflupam†	ORAL: *Adults*—as hypnotic, 15 to 30 mg at bedtime. *Elderly*—15 mg.	Onset: 20 to 45 min. Duration: 7 to 8 hr. Active metabolite is formed with a half-life of 47 to 100 hr, so repeated use leads to cumulation of this metabolite and may impair daytime activity.
Halazepam	Paxipam	ORAL: *Adults*—20 to 40 mg 3 or 4 times daily. *Elderly*—Reduce dose to 20 mg 1 or 2 times daily.	Active metabolite with a long half-life.
Lorazepam	Ativan*	ORAL: *Adults*—for anxiety, 1 to 2 mg 2 to 3 times daily, may increase dose to 10 mg maximum daily; as hypnotic, 2 to 4 mg at bedtime. *Elderly*—½ adult dose. INTRAMUSCULAR: 0.5 mg/kg INTRAVENOUS: 0.044 mg/kg, max 2 mg, administered 15 min prior to surgery for sedation.	Half-life is 15 hr so there is little cumulation. Metabolites are inactive.

Oxazepam	Apo-Oxazepam† Ox-Pam† Serax*	ORAL: *Adults*—for anxiety, 30 to 120 mg daily in 3 to 4 doses. *Elderly*—30 mg in 3 divided doses, increased if necessary to 45 to 60 mg.	Half-life is 3 to 21 hr, so there is little cumulation. Metabolites are inactive.
Prazepam	Centrax	ORAL: *Adults*—20 mg in a single dose, increased to 40 to 60 mg daily in divided doses or once at bedtime. *Elderly*—10 to 15 mg.	Half-life is 30 to 200 hr. Metabolites are active.
Temazepam	Restoril	ORAL: *Adults*—30 mg at bedtime. *Elderly*—reduce dose to 15 mg for elderly patients.	Slowly absorbed. Metabolites are inactive.
Triazolam	Halcion	ORAL: *Adults*—0.25 to 0.5 mg at bedtime. *Elderly*—reduce dose to 0.25 mg for elderly patients.	Metabolites are inactive.

*Available in U.S. and Canada
†Available in Canada only

Nurse Alert for Benzodiazepines

- Benzodiazepines are Schedule IV drugs.
- If dependence occurs, withdrawal symptoms will occur, including depression, insomnia, nightmares, agitation, and psychological distress, lasting up to 6 weeks.
- The sedative effect of benzodiazepines is increased by other CNS depressants, tricyclic antidepressants, alcohol, narcotic analgesics, antipsychotics, and antihistamines.
- Benzodiazepines are contraindicated for women in labor and nursing mothers.
- Benzodiazepines may make glaucoma worse.

Side Effects of Benzodiazepines

Common side effects include daytime sedation, ataxia, dizziness, and headaches; tolerance to these effects develops quickly. The elderly are more likely to experience these to a disabling degree. Less common side effects include blurred or double vision, hypotension, tremor, amnesia, slurred speech, urinary incontinence, and constipation. Jaundice has occasionally been reported.

Nursing Implications for Benzodiazepines

- Benzodiazepines should be used with caution in patients with renal impairment. Urinary retention may occur; monitor the fluid intake and output.
- Blood dyscrasias have been reported in long-term therapy. Instruct the patient to report any sore throat, fever, malaise, jaundice, bruising, or bleeding tendencies.
- Gastrointestinal symptoms may be reduced by taking the medication with meals, immediately after eating, or with a small snack.
- Cimetidine (Tagamet) potentiates the sedative effects of diazepam; the dose of the latter may have to be reduced.
- After long-term therapy, even at relatively low doses, the benzodiazepines should be discontinued slowly. Review with patients the possible withdrawal symptoms and instruct the patient to report signs of withdrawal to the physician. It may be necessary to slow the rate at which the drug is being

Sedative-hypnotics, Antianxiety Agents, and Anti-Alcohol Agents

discontinued. Instruct patients on long-term therapy not to discontinue the drug without physician approval.

- Although overdose with a single preparation of the benzodiazepines may not be fatal, patients who choose to attempt suicide by drug overdose often consume many different drugs and/or alcohol in their attempt. The combined effect of many CNS depressants may quickly be fatal.
- Symptoms of benzodiazepine overdose are somnolence, confusion, coma, and diminished reflexes. In all cases of drug overdose, the vital signs should be carefully monitored and supportive care provided, usually in an acute-care setting. Dialysis is of limited value with this group of drugs.
- Intravenous diazepam: Intravenous diazepam should be given slowly, at a rate not exceeding 5 mg per minute. The drug should not be mixed with other drugs or intravenous solutions; administer as close to the venous insertion site as possible. Monitor respiration, blood pressure, and level of consciousness. Resuscitation equipment and intubation equipment should be readily available.
- Intramuscular chlordiazepoxide: Prepare intramuscular chlordiazepoxide as directed by the manufacturer by using the diluent provided, and administer immediately after it is reconstituted. When prepared with the supplied diluent, it should not be given intravenously. Any unused solution should be discarded.
- Intravenous chlordiazepoxide: Dilute the sterile powder with 5 ml of sterile water for injection or normal saline solution added to 100 mg of powder. Agitate the ampule gently to reconstitute, and administer immediately over at least a minute. Any unused portion should be discarded. When reconstituted with sterile water or normal saline solution, the drug should not be administered intramuscularly.

Other Sedative-hypnotics and Antianxiety Drugs

Chloral hydrate	Methyprylon
Triclofos sodium	Ethchlorvynol

Ethinamate
Glutethimide
Hydroxyzine hydrochloride

Hydroxyzine pamoate
Meprobamate

Actions of Other Sedative-hypnotics and Antianxiety Agents

These other agents more closely resemble the barbiturates than the benzodiazepines in action, with the potential for dependence and withdrawal symptoms.

Indications for Other Sedative-hypnotics and Antianxiety Agents

Chloral hydrate is used as sedative or hypnotic. *Triclofos sodium, methyprylon, ethchlorvynol, ethinamate,* and *glutethimide* are all used as hypnotics. *Hydroxyzine hydrochloride* or *pamoate* is used for anxiety or allergic skin reactions, motion sickness, and as preanesthetic. *Meprobamate* is used for anxiety.

Nurse Alert for Other Sedative-hypnotic and Antianxiety Agents

- Dependence may occur, along with withdrawal symptoms similar to those of barbiturates.
- Methyprylon is a Schedule II substance with a high potential for abuse.
- Glutethimide, a Schedule III substance, is widely abused, with less success in treating overdoses because of high incidence of cardiovascular collapse.

Side Effects of Other Sedative-hypnotics and Antianxiety Agents

Chloral hydrate may cause paradoxical excitement, gastric irritation, and displacement of coumarin anticoagulants from plasma protein. *Ethchlorvynol* may produce an unpleasant aftertaste, exaggerated depression with deep sleep and muscular weakness, or an idiosyncratic CNS-stimulation effect. *Glutethimide* used chronically has atropine-like effects of mydriasis and dry mouth. *Meprobamate* may produce withdrawal symptoms including insomnia, anxiety, hallucinations, and grand mal seizures. Other effects of these agents may include CNS depressant side effects such as ataxia, sedation, visual changes, hangover effects, and allergic reactions.

Nursing Implications for Other Sedative-hypnotics and Antianxiety Agents

- Glutethimide and chloral hydrate should be used with caution in patients taking oral anticoagulants because the dose of the latter may have to be increased to provide adequate anticoagulation.
- Blood dyscrasias have been reported with some of the agents. Caution patients to report sore throat, fever, malaise, bruising, unexplained bleeding, or jaundice.
- Taking the prescribed medication with a small snack may help to reduce gastric irritation.
- Preparations for bed should be completed before taking the medication. Once a drug has been taken to induce sleep, its effects may begin within 15 to 30 minutes.
- Abrupt withdrawal of any of the hypnotic drugs discussed may result in withdrawal symptoms, especially if the patient was receiving large doses or had been on long-term therapy. Instruct patients to discontinue the medications only on the advice of their physicians.

Antialcohol Agent

Disulfiram (Antabuse)

Actions of Disulfiram

Disulfiram blocks the oxidation of acetaldehyde, the product of alcohol metabolism, and thereby causes unpleasant symptoms when alcohol is ingested, including flushing, throbbing headache, respiratory difficulty, nausea, vomiting, sweating, thirst, chest pain, rapid breathing, tachycardia, fainting, weakness, vertigo, blurred vision, and confusion.

20 **Pocket Nurse Guide to Drugs**

Table 1-3 Administration of other sedative-hypnotics and antianxiety agents

Generic Name	Trade Name	Dosage and Administration
Chloral hydrate	Noctec* Novochlor-hydrate† Chloralvan† Oradrate SK-Chloral Hydrate	ORAL, RECTAL: *Adults*—as sedative, 250 mg 3 times daily after meals; as hypnotic, 500 mg to 1 Gm 15 to 30 min before bedtime. *Children*—as sedative, 25 mg/kg in 3 to 4 doses daily; as hypnotic, 50 mg/kg at bedtime, not to exceed 500 mg.
Triclofos sodium	Triclos	ORAL: *Adults*—as hypnotic, 1.5 Gm 15 to 30 min before bedtime. *Children*—over 12 yr, as hypnotic, as for adults; under 12 yr, 20 mg/kg.
Methyprylon	Noludar*	ORAL: *Adults*—for hypnosis, 200 to 400 mg at bedtime. *Children over 3 mo*—50 to 200 mg at bedtime.
Ethchlorvynol	Placidyl*	ORAL: *Adults only*—as hypnotic, 500 mg to 1 Gm at bedtime.
Ethinamate	Valmid	ORAL: *Adults only*—as hypnotic, 500 mg to 1 Gm at bedtime.
Glutethimide	Doriden*	ORAL: *Adults only*—as hypnotic, 250 to 500 mg at bedtime.
Hydroxyzine hydrochloride, hydroxyzine pamoate	Atarax* Vistaril Durrax Orgatrax	ORAL: *Adults*—for anxiety, 75 to 400 mg daily in 4 divided doses.

*Available in U.S. and Canada
†Available in Canada only

Sedative-hypnotics, Antianxiety Agents, and Anti-Alcohol Agents

Table 1-3 Administration of other sedative-hypnotics and antianxiety agents—cont'd.

Generic Name	Trade Name	Dosage and Administration
Hydroxyzine—cont'd. hydrochloride, hydroxyzine pamoate	Vistacen Vistaject E-Vista	For allergic skin reactions: ORAL: *Adults*—25 mg 3 or 4 times daily. *Children under 6 yr*—50 mg daily in 3 to 4 divided doses. INTRAMUSCULAR: *Adults*—for anxiety, 50 to 100 mg every 4-6 hr.
Meprobamate	Apo-Meprobamate† Equanil Meditran† Meprospan Meprospan-400 Miltown* Quietae†	ORAL: *Adults*—for anxiety, 1.2 to 1.6 Gm daily divided into 3 or 4 doses. *Children over 6 yr*—for anxiety, 25 mg/kg daily divided into 2 or 3 doses.

*Available in U.S. and Canada
†Available in Canada only

Indications for Disulfiram

Because of the potential severity of effects, disulfiram is used to treat alcoholism only in well-informed, highly motivated patients and only when accompanied by psychiatric therapy.

Nurse Alert for Disulfiram

- Severe reactions can cause death from cardiovascular collapse or respiratory failure
- Disulfiram is contraindicated in severe myocardial disease and psychosis, and should be used cautiously with patients with diabetes mellitus, epilepsy, nephritis, cirrhosis, hypothyroidism, or cerebral damage
- Disulfiram may cause liver toxicity. Therapy longer than six months should include monitoring of hepatic enzymes.

Administration of Disulfiram

Oral, Adults: Loading dose is 500 mg daily for one week. Maintenance doses are 125-500 mg daily, depending on the individual.

Side Effects of Disulfiram

Transient side effects may include drowsiness, fatigue, impotence, headache, acne, and a metallic or garliclike aftertaste.

Nursing Implications for Disulfiram

- Patients who receive or have recently received metronidazole, paraldehyde, alcohol, or alcohol-containing preparations (e.g., cough syrups, over-the-counter tonics) should not be given disulfiram.
- Patients should be taught about the effects of taking disulfiram and what will happen if alcohol is consumed while on the drug. Possible sources of alcohol ingestion should be reviewed: liquor, beer, wine, sauces used in cooking and desserts, vinegars, and some liquid medications. The effects of a single dose of disulfiram may last as long as 14 days.
- In addition to ingested alcohol, the patient should be instructed to avoid topical applications of alcohol, such as after-shave lotions, back rubs, and some colognes.
- Treatment with disulfiram is not a cure for alcoholism and should be used only with other forms of supportive therapy. Patients should be assessed carefully before this drug is prescribed. Highly motivated, reliable patients may have success with disulfiram, but only when used with other forms of therapy.
- Usually patients are instructed to take their daily dose of disulfiram in the morning, but if the sedation produced by the drug is troublesome, some patients may find that taking the dose in the evening is better.
- Patients being treated with disulfiram should carry an identification card indicating that they are on disulfiram

Sedative-hypnotics, Antianxiety Agents, and Anti-Alcohol Agents 23

therapy and who should be notified in the event of an emergency. These cards can be obtained from the drug manufacturer.

- Treatment of a severe disulfiram reaction may require hospitalization because the patient may go into shock. The patient's family should be instructed in detail about the effects of alcohol consumption while the patient is receiving disulfiram.

Antipsychotic Drugs

2

Phenothiazines
  Aliphatic
    Chlorpromazine
    Triflupromazine
  Piperidine
    Mesoridazine
    Piperacetazine
    Thioridazine
  Piperazine
    Acetophenazine
    Carphenazine
    Fluphenazine
    Perphenazine
    Prochlorperazine
    Trifluoperazine

Thioxanthenes
    Chlorprothixene
    Thiothixene
  Butyrophenone
    Haloperidol
  Dibenzoxazepine
    Loxapine
  Dihydroindolone
    Molidone

Actions of Antipsychotics

The antipsychotics have four primary effects resulting from four main actions. Receptor blockade (probably dopaminergic) in the limbic system causes the antipsychotic effect. Receptor blockade (dopaminergic) in the chemoreceptor trigger zone causes an antiemetic effect. Blockade of neurons (probably cholinergic) from the basal ganglia in the corpus striatum causes extrapyramidal effects. Dopaminergic blockade in the pituitary gland causes endocrine effects.

Indications for Antipsychotics

Chlorpromazine hydrochloride is used for control of psychotic disorders and the control of severe nausea and vomiting, intractable hiccups, tetanus, and acute intermittent porphyria. *Triflupromazine hydrochloride* is used for the management of psychotic disorders and the control of nausea and vomiting. *Thioridazine* is used for psychotic disorders and may be

24

effective in alcohol withdrawal syndrome, intractable pain, and senility. *Mesoridazine besylate, piperacetazine, acetophenazine maleate, promazine,* and *carphenazine maleate* are used to manage psychotic disorders. *Fluphenazine hydrochloride* is potent for use in the treatment of psychotic disorders. *Perphenazine* is used for acute psychotic disorders, and, in lower doses, as an antiemetic. *Prochlorperazine* is most widely used to control severe nausea and vomiting. *Trifluoperazine, chlorprothixene,* and *thiothixene hydrochloride* are used in the management of psychotic disorders. *Haloperidol* is used in the management of psychotic disorders, in severe cases of hyperkinetic retardation, and is drug of choice for Gilles de la Tourette syndrome. *Loxapine succinate* and *molindone hydrochloride* are used for patients refractory to established antipsychotic drugs.

Nurse Alert for Antipsychotics

- Antipsychotics potentiate the actions of CNS depressants, resulting in a higher risk of a toxic overdose.
- With initial therapy, the nurse should observe closely for changes in affect and behavior and should monitor vital signs, level of consciousness, signs of toxic reactions, and seriousness of side effects.
- Chlorpromazine is contraindicated for seizure-prone patients.
- Fluphenazine is not recommended for the elderly or patients who may have difficulty with extrapyramidal reactions.
- Haloperidol is very likely to produce extrapyramidal reactions.

Side Effects of Antipsychotics

The side effects of the antipsychotics are related to the four primary actions of these drugs. *Effects of adrenergic blockade* include sedation and orthostatic hypotension, usually transient.

Effects of cholinergic blockade include atropine-like effects of dry mouth, blurred vision, constipation, and delayed micturition, usually transient.

Text continued on p. 35

Table 2-1   Administration of antipsychotics

Generic Name	Trade Name	Dosage and Administration
Phenothiazines, Aliphatic		
Chlorpromazine hydrochloride	Thorazine Chlor-PZ Promapar Ormazine Chlorprom† Promamyl† Largactil†	Psychiatric outpatients: ORAL: *Adults*—12 to 40 yr, average dose 400 to 800 mg daily; over 40, a limit of 300 mg daily is suggested. Acutely psychotic, hospitalized patients: INTRAMUSCULAR: *Adults*—25 to 100 mg every 1 to 4 hr until symptoms are controlled. *Elderly or debilitated patients*—10 mg every 6 to 8 hr to control acute symptoms. *Children*—maximum of 40 mg for children under 5 years and 75 mg for those under 12 years. INTRAVENOUS: Not recommended because it is highly irritating. Drug must be diluted to at least 1 mg/ml and no more than 1 mg/min given. ORAL: *Adults*—200 to 600 mg daily in divided doses, increased every 2 to 3 days by 100 mg, up to 2 Gm if needed. *Elderly or debilitated patients*—⅓ to ½ of adult dose with 20 to 25 mg increments. *Children*—0.5 mg/kg every 4 to 6 hr. To control nausea and vomiting: ORAL: 25-50 mg every 6 hr.

		INTRAMUSCULAR: 25 mg initially, then 25 to 50 mg every 3 to 4 hr to stop vomiting.
		Other uses:
		ORAL: *Adults*—25 to 50 mg 3 or 4 times daily
		INTRAMUSCULAR: 25 mg every 3 or 4 hr.
Triflupromazine hydrochloride	Vesprin	Psychotic disorders:
		ORAL: *Adults*—50 to 150 mg daily. *Elderly patients*—20 to 30 mg orally daily. *Children over 2½ yr*—0.5 mg/kg, up to 150 mg maximum.
		INTRAMUSCULAR: *Adults*—50 to 150 mg daily. *Elderly patients*—10 to 75 mg daily. *Children over 2½ yr*—0.2 to 0.25 mg/kg up to 10 mg maximum, divided into 3 daily doses.
		Nausea and vomiting:
		INTRAVENOUS: *Adults*—1 mg up to 3 mg.
		INTRAMUSCULAR: *Adults*—5 to 15 mg every 4 hr up to 60 mg daily.
		ORAL: *Adults*—20 to 30 mg total daily.
		ORAL, INTRAMUSCULAR: *Children over 2½ yr*—0.2 mg/kg, up to 10 mg in 3 doses daily.

cont'd. next page

*Available in U.S. and Canada
†Available in Canada only

Table 2-1 Administration of antipsychotics—cont'd.

Generic Name	Trade Name	Dosage and Administration
Promazine	Sparin*	INTRAMUSCULAR: *Adults*—50-150 mg ORAL: *Adults*—10 to 200 mg every 4 to 6 hr. *Children*—10 to 25 mg every 4 to 6 hr for children over 12 yr
Phenothiazines, Piperidine		
Thioridazine	Mellaril* Hydrochloride Novoridazine†	Psychotic disorders: ORAL: *Adults*—50 to 100 mg 3 times daily, increasing up to 800 mg. *Elderly patients*—⅓ to ½ adult dose. *Children over 2 yr*—1 mg/kg in divided doses. Depressive neurosis, alcohol withdrawal syndrome, intractable pain, senility: 10 to 50 mg 2 to 4 times daily.
Mesoridazine besylate	Serentil*	ORAL: *Adults*—150 mg daily initially, increasing by 50 mg increments until symptoms controlled. *Elderly patients*—⅓ to ½ adult dose. INTRAMUSCULAR: *Adults and children over 12 yr*—25 to 175 mg daily in divided doses. Injection may irritate the site.
Piperacetazine	Quide*	ORAL: *Adults and children over 12 yr*—20 to 40 daily, increasing by increments of 10 mg up to 160 mg to control symptoms. *Elderly patients*—⅓ to ½ adult dose.

Antipsychotic Drugs **29**

Phenothiazines, Piperazine

Acetophenazine maleate	Tindal Maleate	ORAL: *Adults*—60 mg daily in divided doses that can be increased in 20 mg increments. Optimal level is usually 80 to 120 mg. Occasionally, severe symptoms require 400 to 600 mg. *Elderly patients*—⅓ to ½ adult dose. *Children*—0.8 to 1.6 mg/kg in divided doses. Maximum, 80 mg daily.
Carphenazine maleate	Proketazine Maleate	ORAL: *Adults*—75 to 150 mg daily in 3 divided doses, increased weekly by 25 to 50 mg; 400 mg maximum. *Elderly patients*—⅓ to ½ adult dose.
Fluphenazine hydrochloride	Apo-Fluphenazine† Prolixin Permitil* Moditen†	ORAL: *Adults*—2.5 to 10 mg initially, reduced to 1 to 5 mg daily for maintenance. *Elderly patients*—⅓ to ½ adult dose. INTRAMUSCULAR: *Adults*—1.25 mg increased gradually to 2.5 to 10 mg daily in 3 or 4 doses. *Elderly patients*—⅓ to ½ adult dose.
Fluphenazine decanoate	Modecate† Decanoate Prolixin Decanoate	INTRAMUSCULAR, SUBCUTANEOUS: *Adults under 50 yr*—12.5 mg initially, then 25 mg every 2 wk. Increase by 12.5 mg amounts if needed. Rarely require more than 100 mg every 2 to 6 wk.
Fluphenazine enanthate	Prolixin Ethanate	

cont'd. next page

*Available in U.S. and Canada
†Available in Canada only

Table 2-1 Administration of antipsychotics—cont'd.

Generic Name	Trade Name	Dosage and Administration
Fluphenazine enanthate—cont'd	Moditen† Enanthate	
Perphenazine	Apo-Perphenazine† Phenazine† Trilafon*	ORAL: *Adults*—16 to 64 mg daily in divided doses. *Elderly patients*—⅓ to ½ adult dose. *Children over 12 yr*—6 to 12 mg daily INTRAMUSCULAR: *Adults*—5 to 10 mg initially, then 5 mg every 6 hr with 15 mg maximum daily in ambulatory and 30 mg daily in hospitalized patients. *Elderly patients*—⅓ to ½ adult dose. *Children over 12 yr*—Lowest adult dose.
Prochlorperazine	Compazine	Psychiatric disorders: ORAL: *Adults*—5 to 10 mg 3 to 4 times daily. Raise dosage every 2 to 3 days as required. Mild cases may require 50 to 75 mg daily; 100 to 150 mg for severe cases. *Elderly patients*—⅓ to ½ adult dosage. *Children over 2 yr*—2.5 mg 2 to 3 times daily up to 20 to 25 mg. Same dosage used rectally.
Prochlorperazine edisylate	Compazine Edisylate	
Prochlorperazine maleate	Compazine Maleate Stemetil†	INTRAMUSCULAR: *Adults*—10 to 20 mg in buttock; repeat every 2 to 4 hr up to 80 mg total. *Elderly patients*—⅓ to ½ adult dose. *Children over 2 yr*—0.06 mg/lb initial dose only, then switch to oral.

Antipsychotic Drugs **31**

Nausea and vomiting:
ORAL: *Adults*—5 to 10 mg 3 or 4 times daily. *Children*—20 to 29 lb, 2.5 mg 1 to 2 times daily; 30 to 39 lb, 2.5 mg 2 to 3 times daily; 40 to 85 lb, 2.5 mg 3 times daily or 5 mg 2 times daily.
INTRAMUSCULAR: *Adults*—5 to 10 mg every 3 to 4 hr. *Children*—0.06 mg/lb.
RECTAL: *Adults*—25 mg twice daily. *Children*—same as oral dosage.

Trifluoperazine	Apo-Trifluoperazine† Novoflurazine† Solazine† Stelazine* Clinatine† Terfluzine†	ORAL: *Adults*—2 to 4 mg daily in divided doses (outpatient), 4 to 10 mg daily (hospitalized). *Elderly or debilitated patients*—⅓ to ½ adult dosage. *Children over 6 yr*—1 mg 1 to 2 times daily, gradually raised to maximum of 15 mg. INTRAMUSCULAR: *Adults*—1 to 2 mg every 4 to 6 hr, maximum 10 mg daily. *Elderly or debilitated patients*—⅓ to ½ adult dose. *Children over 6 yr*—same as oral dosage.
Thioxanthenes		
Chlorprothixene	Taractan Tarasan†	ORAL: *Adults and children over 12 yr*—75 to 200 mg daily in divided doses. Gradually increase if necessary, up to 600 mg daily. *Elderly patients*—½ adult dose. *cont'd. next page*

*Available in U.S. and Canada
†Available in Canada only

Table 2-1 Administration of antipsychotics—cont'd.

Generic Name	Trade Name	Dosage and Administration
Chlorprothixene—cont'd		INTRAMUSCULAR: *Adults and children over 12 yr*—70 to 100 mg daily in divided doses. *Elderly patients*—½ adult dose.
Thiothixene hydrochloride	Navane* Hydrochloride	ORAL: *Adult and children over 12 yr*—6 to 10 mg daily in divided doses. Gradually increase as required, up to 20 to 60 mg daily. *Elderly patients*—⅓ to ½ adult dose.
		INTRAMUSCULAR: *Adults and children over 12 yr*—4 mg 2 to 4 times daily; gradually increase if necessary to a maximum of 30 mg. *Elderly patients*—⅓ to ½ adult dose.
Butyrophenone		
Haloperidol	Apo- Haloperidol† Haldol* Peridol†	Acute psychotic management: ORAL: *Adults and children over 12 yr*—1 to 15 mg in divided doses initially, which can be increased gradually up to 100 mg to bring symptoms under control. Dosage is then gradually reduced. Maintenance dose, usually 2 to 8 mg daily. *Elderly patients and children under 12 yr*—0.5 to 1.5 mg daily initially. Dosage increased by 0.5 mg increments if necessary. Usual maintenance dose, 2 to 4 mg daily.
		INTRAMUSCULAR: *Adults and children over 12 yr*—2 to 5 mg every 4 to 8 hr or every hour if acute state requires. Acute symptoms are usually under control in 72 hr, and 15 mg daily is usually sufficient.

Antipsychotic Drugs **33**

Chronic schizophrenia:

ORAL: *Adults and children over 12 yr*—6 to 16 mg in divided
doses gradually increased to as high as 100 mg to achieve
control. Doses are then gradually reduced to achieve
maintenance of control, usually 15 to 20 mg daily. *Elderly
patients*—0.5 to 1.5 mg initially, increased very gradually.
Maintenance dosage, usually 2 to 8 mg daily.

Mental retardation with hyperkinesia:

ORAL (given after intramuscular treatment as for acute
psychoses): *Adults and children over 12 yr*—80 to 120 mg daily,
gradually reduced to a maintenance dose of about 60 mg daily.
Elderly patients and children under 12 yr—1.5 to 6 mg daily in
divided doses; gradually increase dosage up to 15 mg daily for
control, then reduce dosage for maintenance.

Gilles de la Tourette syndrome:

Initial dosages to achieve control are like those for chronic
schizophrenia. Maintenance dosages: adults and children over
12 yr—9 mg daily; children under 12 yr—1.5 mg daily.

cont'd. next page

* Available in U.S. and Canada
† Available in Canada only

Table 2-1 Administration of antipsychotics—cont'd.

Generic Name	Trade Name	Dosage and Administration
Dibenzoxazepine		
Loxapine succinate	Loxitane Loxapac†	ORAL: *Patients over 16 yr*— 10 to 25 mg twice daily initially, with dosage increased rapidly over 7 to 10 days to achieve control. Dosage reduced for maintenance to 60 to 100 mg daily; maximum, 250 mg daily. *Elderly patients*—⅓ to ½ dose just listed.
Dihydroindolone		
Molindone hydrochloride	Moban	ORAL: *Adults*— 15 to 40 mg daily initially, with increased dosage to control symptoms, up to 225 mg daily. Dosage should then be reduced for maintenance. *Elderly patients*—⅓ to ½ adult dose.

*Available in U.S. and Canada
†Available in Canada only

Effects of endocrine-dopamine blockade include erection problems (men), menstrual irregularities, and unexpected lactation (women), usually transient.

Extrapyramidal effects include acute dystonia common in first few days (neck twisting, facial grimacing, involuntary eye movements), akathisia (restlessness) most common in first few days, parkinsonism (motor retardation, tremor, rigidity, salivation, and shuffling gait) most common after the first week, and tardive dyskinesia (protrusion of tongue, puffing of cheeks, chewing movements, involuntary trunk and extremity movements) most common when dosage is lowered after prolonged therapy. Extrapyramidal effects may require additional drug therapy to reverse. Tardive dyskinesia may be permanent.

Allergic reactions may include photosensitivity, cholestatic hepatitis, and agranulocytosis.

Other side effects may include ECG changes, increased risk of seizures, and blood dyscrasias.

Table 2-2 compares the relative incidence of side effects of antipsychotics in terms of the major groupings of side effects.

Nursing Implications for Antipsychotics

- Caution patients to avoid activities that require mental alertness such as driving or operating machinery. Keep the siderails up on the beds of hospitalized patients. Supervise ambulation and use discretion in supervising other possibly dangerous activities such as smoking.
- Instruct the patient and family that the patient should not take other drugs while receiving antipsychotic drugs unless the drugs and dosages have been approved by the physician. Of particular concern are other drugs causing sedation or hypotension. Remind the patient that over-the-counter medications should be approved by the physician also; many combination products in this latter group contain drugs that may aggravate side effects of the antipsychotic drugs.
- Patients taking antipsychotic drugs should avoid the use of alcohol.

Table 2-2   Side effects of antipsychotics

Drug	Potency Relative to Chlorpromazine	Relative Incidence of Side Effects			
		Sedative Effect	Orthostatic Hypotension	Anticholinergic Effects	Extrapyramidal Symptoms
Phenothiazines					
Aliphatic					
Chlorpromazine	100	High	Moderate-High*	Moderate-High*	Moderate
Triflupromazine	25	High	Moderate	Moderate-High	Moderate-High
Promazine	200	Moderate	Moderate-Low	High	Moderate
Piperidine					
Mesoridazine	50	High	Moderate	Moderate	Low
Piperacetazine	10	Moderate	Low	Low-Moderate	Moderate
Thioridazine	100	High	Moderate-High*	Moderate-High*	Low
Piperazine					
Acetophenazine	20	Moderate	Low	Low	High
Carphenazine	25	Moderate	Low	Low	High
Fluphenazine	2	Low	Low	Low	High

Perphenazine	8	Low	Low	Low	High
Prochlorperazine	10	Moderate	Low	Low	High
Trifluoperazine	4	Moderate	Low	Low	High
Thioxanthenes					
Chlorprothixene	100	High	Moderate-High	Moderate-High	Low-Moderate
Thiothixene	4	Low	Low-Moderate	Low	Moderate-High
Butyrophenone					
Haloperidol	2	Low	Low	Low	High
Dibenzoxazepine					
Loxapine	10-20	Moderate	Low-Moderate	Low-Moderate	Moderate-High
Dihydroindolone					
Molindone	10-20	Moderate	Low-Moderate	Moderate	Moderate

*Depends on route and dose

38 Pocket Nurse Guide to Drugs

- If the patient is hospitalized, monitor the blood pressure every 4 hours until stable. This may require several days to 2 weeks as most of the antipsychotic drugs are cumulative and marked side effects may not appear in the first day or two of therapy. Some physicians may request that blood pressure be checked with the patient in lying, sitting, and standing positions.
- Instruct the patients to move slowly from lying to sitting or standing positions. If orthostatic hypotension should occur, instruct the patient to lie or sit down. Symptoms include dizziness, lightheadedness, visual changes, and occasionally syncope. Hypotension may be accentuated with hot baths or showers; these should be avoided. Having the patient wear elastic stockings may help; consult the physician.
- The patient may be unsteady when ambulating. Supervise and assist with ambulation until the patient is stable and steady. Instruct the patient to call for assistance before getting up, if dizzy or unsteady.
- The anticholinergic effect of dry mouth may be annoying to the patient. Offer fluid frequently. Chewing sugarless mints or gum or sucking on hard candies may help. Encourage frequent oral hygiene including brushing the teeth and rinsing with a pleasant-tasting oral rinse or mouthwash. Keep the lips moist with application of a lip balm or ointment. The use of a commercially prepared saliva substitute may be helpful.
- To monitor for delayed micturition, monitor the fluid intake and output. This problem will be more common in immobilized patients, elderly persons, or men who already have an enlarged prostate gland.
- To counteract constipation keep a record of the frequency of bowel movements and have the patient or the family do the same at home. Maintain an adequate fluid intake (2500 to 3000 ml per day), and encourage the patient to eat a diet that contains a variety of fruits, fiber, and vegetables. Frequent ambulation or exercise may help. If constipation is a frequent or constant problem, the addition of a daily stool softener, bulk-former, or other aid to defecation may be appropriate; check with the physician.

Antipsychotic Drugs **39**

- Instruct the patient to report blurred vision or other visual changes. If blurred vision occurs, it may necessitate reducing the drug dosage or changing drugs. The patient should avoid driving or other potentially dangerous activities until the vision improves. Because long-term therapy has been associated with ocular changes, patients receiving antipsychotic drugs on a long-term basis should be encouraged to have regular eye examinations.
- The possible endocrine impairments and side effects should be explained to the patient and appropriate family members. Both the patient and spouse may need emotional support if impotence should occur. The patient should be asked to report the onset of amenorrhea, galactorrhea, gynecomastia, or menstrual irregularities. The institutionalized patient should be monitored for endocrine changes on a regular basis. For some patients the endocrine abnormalities are so disturbing as to cause the patient to want to discontinue therapy with the particular drug.
- Weigh the patient regularly. This may mean weekly for the outpatient (the patient could do this at home and keep a record) or monthly for patients in the long-term care facility. Antipsychotics may contribute to fluid retention and/or increased appetite.
- Explain to the patient and family that various extrapyramidal symptoms may occur and instruct the patient to report them if they do. For some patients the extrapyramidal symptoms may be the most bothersome side effects; emotional support of the entire family may be necessary. If other drugs are prescribed to alleviate some of the extrapyramidal symptoms, the use and side effects of these drugs should also be explained to the patient.
- Evaluate the appearance of new behaviors and of new signs and symptoms in the patient carefully. What may appear to be increased agitation may be akathisia or what may resemble anxiety may be early parkinsonian-type side effects. The decision to increase the dose of antipsychotic drug or add additional drugs to the patient's regimen should be made carefully and after thoughtful patient evaluation.
- It is important to monitor the patient frequently for symptoms of tardive dyskinesia. Since there is no effective

Pocket Nurse Guide to Drugs

treatment for this unpleasant side effect, its early detection is imperative. Fine vermicular (wormlike) movements of the tongue have been cited as a possible early sign of tardive dyskinesia.

- Photosensitivity may be a side effect. Caution patients to avoid exposure to the sun or ultraviolet light or use an appropriate sun screen. The appearance of any skin changes or discoloration should be reported. Hyperpyrexia has been reported in some patients receiving phenothiazines; caution patients to avoid excessive heat.
- Cholestatic hepatitis can occur. Instruct the patient to report any skin color changes (jaundice), right upper quadrant abdominal pain, fever, or change in the color or consistency of stools.
- Instruct the patient to report any fever, sore throat, general malaise; these are symptoms of agranulocytosis.
- Contact dermatitis with the phenothiazines has been reported. Personnel preparing and administering these drugs should be careful to avoid letting the drugs make contact with their skin, and they should wash the area carefully if contact should occur. It may be appropriate to have personnel wear gloves if they must work frequently with these drugs.
- Women of childbearing age may wish to consider the use of birth control measures when taking antipsychotic drugs. Women should consult their physicians for appropriate advice about possible pregnancy. While fetal malformations have not been associated with antipsychotic drugs, these drugs do cross the placenta. Extrapyramidal effects may be seen in infant also.
- Antipsychotic drugs have been associated with hyperglycemia and hypoglycemia. Patients with diabetes mellitus may require readjustment of diet and of drug therapy (insulin or oral hypoglycemics). Caution these patients to monitor their urine glucose concentration carefully and to report frequent episodes of hypoglycemia or excessive spilling of sugar in their urine.
- Supervise the psychiatric patient carefully to ascertain that any dose of medication is actually swallowed and not

Antipsychotic Drugs 41

hidden in the mouth to be discarded later or stored by the patient. Some of the antipsychotic drugs are available in syrup, injection, or depot injection forms to help ensure that the patient receives the prescribed dose. On an outpatient basis it may be necessary for a responsible family member to supervise the taking of medications.

- Antipsychotic drugs should be used with extreme caution in children or adolescents who display signs or symptoms suggestive of Reye's disease.
- Many antipsychotic drugs have some pulmonary side effects. For this reason they should be used cautiously in patients with chronic obstructive lung disease, emphysema, or asthma; elderly persons; postoperative patients; individuals confined to bed; or anyone with a decreased level of consciousness.
- Monitor patients with a history of seizures carefully when administering an antipsychotic drug.
- Antipsychotic drugs may produce false results (positives) in pregnancy tests. If there is a possibility of pregnancy, women should consult their physicians.
- Although hypotension is the much more frequent side effect, chlorpromazine may counteract the antihypertensive effects of guanethidine. Monitor the blood pressure frequently.
- There are concentrated oral forms of most of the antipsychotic drugs available for institutional use. The dose should be diluted to at least 60 ml in one of the diluents suggested by the manufacturer. Note that coffee and tea are listed by some manufacturers as acceptable diluents, although these may cause the drugs to precipitate.
- Apparent treatment failures require thoughtful investigation.
- Antipsychotic drugs should not be discontinued suddenly. Encourage patients receiving long-term therapy to continue the ordered drugs, to report complaints about the drugs to the physician, and to report the appearance of new side effects.
- Intramuscular injection of non-depot forms of phenothiazines may cause marked hypotension. For the same

42   **Pocket Nurse Guide to Drugs**

reason, most phenothiazines are not given FV. The patient should be kept lying down for ½ to 1 hour, the blood pressure monitored, and the patient allowed to get up slowly. For rare severe reactions, levarterenol (Levophed) and phenylephrine (Neo-Synephrine) are the vasoconstrictors of choice; epinephrine and other agents should not be used.

- With the exception of mild sedation, mild hypotension, and occasionally dry mouth, side effects are rare when the antipsychotic drugs are used for their antiemetic effects. On the other hand, any of the side effects can occur in rare individuals who are extremely sensitive to the drug, so health care personnel should be alert to possible side effects. Remember that when the antipsychotic drugs are given with narcotic analgesics, they may potentiate the effects of the analgesics, including sedation and hypotension.

- Mesoridazine (Serentil) contains a specific coloring, FD&C yellow number 5 (tartrazine) which may cause allergic-type reactions in some individuals. This allergic-type reaction is seen more often in individuals with aspirin hypersensitivity.

Antidepressant Drugs

3

Tricyclic antidepressants
    Amitriptyline hydrochloride
    Desipramine hydrochloride
    Doxepin hydrochloride
    Imipramine hydrochloride
    Imipramine pamoate
    Nortriptyline hydrochloride
    Protriptyline hydrochloride
    Trimipramine maleate
Second generation antidepressants
    Amoxapine
    Maprotiline
    Trazodone

Monoamine oxidase (MAO) inhibitors
    Isocarboxazid
    Phenelzine sulfate
    Tranylcypromine sulfate
Lithium
    Lithium carbonate
    Lithium citrate

Tricyclic Antidepressants

Actions of Tricyclic Antidepressants

These drugs block the reuptake of norepinephrine and/or serotonin into presynaptic neurons and also are thought to alter the sensitivity of brain tissue to actions of norepinephrine and serotonin.

Indications for Tricyclic Antidepressants

Tricyclic antidepressants are used to treat endogenous depression, but not reactive depression, manic-depressive disorder, or depression resulting as a drug side effect. *Doxepin* is indicated when cardiac function must be considered. *Protriptyline* is most useful for patients physically immobilized by depression or who sleep excessively. *Imipramine* is also used occasionally to treat enuresis in older children or adults.

Nurse Alert for Tricyclic Antidepressants

- Because of sedative effects, the patient should be cautioned to avoid activities requiring mental alertness until the drug's effects have been evaluated.
- The anticholinergic effects of these drugs may worsen the condition of patients with glaucoma or urinary retention, particularly the elderly.
- These drugs are contraindicated for patients with a recent myocardial infarction and should be used cautiously in patients with cardiac disease or hyperthyroidism.
- A major problem is the toxicity of tricyclic antidepressants in patients taking an overdose in a suicide attempt.
- Antidepressants should be used cautiously in women of childbearing age because of the potential for congenital anomalies.

Side Effects of Tricyclic Antidepressants

Tricyclic antidepressants cause sedation and anticholinergic side effects. Anticholinergic effects include dry mouth, blurred vision, constipation, urinary retention, temporary confusion, and speech blockage. The sedation and the anticholinergic effects are more prominent with amitriptyline and doxepin, and less so with desipramine and imipramine. The sedative effect of trimipramine is strong, that of nortriptyline is moderate, and that of protriptyline is high. The anticholinergic effects of the three are moderate. Complex cardiac effects may also result. Other side effects may include urinary retention, hypotension or orthostatic hypotension, changes in blood glucose levels, photosensitivity, and rarely agranulocytosis or thrombocytopenia. Imipramine used in children for enuresis may cause nervousness, sleep disorders, and gastrointestinal upset. Toxic levels may produce confusion, inability to concentrate, hallucinations, delirium, seizures, coma, respiratory depression, and tachycardia or bradycardia.

General Nursing Implications for All Antidepressants

- While some side effects may persist, reassure patients and families that many of the side effects resulting from the antidepressants may diminish or disappear with continued use of the drug.

- Several weeks of drug therapy are often needed to produce improvement.
- Medications should be taken only as ordered. The persistent blood level of the drug produces the improvement.
- The risk of suicide is present in seriously depressed patients and may persist for several weeks after the patient starts antidepressant therapy.
- Because of the possibility of drug interactions, patients should be cautioned to keep all their health care providers informed of all medications they are receiving.
- Caution the patient to avoid over-the-counter preparations unless they are first cleared with the physician.
- As the patient's mood improves, there may be a significant improvement in appetite and some patients will find weight gain to be a problem.
- Development of heart conditions in the patient may alter the patient's ability to tolerate antidepressants because of the effects of the drugs on the myocardium.
- Caution patients to discontinue antidepressant therapy only on the advice of the physician.

Nursing Implications for Tricyclic and Second Generation Antidepressants

- If dry mouth is a problem, chewing gum or taking sugarless mints or candies, or using a commercially prepared saliva subsitute may make it more tolerable.
- The patient should be instructed to report blurred vision immediately.
- Encourage the patient to have regular checks for glaucoma.
- Hospitalized patients should have their blood pressure and pulse monitored twice a day until stable.
- Patients receiving tricyclic antidepressants should avoid ethclorvynol (Placidyl), delirium may be precipitated.
- Tofranil and Norpramin both contain FD&C number 5 coloring (tartrazine), which in a few susceptible individuals can cause an allergic response, including an asthmalike reaction. This response is rare, but is seen most often in patients who also have a hypersensitivity to aspirin.

Table 3-1 Administration of tricyclic antidepressants

Generic Name	Trade Name	Dosage and Administration
Tricyclic Antidepressants		
Amitriptyline hydrochloride	Amitril Elavil* Endep Amiline† Deprex† Levate† Novotriptyn†	ORAL: *Adults* — begin with 50 mg at bedtime, increase dosage by 25 to 50 mg if necessary to 150 mg. Alternatively, start with 25 mg 3 times daily, increase to 50 mg 3 times daily; maximum 300 mg daily. Maintenance doses are usually 50 to 100 mg at bedtime. These are outpatient dosages; inpatient dosages may be twice as much. *Adolescents and elderly* — 10 mg 3 times daily plus 20 mg at bedtime (50 mg total). INTRAMUSCULAR: 20 to 30 mg 4 times daily.
Desipramine hydrochloride	Norpramin* Pertofrane*	ORAL: *Adults* — begin with 25 mg 3 times daily, increase gradually to a total of 200 mg daily; maximum 300 mg daily; maintenance dosages usually 50 to 200 mg taken at bedtime. *Adolescents and elderly:* 25 to 50 mg daily; increased to 100 mg in divided doses if necessary.
Doxepin hydrochloride	Adapin Sinequan*	ORAL: *Adults* — 75 mg, increased to 150 mg in divided doses or at bedtime; maintenance dose usually 25 to 150 mg daily; maximum 300 mg daily.

Drug	Trade names	Dosage
Imipramine hydrochloride Imipramine pamoate	Apo-Imipramine† SK-Pramine Impril† Novopramine† Tofranil* Tofranil-PM	ORAL: *Adults* — 75 mg daily in divided doses or at bedtime. Dose may be increased up to 200 mg daily if required. These are outpatient doses; inpatient doses are ⅓ higher. *Adolescents and elderly* — 30 to 40 mg daily, increased to a maximum of 100 mg/day. *Children* — over 6, for bed-wetting, 25 mg, 1 hr before bedtime; if no response in 1 week, increase to 50 mg; over 12, may receive up to 75 mg.
Nortriptyline hydrochloride	Aventyl* Pamelor	ORAL: *Adults* — initially, 40 mg in divided doses or at bedtime; maximum dose 100 to 150 mg daily. *Adolescents and children* — 30 to 50 mg daily in divided doses.
Protriptyline hydrochloride	Vivactil Triptil†	ORAL: *Adults* — 15 to 40 mg daily divided in 3 to 4 doses; maximum dose 60 mg daily. Increments are added to the morning dose. *Adolescents and elderly* — 15 mg daily in 3 doses; maximum 20 mg total.
Trimipramine maleate	Surmontil*	ORAL: *Adults* — 75 mg daily increased to 150 mg in divided doses or at bedtime. These are outpatient dosages; inpatient dosages 100 mg daily increased to 200 mg daily with a maximum of 300 mg daily. *Adolescents and elderly* — 50 mg daily increased to no more than 100 mg daily as required.

*Available in U.S. and Canada
†Available in Canada only

Pocket Nurse Guide to Drugs

Second Generation Antidepressants

Amoxapine
Maprotiline
Trazodone

Actions of Second Generation Antidepressants

Amoxapine inhibits the neuronal uptake of biogenic amines and is a more potent inhibitor of norepinephrine uptake than of serotonin uptake. Maprotiline inhibits norepinephrine uptake but not serotonin uptake. Trazodone inhibits serotonin uptake.

Table 3-2 Administration of second generation antidepressants

Generic Name	Trade Name	Dosage and Administration
Amoxapine	Ascendin	ORAL: *Adults*—75 mg initially, increase to 100 mg daily in divided doses. If no improvement in 3 weeks, increase dosage 50 mg daily, every other week to a maximum of 300 mg.
Maprotiline	Ludiomil	ORAL: *Adults*—75 mg, increased to 150 mg daily in divided doses. If no improvement in 3 weeks, increase dosage 50 mg daily, every other week to a maximum of 300 mg. ORAL: *Elderly and adolescents* —Decrease dosage by $\frac{1}{3}$.
Trazodone	Desyrel	ORAL: *Adults*—75-150 mg initially, increased by 50 mg daily every 3-4 days to 300 mg if necessary. If no improvement in 3 weeks, increase dosage 50 mg daily, every other week to a maximum of 400 mg. for outpatients, 600 mg for inpatients.

Indications for Second Generation Antidepressants

The second generation antidepressants are alternatives to the tricyclic antidepressants for endogenous depression. Amoxapine is used to treat major depression and relieve anxiety and agitation associated with depression.

Nurse Alert for Second Generation Antidepressants

- Because of sedative effects, the patient should be cautioned to avoid activities requiring mental alertness until the drug's effects have been evaluated.
- These drugs should be used cautiously in women of childbearing age who may become pregnant.

Side Effects of Second Generation Antidepressants

All the second generation antidepressants may cause anticholinergic, sedative, and cardiovascular side effects, but with a lower incidence and intensity than with the tricyclic antidepressants. Trazodone may cause drowsiness.

Nursing Implications for Second Generation Antidepressants

- See general nursing implications for antidepressants (pp. 44-45).
- See nursing implications for tricyclic antidepressants (p. 45).

MAO Inhibitors

    Isocarboxazid
    Phenelzine sulfate
    Tranylcypromine sulfate

Actions of MAO Inhibitors

The MAO inhibitors irreversibly inhibit the enzyme monoamine oxidase and prevent the degradation of norepinephrine and serotonin.

Indications for MAO Inhibitors

The MAO inhibitors are not as effective as tricyclic antidepressants or second generation antidepressants in treating endogenous depression, but are more effective in treating depressions exhibited as phobias.

Nurse Alert for MAO Inhibitors

- MAO inhibitors interact with many common foods and medication to produce clinically significant problems. Significant drug interactions include hypertensive crisis with sympathomimetics or tricyclic antidepressants; CNS depression with alcohol, meriperidine, sedatives and hypnotics, and antihistamines; orthostatic hypotension with antihypertensive drugs and diuretics; hypoglycemia with insulin or oral hypoglycemic drugs. Foods containing tyramine can cause a hypertensive crisis if ingested while being treated with MAO inhibitors.

Table 3-3 Administration of MAO inhibitors

Generic Name	Trade Name	Dosage and Administration
Isocarboxazid	Marplan*	ORAL: *Adults*—20 to 30 mg daily in divided doses; maintenance dose usually 10 to 20 mg daily.
Phenelzine sulfate	Nardil*	ORAL: *Adults*—45 to 75 mg daily in 3 doses or 1 mg/kg body weight in divided doses. Daily dosage should not exceed 90 mg.
Tranylcypromine sulfate	Parnate*	ORAL: *Adults*—20 to 40 mg daily in 2 doses for 2 weeks. Dosage is reduced after a response is obtained. Usually the maintenance dose is below 30 mg. Higher doses are not advised for out-patients.

*Available in U.S. and Canada

Antidepressant Drugs 51

- These drugs should be used with caution in patients with a history of seizures or diabetes mellitus.

Side Effects of MAO Inhibitors

Tranylcypromine may cause psychomotor stimulant activity characteristic of amphetamine. The *MAO inhibitors* may result in sedation, anticholinergic effects, and orthostatic hypotension. Toxic levels may cause restlessness, anxiety, insomnia, rapid heart rate, dizziness, high fever, and convulsions.

Nursing Implications for MAO Inhibitors

- See general nursing implications for antidepressants (pp. 44-45).
- Patient care implications related to anticholinergic effects, sedation, and hypotension are discussed under tricyclic antidepressants on p. 44.
- Review the necessary dietary restriction with the patient and family.
- Symptoms of hypertensive crisis that might occur after ingestion of tyramine-rich foods include headache, palpitations, visual changes, neck stiffness or soreness, nausea, vomiting, sweating, photophobia, pupillary changes, and bradycardia or tachycardia. Hypertensive crisis is an emergency, and the patient should seek medical assistance if these symptoms occur.
- Phentolamine is used to reduce the blood pressure in hypertensive crisis.
- When possible, monoamine oxidase (MAO) inhibitors should be discontinued 10 days to 2 weeks before elective surgery.
- Instruct the patient to report any jaundice, change in skin color, right upper quadrant abdominal pain, or change in the color of stools because these symptoms may indicate liver dysfunction.

Lithium

Lithium carbonate
Lithium citrate

Actions of Lithium

Lithium lowers concentrations of norepinephrine and serotonin in the brain by inhibiting their release and enhancing their reuptake by neurons.

Indications for Lithium

Lithium is indicated for treating the manic phase of bipolar disorder and as prophylaxis for recurrent mania.

Nurse Alert for Lithium

- Lithium is contraindicated in pregnancy because of the risk of congenital malformations.
- Lithium potentiates the effects of haloperidol, tricyclic antidepressants, and other drugs; see interaction chart in Appendix A.
- Lithium is contraindicated for patients on a sodium- or fluid-restricted diet (patients with renal, cardiovascular, or hypertensive disease).

Table 3-4 Administration of lithium

Generic Name	Trade Name	Dosage and Administration

Lithium carbonate	Eskalith
	Lithane*
	Lithonate
	Lithotabs
	Lithizine†
	Eskalith-CR
	  Sustained
	  release forms
	Lithobid
		ORAL: *Adults*—initially 0.6 to 2.1 Gm daily divided into 3 doses. Increase or decrease dose by 0.3 Gm/day to obtain a blood level of 0.8 to 1.5 mEq/L.

Lithium citrate	Lithonate-S	Maintenance dose usually 0.9 to 1.2 Gm daily in divided doses.

*Available in U.S. & Canada
†Available in Canada only

Side Effects of Lithium

Common side effects include mild nausea, dry mouth, increased thirst, polyuria, and fine tremor of the hands. The thyroid gland may become enlarged, nephrogenic diabetes insipidus may develop, or permanent renal damage may occur with long-term lithium therapy. Additional side effects include excessive weight gain or edematous swelling of wrists and ankles, and a metallic taste in the mouth. Toxic effects may include fasciculations, ataxia, confusion or stupor, dizziness, anorexia, nausea, vomiting, glycosuria, sedation, and blurred vision.

Nursing Implications for Lithium

- See general nursing implications for antidepressants (pp. 44-45)
- Taking lithium with meals may decrease nausea associated with the drug.
- Instruct patients to report any change in size of the thyroid gland.
- Some patients will find the fine hand tremor that lithium produces to be embarrassing; provide appropriate reassurance and support.
- Remind patients to return for follow-up visits to have their serum lithium levels monitored until the dose is stabilized.
- Polyuria may be a nuisance to the patient but may decrease with continued therapy. If polyuria persists, evaluate patient for diabetes insipidus: polyuria of copious amounts of dilute urine, specific gravity, 1.000 to 1.005.
- If the patient develops diarrhea, the physician should be notified; electrolyte depletion may promote lithium toxicity.

Central Nervous System Stimulants

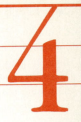

CNS stimulants for narcolepsy and hyperkinesis
- Amphetamine sulfate
- Dextroamphetamine sulfate
- Methamphetamine hydrochloride
- Methylphenidate hydrochloride
- Pemoline
- Deanol

CNS stimulants to suppress appetite
- Benzphetamine hydrochloride
- Clortermine hydrochloride
- Diethylpropion hydrochloride
- Fenfluramine hydrochloride
- Mazindol
- Phendimetrazine tartrate
- Phentermine
- Phenylpropanolamine hydrochloride

CNS stimulants for respiratory stimulation
- Citrated caffeine
- Caffeine sodium benzoate
- Doxapram
- Theophylline

General Actions of CNS Stimulants

Stimulants of the central nervous system produce their effects either by promoting excessive activity or excitatory neurons or by blockade of inhibitory neurons.

General Indications for CNS Stimulants

Central nervous system stimulants are acceptable only for the treatment of narcolepsy, hyperkinetic behavior in children, obesity, stimulation of respiratory function, and occasionally depression in geriatric patients.

General Nursing Implications for CNS Stimulants

- See specific nursing implications for stimulants for narcolepsy and hyperkinesis (pp. 57, 62), to suppress appetite (pp. 63, 66), and for respiratory stimulation (pp. 68, 70).
- Review with patients, parents of children, or other appropriate family members, the possible side effects of drug therapy. Significant alterations in mood, irritability, agitation, hallucinations, or any other behavioral change may represent poor patient tolerance to the prescribed drug(s) or inappropriate dosage, and the physician should be notified.
- Because of the potential for abuse, many of these drugs are dispensed in small quantities, requiring the patient to return to the physician for refills.
- These drugs should be taken only as directed. Patients should not try to "catch up" if a dose is missed.
- Keep these and all medications out of the reach of children. Parents should supervise medication administration in children with hyperkinesis.
- Remind patients to keep all health care professionals informed of all medications being taken, including over-the-counter preparations. Instruct patients to avoid taking any medications unless the drug and dose have been cleared by the physician.
- After prolonged administration these drugs should be discontinued slowly and with the advice of a physician.
- None of these drugs is appropriate for treatment of general fatigue.
- Insomnia may decrease with continued use of a specific drug but may be better treated by eliminating the last dose of medication during the day; check with the physician.
- Sucking on hard candy, chewing sugarless gum, or using a commercially prepared saliva substitute may help relieve dry mouth if it is a problem.
- The hospitalized patient should have the blood pressure and pulse checked every 4 hours until the effects of the drug can be ascertained.
- Instruct patients to report any rash, skin changes, unusual bruising, diarrhea, constipation, impotence, visual disturbances, or any unusual sign or symptom.

56 Pocket Nurse Guide to Drugs

- Caution diabetic patients to monitor their urine sugar concentration carefully as it may be necessary to change insulin and/or diet requirements while receiving amphetamines or appetite suppressants.
- Warn patients that there may be impairment of ability to engage in hazardous activities such as driving or operating machinery.
- Except for treatment of hyperkinesis, the use of any of these drugs in children is not recommended.
- The use of these drugs during pregnancy is not recommended. Some women may wish to consider the use of birth control measures while receiving any of these drugs. Consult with the physician.

CNS Stimulants for Narcolepsy and Hyperkinesis

Amphetamine sulfate
Dextroamphetamine sulfate
Methamphetamine hydrochloride
Methylphenidate hydrochloride
Pemoline
Deanol

Actions of CNS Stimulants for Narcolepsy and Hyperkinesis

Amphetamines increase the release and effectiveness of catecholamine neurotransmitters in the brain and peripheral nerves and block the reuptake of catecholamine neurotransmitters into the presynaptic neuron. Amphetamines stimulate the reticular formation, creating increased alertness and sensitivity to stimuli, and the medial forebrain bundle, creating sensations of pleasure. *Methylphenidate* blocks the neuronal uptake of catecholamines and has effects similar to the amphetamines. The exact mechanism of *pemoline* is unknown, but the effects are similar to amphetamines, except that the sympathomimetic effects are less pronounced. *Deanol* is a precursor of acetylcholine with central nervous system effects, differing from other CNS stimulants in that it does not produce excessive stimulation, jitteriness, or appetite suppression.

Indications for CNS Stimulants for Narcolepsy and Hyperkinesis

See the "Administration" table below for the indications for each of these drugs.

Nurse Alert for CNS Stimulants for Narcolepsy and Hyperkinesis

Amphetamines

- Amphetamines should not be used in patients with significant cardiovascular disease, hypertension, hyperthyroidism, or glaucoma.

Methylphenidate

- Methylphenidate may lower the seizure threshold in individuals with a history of seizures. Observe these patients carefully when therapy is initiated.
- Methylphenidate is usually contraindicated in patients with tourette syndrome or a history of tics.

Pemoline

- Pemoline should be used cautiously in patients with significant renal or hepatic impairment.
- Signs of dyskinesia, a possible side effect of pemoline, include uncontrolled movements of the tongue, lips, face, and extremities.

Side Effects of CNS Stimulants for Narcolepsy and Hyperkinesis

Amphetamines

Gastrointestinal effects include vomiting, diarrhea, abdominal cramps, dry mouth, anorexia. *Central nervous system* effects may include restless behavior, tremor, irritability, talkativeness, insomnia, mood changes, and possibly aggressiveness,

Text continued on p. 62

Table 4-1 Administration of CNS stimulants for narcolepsy and hyperkinesis

Generic Name	Trade Name	Medical Use	Dosage and Administration	Comments
Amphetamine sulfate (also called racemic or dl-amphetamine sulfate)	Benzedrine*	Narcolepsy	ORAL: *Adults and children over 6 — 5 to 60 mg daily in divided doses.* Sustained action formulations may be given once daily.	Dosage is adjusted according to patient's needs and tolerance. Sympathomimetic effects on cardiovascular system and central nervous system toxicity may be noted with long-term use.
		Hyperkinesis	ORAL: *Children — 3 to 5 yr,* 2.5 mg daily and increase by 2.5 mg increments weekly to achieve desired effect; *6 yr and older,* initially 5 mg daily and increase by 5 mg increments weekly up to a maximum daily dose of 40 mg.	Dosage should be minimal required for control of symptoms. Long-term continuous use should be avoided to prevent growth inhibition. Drugs may be withdrawn during less stressful periods, such as summer holidays. Schedule II substance.

Dextroamphetamine sulfate	Dexampex Dexedrine* Ferndex	Narcolepsy Hyperkinesis	Same as for amphetamine sulfate. Same as for amphetamine sulfate.	Same as for amphetamine sulfate, except less tendency to produce cardiovascular toxicity. Schedule II substance.
Methamphetamine hydrochloride	Desoxyn Methampex	Hyperkinesis	ORAL: *Children 6 yr and older* — 2.5 to 5 mg once or twice daily; increase by 5 mg increments at weekly intervals to optimal dosage, usually 20 to 25 mg.	Has central nervous system and cardiovascular toxicity. Schedule II substance.
Methylphenidate hydrochloride	Methidate† Ritalin*	Hyperkinesis	ORAL: *Children 6 yr and older* — 5 mg before breakfast and lunch; increase by 5 to 10 mg at weekly intervals up to 0.3 to	Drug of choice for most hyperkinetic children. Schedule II substance. *cont'd. next page*

*Available in U.S. and Canada
†Available in Canada only

Pocket Nurse Guide to Drugs

Table 4-1 Administration of CNS stimulants for narcolepsy and hyperkinesis—cont'd.

Generic Name	Trade Name	Medical Use	Dosage and Administration	Comments
Methylphenidate hydrochloride—cont'd.			0.5 mg/kg. Special cases may rarely require doses up to 2 mg/kg.	
		Narcolepsy	ORAL: *Adults* — 10 to 60 mg daily. Common dose is 10 mg twice or 3 times daily.	May be used with imipramine to treat narcolepsy. Schedule II substance.
Pemoline	Cylert	Hyperkinesis	ORAL: *Children 6 and older* — 37.5 mg daily in a single dose; increase weekly by 18.75 mg increments until response is obtained. Effective dosage range usually 56 to 75 mg daily. Do not exceed 112.5 mg daily.	Clinical effects develop over 3 to 4 wk period. Schedule IV substance.

| Deanol | Deaner | Hyperkinesis, some learning disorders | ORAL: *Children 6 and older* — 500 mg daily, reduced to 250 mg daily as response allows. | Less effect on central nervous system stimulation, basal metabolic rate, blood pressure, or pulse rate. |

*Available in U.S. and Canada
†Available in Canada only

Pocket Nurse Guide to Drugs

confusion, panic, or increased libido. Rarely, a schizophrenia-like syndrome may occur, with delirium or hallucinations. *Cardiovascular* effects include headache chilliness, palpitations, pallor or flushing, precipitation of angina or arrhythmias: hypertension or hypotension may occur during drug intoxication, with circulatory collapse with severe intoxication. Children may experience growth retardation.

Methylphenidate

Nervousness and insomnia. Gastrointestinal, central nervous system, and cardiovascular side effects are similar to those of amphetamines (see above). Temporary slowing of growth may occur in prepubertal children.

Pemoline

Seldom causes serious toxic reactions. May cause transient insomnia. May cause anorexia, stomache ache, and nausea. Allergic reactions may produce skin rashes and altered liver function tests. Central nervous system effects may include irritability, mild depression, dizziness, headache, and hallucinations. Overdose usually results in tachycardia and agitation.

Additional Nursing Implications for CNS Stimulants for Narcolepsy and Hyperkinesis

- See also general nursing implications, pp. 55-56.
- When therapy is being initiated with these drugs, the patient should be weighed two to three times per week until the effects of the drug can be evaluated.
- Although not being given for the purpose of weight reduction, most of these drugs will suppress the appetite.
- Careful weight and height records should be kept on a weekly or monthly basis for children being treated for hyperkinesis. Parents can be instructed to do this at home.
- Caution parents that several weeks of therapy may be necessary in some cases before the results can be seen.
- Drug therapy for hyperkinesis or narcolepsy should be accompanied by appropriate family and patient teaching, counseling, and support.

CNS Stimulants to Suppress Appetite

Benzphetamine hydrochloride
Clortermine hydrochloride
Diethylpropion hydrochloride
Fenfluramine hydrochloride
Mazindol
Phendimetrazine tartrate
Phentermine
Phenylpropanolamine hydrochloride

Actions of CNS Stimulants to Suppress Appetite

Many CNS stimulants suppress appetite even while stimulating other CNS functions. These are termed anorexiants. Most anorexiants cause less stimulation of the CNS than the amphetamines. Benzphetamine, phenmetrazine, and mazindol resemble the amphetamines in action but produce less severe reactions. Diethylpropion, clortermine, and phendimetrazine produce little significant cardiovascular stimulation. Fenfluramine depresses the CNS while suppressing appetite.

Indications for CNS Stimulants for Appetite Suppression

The use of appetite suppressants in the treatment of obesity remains controversial because of the side effects, risks, and potential for abuse and psychological dependence. They should be used only temporarily (less than 12 weeks), and only with supervision.

Nurse Alert for CNS Stimulants for Appetite Suppression

- Not proven safe during pregnancy or lactation.
- May precipitate psychotic reactions with prolonged use or overdose.
- Fenfluramine is contraindicated for patients with history of depression or suicidal tendencies.

Table 4-2 Administration of CNS stimulants for appetite suppression

Generic Name	Trade Name	Dosage and Administration	Comments
Benzphetamine hydrochloride	Didrex	ORAL: *Adults*—25 to 50 mg once daily; may be increased as needed up to 3 doses daily.	Similar to amphetamine. Schedule III substance.
Clortermine hydrochloride	Voranil	ORAL: *Adults*—50 mg daily at midmorning.	Insomnia is common reaction. Schedule III substance.
Diethylpropion hydrochloride	Depletite Tenuate* Tepanil	ORAL: *Adults*—25 mg 1 hr before morning, noon, and evening meals and at mid-evening if needed. Timed-release formulations (75 mg) are taken once daily.	Safest anorexiant for use in patients with mild cardiovascular disease. Dry mouth and constipation are common reactions. Schedule IV substance.
Fenfluramine hydrochloride	Pondimin* Ponderal†	ORAL: *Adults*—20 mg 3 times daily before meals. Dosage may be doubled if required.	Only anorexiant that depresses central nervous system activity. Schedule IV substance.
Mazindol	Mazanor Sanorex* Teronac†	ORAL: *Adults*—Doses range from 1 mg daily at breakfast to 1 mg 3 times daily with meals. Minimum dose should be used.	May be used in patients with mild cardiovascular disease. Insomnia, dizziness, and agitation occur. Schedule III substance.

Phendimetrazine tartrate	Anorex Bacarate Ex-Obese Limit Melfiat Plegine Statobex	ORAL: *Adults*—35 mg 2 or 3 times daily taken before meals. Sustained release, 105 mg taken once in the morning.	Stimulates the central nervous system in the same manner as the amphetamines. Gastrointestinal distress may occur. Schedule III substance.
Phentermine	Adipex Fastin Ionamin Tora	ORAL: *Adults*—8 mg 3 times daily before meals or single dose of 15 or 37.5 mg may be taken 2 hr after breakfast.	Commonly causes insomnia and cardiovascular effects. Schedule IV substance.
Phenylpropanolamine hydrochloride	Control Dex-A-Diet II Dexatrim Diadax Dietac Prolamine	ORAL: *Adults*—35 mg 3 times daily before meals or 50 to 75 mg of sustained-action formulation once daily at midmorning.	Widely used as a nasal decongestant. Blood pressure increases occur. These diet preparations should never be used with cold or allergy medications. Nonprescription.

*Available in U.S. and Canada
†Available in Canada only

66   Pocket Nurse Guide to Drugs

- Patients should be cautioned to avoid cold remedies, allergy medications, and nasal decongestants that include sympathomimetic agents, because of heightened effects. Not for use in children under age 12 because of possible growth retardation.

Side Effects of CNS Stimulants for Appetite Suppression

Psychological dependence, psychotic reactions in toxic doses, gastrointestinal distress, dry mouth, blurred vision, heart palpitations, hypertension.

Table 4-3 lists systemic effects of the anorexiants.

Additional Nursing Implications for CNS Stimulants for Appetite Suppression

- See also the general nursing implications for CNS stimulants (pp. 55-56).
- Although weight reduction will usually occur while patients are taking appetite suppressants, long-term weight reduction requires the concomitant use of patient counseling and patient alteration of dietary habits.
- Weight reduction will occur rapidly during the first couple of weeks of therapy, but will slow after that.
- These drugs may alter the seizure threshold. Observe patients with a history of seizures when initiating therapy.
- If tolerance to the loss of appetite effects occurs after several weeks, the patient should be instructed to notify the physician. The treatment is to discontinue therapy rather than to increase the dose of the drug.
- Fenfluramine should not be given to patients with a history of depression or suicidal tendencies, or to patients with a history of alcohol abuse.

CNS Stimulants for Respiratory Stimulation

Citrated caffeine   Doxapram
Caffeine sodium benzoate   Theophylline

Table 4-3   Systemic effects of the anorexiants

Generic Name	Effects On				
	Mood	Motor Activity	Heart Rate	Blood Pressure	Abuse Potential
Amphetamine sulfate	Highly elevated	Increased	Increased	Increased	Very high
Benzphetamine	Elevated	May increase	May increase	May increase	High
Clortermine	May be elevated	May increase	Unchanged	Unchanged	High
Diethylpropion	May be elevated	May increase	Unchanged	Unchanged	Relatively low
Fenfluramine	Depressed	Depressed	Usually no change	May increase	Relatively low
Mazindol	May be elevated	May increase	Increased	Usually no change	High
Phendimetrazine	Highly elevated	Increased	Usually no change	Usually no change	High
Phenmetrazine	Highly elevated	Increased	Increased	Increased	Very high
Phentermine	Usually no change	May increase	Increased	Increased	Relatively low
Phenylpropanolamine	Usually no change	Usually no change	May increase	May increase	None

Actions of CNS Stimulants for Respiratory Stimulation

Methylxanthines (caffeine and theophylline) block the destruction of cyclic AMP, which mediates the effects of beta adrenergic stimulation, thus affecting many body systems. Depending on dose, caffeine stimulates all levels of the CNS, including the medullary centers controlling respiration, vasomotor tone, and vagal tone; very high doses may stimulate the spinal cord and cause convulsion. Theophylline produces similar effects with greater action on the heart.

At low doses, *doxapram* seems to stimulate peripheral carotid chemoreceptors, increasing the impulse to breathe. At higher doses it stimulates the medullary centers controlling respiration.

Indications for CNS Stimulants for Respiratory Stimulation

Used to stimulate respiration, but the use of these drugs is less common because of modern ventilatory therapy techniques.

Theophylline is most often used to relax bronchial smooth muscle, to treat chronic obstructive pulmonary disease (COPD) and asthma, and to stimulate respiration in newborn infants.

Nurse Alert for CNS Stimulants for Respiratory Stimulation

- Must be used cautiously because of nonspecific stimulation of CNS that may produce unwanted effects. In high doses may produce convulsion in predisposed patients.
- Doxapram is contraindiated in patients receiving other medication to raise blood pressure and in patients on inhalation anesthetics such as halothane, cyclopropane, and enflurane.

Side Effects of CNS Stimulants for Respiratory Stimulation

Methylxanthines irritate the GI tract and may product bleeding, nausea, vomiting. Normal doses may produce nervous-

Table 4-4 Administration of CNS stimulants for respiratory stimulation

Generic Name	Trade Name	Dosage and Administration	Comments
Caffeine (citrated caffeine)		ORAL, NASOGASTRIC TUBE: 10 mg/kg initially, then 2.5 mg/kg daily.	Used especially in newborn infants.
Caffeine sodium benzoate injection		INTRAMUSCULAR, INTRAVENOUS: 500 mg as necessary.	Care must be taken to avoid overdosage.
Doxapram	Dopram*	INTRAVENOUS: *Adults*—0.5 to 2 mg/kg intermittently as needed. For chronic obstructive pulmonary disease, 1 to 2 mg/min infusion for 2 hr.	Rapidly acting drug whose action is over within 12 min.
Theophylline		ORAL, NASOGASTRIC TUBE: 6 mg/kg initial dose, then 2 mg/kg every 12 hr. INTRAVENOUS: Aminophylline, the only form for parenteral use, contains 79-85% theophylline. Doses are 5.5 mg/kg initially, then infusion of 1.1 mg/kg until proper plasma level of theophylline is reached.	Most commonly used to treat asthma but is also used to treat apnea in newborn infants. Effective plasma concentrations range from 5 to 12 μg/ml with toxicity expected above 20 μg/ml.

*Available in U.S. and Canada

70 **Pocket Nurse Guide to Drugs**

ness, or jitteriness, with excessive CNS stimulation and convulsions at high doses. Theophylline commonly causes tachycardia, and may precipitate other arrhythmias or hypotension. Diuresis may occur with these agents. *Doxapram* may cause dizziness, apprehension, disorientation, involuntary muscle activity, increased reflexes, warmth with flushing and sweating, elevated blood pressure, chest pains and cardiac arrhythmias; overdose may cause extreme agitation, hallucinations, and convulsions.

Additional Nursing Implications for CNS Stimulants for Respiratory Stimulation

- See also general nursing implications for CNS stimulants, pp. 55-56.
- Seizures may occur as a result of using these drugs. Have a suction machine at the bedside. Keep siderails, up, use padded siderails, or by other means make certain that the patient cannot fall. The patient should not be left unattended.
- Oxygen and resuscitation equipment should be readily available.
- Monitor pulse, blood pressure, and respiration frequently. This may mean every 3 to 5 minutes with intravenous adminstration of a drug, to every 15 to 30 minutes with nasogastric adminstration.
- The patient should be attached to a cardiac monitor.
- Monitor the patient's temperature when using doxapram.
- Short-acting barbiturates (e.g., pentobarbital sodium) should be available to counteract the central nervous system stimulant effects of these drugs.
- See the manufacturer's literature for specific guidelines about drug dilution, dose, and rate of administration for doxapram.

Narcotic Analgesics and Antagonists

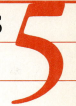

Narcotic analgesics
  Alphaprodine hydrochloride
  Buprenorphine hydrochloride
  Butorphanol tartrate
  Codeine sulfate
  Codeine phosphate
  Fentanyl
  Hydromorphone hydrochloride
  Levorphanol tartrate
  Meperidine hydrochloride
  Methadone hydrochloride
  Morphine sulfate
  Nalbuphine hydrochloride
  Oxycodone
  Oxymorphone hydrochloride
  Pentazocine hydrochloride
  Pentazocine lactate
  Propoxyphene hydrochloride
  Propoxyphene napsylate
  Sufentanil citrate

Narcotic antagonists
  Levallorphan tartrate
  Naloxone hydrochloride
  Naltrexone

Narcotic Analgesics

Actions of Narcotic Analgesics

Narcotic analgesics mimic endorphins; they act at brain sites to modify pain perception and reaction, and to depress medullary centers including the respiratory center, and the chemoreceptor trigger zone.

Indications for Narcotic Analgesics

Narcotic analgesics are used in the management of pain, and for preanesthetic medication and surgical anesthesia. Table

5-1 compares the narcotic analgesics as indicated for different pain levels, including onset and duration. Morphine is also the narcotic of choice for pulmonary edema or myocardial infarct patients. Methadone is also used as a replacement drug for opiate dependence or to facilitate withdrawal. Buprenorphine is an investigational drug administered for analgesia.

Nurse Alert for Narcotic Analgesics

- Opiates should be used cautiously if at all in patients with impaired respiratory function, asthma, or head injuries; in nursing mothers, and pregnant women.
- Opiates should be used cautiously in patients with shock, blood loss, or chronic obstructive lung disease
- Drug tolerance and dependency may result with any of the opioids
- The opioid withdrawal syndrome includes symptoms of rhinorrhea, lacrimation, sweating, yawning, and less reactive pupils in the first 16 hours, followed by restlessness, insomnia, hot and cold flashes, and abdominal cramps over the next 20 hours, with nausea, vomiting, and diarrhea occurring by 36 hours.
- If opioids are given intravenously or in high doses, antagonists and resuscitation equipment should be available.
- Meperidine in high doses is excitatory and may cause convulsions, especially in renally impaired patients, due to accumulation of its metabolite, normeperidine.
- Butorphanol increases pulmonary artery pressure and cardiac work load and is contraindicated for the pain of myocardial infarction or pulmonary edema.
- Pentazocine is less desirable for myocardial infarction and pulmonary hypertension; it causes dysphoria rather than euphoria, including nightmares, hallucinations, and seizures in large doses.
- Narcotic overdose is manifested by respiratory depression, slower breathing, Cheyne-Stokes respirations, cyanosis, sleepiness progressing to stupor or coma, hypotension, and skeletal muscle flaccidity.

Text continued on p. 77

Table 5-1 Narcotic analgesics

Level of Pain	Drug	Equivalent Analgesic Dose (mg) Given IM or SC	Time for Peak Effect (min)	Duration (hr)
Severe	Morphine	10	30 to 90	4 to 6
	Hydromorphone hydrochloride (Dilaudid)	1.5	30 to 90	4 to 5
	Oxymorphone (Numorphan)	1 to 1.5	30 to 90	3 to 6
	Levorphanol tartrate (Levo-Dromoran)	2 to 3	60 to 90	4 to 8
	Methadone (Dolophine)	7.5 to 10	60 to 120	4 to 6*
Moderate to severe	Alphaprodine (Nisentil)	40 to 60	30	1 to 2
	Buprenorphine (Buprenex)	0.3 to 0.6		
	Butorphanol (Stadol)	1.5 to 3.5	30	3 to 4
	Meperidine (Demerol)	75 to 100	30 to 60	2 to 4
	Nalbuphine (Nubain)	10	30	3 to 6
	Pentazocine (Talwin)	40 to 60	30 to 60	2 to 3
	Oxycodone	15 PO	60 to 90	4 to 6
Mild to moderate	Codeine phosphate	120	60 to 90	4 to 6
	Propoxyphene (Darvon)	180 to 240 PO	60	4 to 6
	Fentanyl	0.1	5 to 30	1 to 2
	Sufentanil	0.02 to 0.14	5 to 30	1

*Increases with prolonged, repeated use due to accumulation.

Table 5-2 Administration of narcotic analgesics

Generic Name	Trade Name	Dosage and Administration
Alphaprodine hydrochloride	Nisentil*	SUBCUTANEOUS: *Adults and children over 12 yr*—0.4 to 1.2 mg/kg not to exceed 240 mg in 24 hr. INTRAVENOUS: *Adults and children over 12 yr*—0.4 to 0.6 mg/kg not to exceed 240 mg in 24 hr. Not for children under 12 yr.
Buprenorphine hydrochloride	Buprenex	INTRAMUSCULAR: *Adults*—0.3 to 0.6 mg, repeat every 6 to 8 hours as required.
Butorphanol tartrate	Stadol	INTRAMUSCULAR: *Adults*—1 to 4 mg every 4 hr. INTRAVENOUS: *Adults*—0.5 to 2 mg every 4 hr.
Codeine sulfate, codeine phosphate		ORAL, INTRAMUSCULAR, SUBCUTANEOUS: *Adults*—30 to 60 mg every 4 to 6 hr. *Children*—0.5 mg/kg every 4 to 6 hr.
Fentanyl	Sublimaze	INTRAMUSCULAR, INTRAVENOUS: 0.025 to 0.1 mg
Hydromorphone hydrochloride	Dilaudid*	ORAL: *Adult*—2 mg every 4 to 6 hr. INTRAMUSCULAR, SUBCUTANEOUS: *Adult*—1 to 1.5 mg every 4 to 6 hr. May be given by slow intravenous injection or as a suppository.
Levorphanol tartrate	Levo-Dromoran*	ORAL, SUBCUTANEOUS: *Adults*—2 mg every 6 to 8 hours

Meperidine hydrochloride	Demerol* Pethidine HCL†	ORAL, INTRAMUSCULAR, SUBCUTANEOUS, SLOW INTRAVENOUS: *Adults*—50 to 150 mg every 3 to 4 hr. *Children*—1 to 1.5 mg/kg up to 100 mg, every 3 to 4 hr.
Methadone hydrochloride	Dolophine	ORAL, INTRAMUSCULAR, SUBCUTANEOUS: *Adults*—2.5 to 10 mg. For pain relief, repeat every 6 to 12 hours.
Morphine sulfate		ORAL: *Adults*—10 to 30 mg every 4 to 6 hours. INTRAMUSCULAR, SUBCUTANEOUS: *Adults*—5 to 20 mg every 4 hr. *Children* (subcutaneous only)—0.1 to 0.2 mg/kg up to 15 mg. INTRAVENOUS: *Adults*—2.5 to 15 mg in 5 ml water, injected over 4 to 5 min. *Children*—0.1 to 0.2 mg/kg.
Nalbuphine hydrochloride	Nubain*	INTRAMUSCULAR, SUBCUTANEOUS, INTRAVENOUS: *Adults*—10 mg every 4 to 6 hr, maximum single dose 20 mg and maximum daily dose 160 mg.
Oxycodone		ORAL: *Adults*—5-10 mg every 6 hours
Oxymorphone hydrochloride	Numorphan*	INTRAMUSCULAR, SUBCUTANEOUS: *Adults*—1 to 1.5 mg every 6 hr. INTRAVENOUS: *Adults*—0.5 mg. RECTAL: *Adults*—5 mg every 4 to 6 hr.

cont'd. next page

*Available in U.S. and Canada
†Available in Canada only

Table 5-2   Administration of narcotic analgesics—cont'd.

Generic Name	Trade Name	Dosage and Administration
Pentazocine hydrochloride	Talwin NX*	ORAL: *Adults*—50 mg every 4 hr, up to 600 mg daily. Every 50 mg of oral pentazocine is now formulated with 0.5 mg naloxone to curb drug abuse.
Pentazocine lactate	Talwin Lactate*	INTRAMUSCULAR, SUBCUTANEOUS, INTRAVENOUS: *Adults*—30 mg every 3 to 4 hr. Subcutaneous route is not recommended, may cause tissue damage
Propoxyphene hydrochloride	Darvon Dolene SK65	ORAL: *Adults*—65 mg every 6 to 8 hr.
Propoxyphene napsylate	Darvon-N*	ORAL: *Adults*—100 mg every 6 to 8 hr.
Sufentanil citrate	Sufenta	INTRAMUSCULAR, INTRAVENOUS: 1 to 2 μg/kg

*Available in U.S. and Canada
†Available in Canada only

Narcotic Analgesics and Antagonists **77**

- Pentazocine, butorphanol, and nalbuphine should be used with caution in narcotic-dependent patients, because withdrawal symptoms may be precipitated.
- Meperidine is contraindicated in patients taking monoamine oxidase inhibitors.
- Meperidine is preferred over morphine in pancreatitis patients because it is less likely to cause biliary tract spasms.

Side Effects of Narcotic Analgesics

Side effects include respiratory depression, nausea and vomiting, constipation, urinary retention, itching, hypotension, inhibition of gastric, biliary, and pancreatic secretions, and reduction in pupil size. Additional side effects may include flushing, palpitations, syncope, pruritus, rashes, uticaria, dry mouth, anorexia, and central nervous system effects such as euphoria, dysphoria, headache, insomnia, agitation, disorientation, and visual disturbances.

Nursing Implications for Narcotic Analgesics

- Narcotic analgesics are drugs with the potential for serious undesirable side effects and abuse. Because most narcotic analgesics are ordered on an "as needed" (p.r.n.) basis, it is important that health care personnel learn to assess each patient with sensitivity and objectivity. In addition, knowledge of the effects of each individual medication the patient is receiving should assist health care personnel in making the decision whether to administer a medication.
- Too often, a narcotic drug is unnecessarily substituted for other comfort measures. Other activities for providing comfort such as repositioning patient, offering food, drink or reassurance may be appropriate.
- Pain in the nonalert patient may be manifested by restlessness, increase in blood pressure or pulse, sweating, and facial grimaces.
- Explain to the patient what results can reasonably be expected from the medications being taken and enlist the patient's aid in determining the best combination of drugs to be used in any anticipated situation. Patients should not be

Pocket Nurse Guide to Drugs

denied appropriate pharmacological help, but neither should health care personnel overmedicate a patient through poor planning or lack of knowledge.

- Pain is a warning signal, and its unexpected persistence should be investigated. If it is suspected that the patient receiving narcotic analgesics is becoming addicted, the health care team should plan as a group an individualized approach to the problem.
- Postoperative patients who fear addiction should be reassured that use of narcotics in decreasing amounts over 3 or 4 days will not cause addiction and that recovery will be easier if severe pain can be lessened.
- If and when a patient with cancer begins to have pain, the choice of analgesic should be based on individual patient assessment and should begin with nonnarcotic analgesics, if possible. For many patients, high doses of aspirin may be adequate initially, and as this becomes ineffective, combination products with aspirin or acetaminophen and a mild narcotic (e.g., propoxyphene combinations, oxycodone combinations) can be tried. Finally, potent narcotic analgesics, either alone or in combination with antiemetics or tranquilizers, may be used.
- The goal for the use of analgesics with terminal cancer patients should be pain relief, or lessening of the pain, without serious side effects or marked sedation. Thus narcotic analgesics may relieve the pain, but their early use in the course of cancer treatment can cause an otherwise functional and active patient to become markedly sedated, to require higher and higher doses of narcotics, and to become less independent and functional.
- Health care personnel should be knowledgeable about the component parts of all analgesic preparations they administer. For example, Tylox and Percocet both contain acetaminophen and oxycodone.
- Narcotic analgesics provide better pain relief if taken before pain becomes severe. For this reason, a pain medication is more effective if taken 30 to 60 minutes before a dressing change, ambulation, wound debridement, or other painful activity.

Narcotic Analgesics and Antagonists **79**

- Because pain interferes with sleep and rest, can increase anxiety, and can decrease a patient's willingness to perform needed postoperative activities (turning, coughing, deep breathing), narcotics should be given every 4 hours (or as ordered) around the clock during the first 24 hours after major surgery. This decision, of course, should still be based on the individual patient's response.
- Because of cough suppression and respiratory depression caused by anesthesia and narcotic analgesics, postoperative patients should be turned and made to cough and breathe deeply every 2 hours to prevent pulmonary complications.
- If nausea and vomiting occur, it may be possible to administer an antiemetic with the analgesic. Although this reduces nausea, it may also potentiate hypotension and sedation.
- Constipation can be a severe problem for patients taking narcotic analgesics. When possible, patients should be ambulated as soon as possible and frequently. Fluid intake should be increased to 2500 to 3000 ml per day. The diet should include a variety of vegetables, fruits, and fiber, if possible. It may be necessary to use cathartics and/or stool softeners in patients receiving narcotics on a long-term basis.
- The elderly or patients receiving narcotic analgesics in moderate to large doses should be assisted to ambulate, and the blood pressure should be monitored every 4 hours. Keep the siderails up while the patient is in bed.
- Patients receiving narcotic analgesics may have a decreased urge to void. Monitor the intake and output. Remind patients to void every 4 hours if they have not. Notify the physician if a patient with an adequate intake is unable to void in 8 hours.
- For the hospitalized patient in severe pain, narcotics are sometimes ordered IV. In some situations, it is desirable to administer the dose via direct intravenous injection (IV push), such as for morphine in a patient experiencing an acute myocardial infarction. Often it may be desirable to infuse the medication slowly over 30 or more minutes. For slow infusion, dilute the medication as directed by the

80 Pocket Nurse Guide to Drugs

pharmacy, use a microdrip infusion set and/or a volume control device, and if appropriate, consider the use of an electronic infusion monitoring device. Calculation of the infusion rate is important. Too rapid infusion of a narcotic, whether by direct infusion or diluted, may produce marked sedation, hypotension, respiratory depression, circulatory collapse, and death. Monitor the vital signs, and slow or stop the infusion if undesirable side effects begin to occur. If an ordered dose for intravenous infusion seems excessively high, do not hesitate to question the physician.

- Discharge teaching for any patient being sent home while taking analgesics needs to be individualized. The patient should be taught the name of the drug, the frequency with which it may be taken, what side effects may occur and what to do about them, and what to do if the pain worsens.
- It is especially important that adults keep narcotic analgesics out of the reach of children to avoid overdose and death.
- Narcotic analgesics may cause drowsiness and should be used with caution when it is necessary to be alert, such as for driving or operating machinery.
- Patients should avoid the use of the central nervous system depressants (including tranquilizers, sedative-hypnotics, narcotic analgesics, and alcohol) while taking narcotic analgesics.
- Meperidine syrup should be taken in a glass of water, because when undiluted, the syrup may cause temporary mucous membrane anesthesia.

Narcotic Antagonists

Levallorphan tartrate
Naloxone hydrochloride
Naltrexone

Actions of Narcotic Antagonists

Narcotic antagonists replace opioids at receptor sites and reverse the effects of narcotics with minimal or no effects.

Indications for Narcotic Antagonists

Levallorphan is used to reverse respiratory depression resulting from narcotic overdose. *Naloxone* is the drug of choice to reverse respiratory depression resulting from narcotic overdose, and is used to reverse narcotic respiratory depression following surgery and to diagnose suspected narcotic overdose. *Naltrexone* is a long-acting antagonist that can be taken orally to block the euphoric physiologic effects of abused opioids as an adjunct in a rehabilitation program.

Table 5-3 Administration of narcotic antagonists

Generic Name	Trade Name	Dosage and Administration
Levallorphan tartrate	Lorfan*	INTRAVENOUS: *Adults*—1 mg followed by 1 or 2 doses of 0.5 mg spaced every 10 to 15 min. *Neonates*—0.05 to 0.1 mg into umbilical vein on delivery.
Naloxone hydrochloride	Narcan*	INTRAVENOUS, INTRAMUSCULAR, SUBCUTANEOUS: *Adults*—0.4 mg for respiratory depression caused by narcotic overdose. Repeated in a few minutes if necessary up to 3 doses. For narcotic depression of respiration after surgery: 0.1 to 0.2 mg every few minutes as necessary. INTRAVENOUS: *Neonates*—0.01 mg/kg.
Naltrexone	Trexan	ORAL: *Adults*—50 mg daily. May be given as 100 mg every other day or 150 mg every three days.

*Available in U.S. and Canada

Nurse Alert for Narcotic Antagonists

- Because naloxone has a short duration of action, monitor the patient to be sure the overdose effects do not return when the naloxone wears off. Patients who have overdosed with long-acting narcotics such as methadone may require repeated injections of naloxone throughout the day.
- Because levallorphan causes respiratory depression (although less than narcotics) it may worsen the patient's respiratory depression if it is not caused by a narcotic. Naltrexone should not be given to a patient with a history of hepatitis or liver failure or to a patient in acute opioid withdrawal.

Side Effects of Narcotic Antagonists

Levallorphan may cause dysphoria and respiratory depression if opioid drug is not present. *Naloxone* may cause hypertension, tachycardia, hyperventilation, and nausea.

Nursing Implications for Narcotic Antagonists

- Monitor the vital signs frequently (every 5 to 15 minutes) until the patient's condition stabilizes after administration of a narcotic antagonist. The patient should not be left unattended. The effects of the narcotic antagonist may wear off before the effects of the narcotic does, and it may be necessary to repeat the dose.
- No drug overdose should be treated lightly. Monitor vital signs, intake and output. Attach patient to cardiac monitor. Intubation and suctioning equipment should be nearby.

General Anesthetics

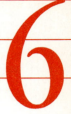

Inhalation anesthetics
  Enflurane
  Halothane
  Isoflurane
  Methoxyflurane
  Nitrous oxide

Intravenous anesthetics
  Barbiturates
    Methohexital sodium
    Thiamylal sodium
    Thiopental sodium
  Benzodiazepines
    Diazepam
    Flunitrazepam
  Miscellaneous
    Ketamine
    Fentanyl citrate
    Droperidol & Fentanyl
    Etomidate

Inhalation Anesthetics

Actions of Inhalation Anesthetics

General anesthetics act on the central nervous system to abolish the perception of pain and reaction to painful stimuli, apparently not by receptor mechanisms but by altering cell membranes in the neurons.

Indications for Inhalation Anesthetics

Halothane is the most widely used of volatile liquid anesthetics. *Isoflurane* is gaining in use as a depressant anesthetic because of fewer side effects. *Methoxyflurane* produces analgesia for dentistry and obstetrics. *Nitrous oxide* is used by itself for dental and obstetrical procedures, and with other anesthetics for surgical anesthesia. *Enflurane* is supplanting halothane because enflurane produces a lesser incidence of liver damage and better skeletal muscle relaxation than halothane.

Nurse Alert for Inhalation Anesthetics

- Preoperative medications are an integral part of anesthesia and must be administered properly.
- Monitor vital signs frequently postoperatively.
- Keep patients on their sides postoperatively, or supervise carefully, to prevent aspiration if vomiting occurs; medicate with an antiemetic if necessary, and keep suctioning equipment available.

Administration of Inhalation Anesthetics

Potency of inhalation anesthetics is determined by the agent's minimum alveolar concentration (MAC) that produces anesthesia, with surgery being conducted at about 1.4 times the MAC value.

Side Effects of Inhalation Anesthetics

Enflurane causes a decrease in blood pressure, low body temperature, hypothermia, and shivering. *Halothane* may cause reduction in cardiac output, hypotension, and possible hepatic dysfunction, especially in patients with liver disease. *Isoflurane* causes a decrease in blood pressure. *Methoxyflurane* causes lowered blood pressure, and in prolonged

Table 6-1 Administration of inhalation anesthetics

Drug	Physical Properties	Onset	MAC
Enflurane (Ethrane)	Nonflammable liquid	Rapid	1.68%
Halothane (Fluothane)	Nonflammable liquid	Rapid	0.77%
Isoflurane (Forane)	Nonflammable liquid	Rapid	1.3%
Methoxyflurane (Penthrane)	Nonflammable liquid	Slow	0.16%
Nitrous oxide	Nonflammable gas	Very rapid	101%

anesthesia may cause high-output reversible renal failure. *Nitrous oxide* increases the incidence of spontaneous abortion and may decrease spermatogenesis. All of the inhalation anesthetics can trigger malignant hyperthermia.

Nursing Implications for General Anesthetics

- Preparation for surgery should include an opportunity for the patient to discuss questions and concerns about anesthesia with the anesthesiologist or nurse anesthetist.
- Anticipate possible patient fears related to the surgery, and other questions; answer them if possible, or refer them to the nurse anesthetist or anesthesiologist.
- The patient should be taught how to cough preoperatively, and told that it will be necessary to do this regularly and frequently postoperatively to prevent respiratory complications.
- Whether the patient is intubated or not, the respiratory function must be monitored closely in terms of rate, depth, and ability to handle secretions. After major surgery, measurement of arterial blood gases may be necessary to assist in the respiratory management. Suctioning equipment should be at the bedside, and ventilatory support equipment should be available.
- Each patient should be evaluated individually in deciding how soon to medicate a patient for pain in the immediate postoperative period (the first 2 to 4 hours after surgery). The evaluation involves considering such parameters as the patient's blood pressure, pulse, respirations, anesthetic agent, length of anesthesia, level of consciousness, and the effects the analgesic may have on these parameters. Often the decision is made to medicate the patient for pain the first time using one-fourth to one-half of the ordered dose of analgesic. Note that the decision to give a reduced dose should be made only with the approval of the physician. It is specifically recommended that when Innovar is used the first dose of postoperative analgesic be a small dose.
- Unless specifically contraindicated, postoperative patients should be encouraged to breathe deeply and to cough

86 Pocket Nurse Guide to Drugs

several times every 2 hours. In addition, other treatments such as blow bottles or *I*ntermittent *P*ositive *P*ressure *B*reathing (IPPB) may be ordered to prevent pulmonary complications, and these should be administered as ordered.

- Effects of anesthesia persist even after the patient appears to be alert and awake. If it is necessary to give instructions about activity, diet, or medications (as it might be in the outpatient or day surgery setting), they should be given both verbally and in writing to the patient and reviewed with family members if present.
- Patients who have a severe reaction or response to any anesthetic should be cautioned to carry with them the name of the particular agent and, if surgery is ever again needed, to inform the anesthesiologist of the previous agent used and the poor response.

Intravenous Anesthetics

Barbiturates
    Methohexital sodium
    Thiamylal sodium
    Thiopental sodium
Benzodiazepines
    Diazepam
    Flunitrazepam

Miscellaneous
    Ketamine
    Fentanyl citrate
    Droperidol & Fentanyl citrate
    Etomidate

Actions of Intravenous Anesthetics

Of these drugs, only ketamine is a true anesthetic that abolishes the perception of and reaction to pain. Barbiturates provide no analgesia.

Indications for Intravenous Anesthetics

The barbiturates are used to induce rapid anesthesia. The benzodiazepines are used occasionally to induce anesthesia but more commonly to sedate patients for cardioversion or endoscopic or dental procedures. Ketamine is used to produce a cataleptic anesthesia (dissociative anesthesia). Fentanyl citrate with droperidol is used to produce neuroleptanesthesia. Various narcotic analgesics are often used for balanced anesthesia. Etomidate is used to induce surgical anesthesia.

Nurse Alert for Intravenous Anesthetics

- Preoperative medications are an integral part of anesthesia and must be administered properly.
- Monitor vital signs frequently postoperatively.
- Keep patients on their sides postoperatively or supervise carefully, to prevent aspiration if vomiting occurs; medicate with an antiemetic if necessary, and keep suctioning equipment available.
- Ketamine should be used cautiously in patients with convulsive disorders, psychosis, mild hypertension, or undergoing eye surgery; it is contraindicated for patients with coronary artery disease, severe hypertension, stroke, or treated hyperthyroidism.
- Diazepam should not be mixed with other liquids for intravenous injection.

Side Effects of Intravenous Anesthetics

Barbiturates depress respiration and may cause yawning, coughing, or laryngospasm (see also Ch. 1). *Methohexital* can cause hiccups. The side effects of *diazepam* are described in Chapter 1; *flunitrazepam* has similar effects. *Ketamine* enhances muscle tone, increases blood pressure, heart rate, and respiratory secretions, and may cause vivid nightmares or hallucinations, vomiting, and shivering. *Droperidol* may cause extrapyramidal symptoms. *Etomidate* may cause pain at the injection site and transient myoclonic skeletal muscle movements.

Nursing Implications for Intravenous Anesthetics for Ketamine

- Psychic disturbances are relatively common and include unpleasant dreams, emergence delirium, irrational behavior, disorientation, and hallucinations. The occurrence of these

Table 6-2 Administration of intravenous anesthetics

Generic Name	Trade Name	Dosage and Administration
Barbiturates		
Methohexital sodium	Brevital Sodium, Brietal Sodium†	INTRAVENOUS: *Adults*—for induction, 5 to 12 ml of 1% solution no faster than 1 ml every 5 sec. Maintenance, 2 to 4 ml of 1% solution as required.
Thiamylal sodium	Surital*	INTRAVENOUS: *Adults*—for induction, 2 to 4 ml of 2.5% solution every 30 to 40 sec, up to 3 to 5 mg/kg maximum. Maintenance, 2 to 4 ml of 2.5% solution as required.
Thiopental sodium	Pentothal*	INTRAVENOUS: *Adults*—for induction, 50 to 100 mg (2 to 4 ml) in 2.5% solution every 30 to 40 sec or 3 to 5 mg/kg. Maintenance, 2 to 4 ml of 2.5% solution as required. *Children*—3 to 5 mg/kg as described for adults.
Benzodiazepines		
Diazepam	Apo-Diazepam†, E-Pam†, Meval†, Novodipam†, Valium*	INTRAVENOUS: *Adults*—0.1 to 0.2 mg/kg body weight to induce sleep. Basal sedation requires only 5 to 30 mg, so 2.5 to 5 mg is injected every 30 sec until a light sleep or slurred speech is produced.

General Anesthetics 89

Flunitrazepam	Rohypnol	INTRAVENOUS: *Adults*—for induction, 36 to 50 μg/kg over a period of 20 to 40 sec. Maintenance, 10 μg/kg as needed.
Miscellaneous		
Ketamine	Ketaject Ketalar*	INTRAVENOUS: *Adults and children*—1 to 4.5 mg/kg over a period of 60 sec., ½ of initial dose used for maintenance as needed. INTRAMUSCULAR: *Adults and children*—6.5 to 13 mg/kg, ½ of initial dose for maintenance as needed.
Fentanyl citrate	Sublimaze*	INTRAVENOUS: *Adults and children over 2 yr*—0.002 to 0.003 mg/kg in divided doses over a period of 6 to 8 min. Maintenance, 0.05 to 0.1 mg every 30 to 60 min. Onset: 1 to 2 min.
Droperidol	Inapsine*	INTRAVENOUS: *Adults and children over 2 yr*—0.15 mg/kg. Onset: 10 to 15 min. Duration: 3 to 6 hr.
Etomidate	Amidate Hypnomidate	INTRAVENOUS: *Adults and children over 10 years*—usual dose is 0.3 mg/kg injected over 30-60 seconds. Dose may vary between 0.2 and 0.6 mg/kg

*Available in U.S. and Canada
†Available in Canada only

90   **Pocket Nurse Guide to Drugs**

side effects may be lessened by providing the patient with a quiet wake-up period, perhaps in the quietest corner of the recovery room. Excessive stimulation should be avoided, although vital signs must still be monitored.

- If psychic side effects occur, provide calm reassurance and reorientation to the patient. Rarely a small hypnotic dose of a short-acting barbiturate may be needed to help terminate a severe reaction. If side effects occur, the patient should not be left unattended. If the patient is returned to the patient care unit from the recovery room, the room should be kept dimly lit and noise and stimulation kept to a minimum. Inform family members of the probable cause of behavior and enlist their aid in patient reorientation and reassurance.

Other Intravenous Anesthetics

See "Nursing implications for general anesthetics" on pp. 85-86.

Anticonvulsants

Barbiturates
   Phenobarbital
   Mephobarbital
   Primidone
Hydantoins
   Phenytoin
   Mephenytoin
   Ethotoin
Succinimides
   Ethosuximide
   Methsuximide
   Phensuximide
Oxazolidinedione
   Paramethadione
   Trimethadione
Benzodiazepines
   Diazepam
   Clonazepam
   Chlorazapate
Miscellaneous
   Acetazolamide
   Carbamazepine
   Lidocaine hydrochloride
   Paraldehyde
   Valproic acid

Actions of Anticonvulsants

The mechanism of action of anticonvulsants is not fully understood, but in general these drugs depress the excitability of neurons and thereby prevent the spread of seizure discharges, presumably by modifying molecular movements across the neuronal membrane or by modifying the neuronal release or uptake of neurotransmitters.

Indications for Anticonvulsants

Of the several drugs available for control of epileptic seizures, the specific indications depend on the seizure patterns and the tolerance and response of the patient to the drug. Table 7-1 compares the drugs most commonly used to treat seizures.

Nurse Alert for Anticonvulsants

- Anticonvulsants, particularly phenytoin and phenobarbital, carry a greater risk for congenital defects when the mother takes the drug during pregnancy; trimethadione is asso-

Text continued on p. 101

Table 7-1   Drugs used to treat seizures

Seizure Type	First-choice Drugs*	Additional Drugs for Second-choice Drugs†	Refractory Cases
General: tonic-clonic (grand mal) Partial: cortical focal (including jacksonian)	Alone or in combination: 1. Phenytoin (Dilantin)— adults 2. Phenobarbital (Luminal)— children 3. Carbamazepine (Tegretol)	1. Other barbiturates: primidone (Mysoline) or mephobarbital (Mebaral) 2. Valproic acid (Depakene)	1. Acetazolamide (Diamox)
General: absence (petit mal)	Alone 1. Ethosuximide (Zarontin) 2. Valproic acid (Depakene)	1. Other succinimides: methsuximide (Celontin) or phensuximide (Milontin) 2. Benzodiazepines: diazepam (Valium) or clonazepam (Clonopin)	1. Trimethadione (Tridione) 2. Acetazolamide (Diamox)
General: myoclonus (intentional or progressive)	1. Valproic acid (Depakene)	1. Clonazepam (Clonopin) 2. 1,5,-Hydroxytryptophan and carbidopa (experimental)	1. Ethosuximide (Zarontin) 2. Diazepam (Valium)
General: infantile spasms	1. ACTH	1. Clonazepam (Clonopin)	

Partial: complex (temporal lobe, psychomotor)	1. Carbamazepine (Tegretol) 2. Phenytoin (Dilantin)	1. Primidone (Mysoline) 2. Chlorezepate	1. Phensuximide (Milontin)
Status epilepticus: continuous tonic-clonic	1. Intravenous diazepam (Valium) 2. Intravenous phenytoin sodium (Dilantin) 3. Intravenous phenobarbital sodium (Luminal Sodium)	1. Rectal paraldehyde 2. Intravenous amobarbital sodium (Amytal Sodium)	1. Lidocaine (Xylocaine)

*First-choice drugs are those which are generally effective for most patients with the least incidence of toxic effects.

†Second-choice drugs are those which are sometimes effective when the first-choice drugs are not effective alone or which are associated with a higher incidence of side effects.

Table 7-2   Administration of anticonvulsants

Generic Name	Trade Name	Dosage and Administration	Comments
Long-acting Barbiturates			
Phenobarbital	Luminal*	ORAL: *Adults*—50 to 100 mg 2 to 3 times daily. *Children*—15 to 50 mg 2 to 3 times daily.	May begin at twice usual dose for the first 4 days to raise plasma concentration rapidly. Multiple daily doses minimize sedation. Effective serum concentration, 15 to 40 μg/ml. In addition to its use for epileptic seizures, phenobarbital is used prophylactically for febrile seizures in children.
	Luminal Sodium*	INTRAMUSCULAR, INTRAVENOUS (SLOW): *Adults*—200 to 320 mg, can repeat after 6 hr. INTRAMUSCULAR: *Children*—3 to 5 mg/kg body weight.	For status epilepticus. Sodium salt must be used for injection.
Mephobarbital	Mebaral*	ORAL: *Adults*—400 to 600 mg daily in divided doses. *Children*—over 5 yr; 32 to 64 mg	Mephobarbital is metabolized to phenobarbital.

Anticonvulsants 95

		given 3 to 4 times daily; under 5 yr, 16 to 32 mg given 3 to 4 times daily.	Effective serum concentrations, 5 to 10 µg/ml.
Primidone	Apo-Primidone† Mysoline* Sertan†	ORAL: *Adults*—250 mg daily at bedtime or up to 2 Gm daily in divided doses. *Children*—over 8 yr, as for adults; under 8 yr, ½ adult dosage.	
Hydantoins Phenytoin	Dilantin*	ORAL: *Adults*—300 mg daily in 3 doses. Maintenance dose, 300 to 600 mg daily. *Children*—5 mg/kg daily in 2 to 3 doses. Maximum dose, 300 mg daily.	May be given once a day to improve compliance. Effective serum concentration, 10 to 20 µg/ml. Brand name should be specified because of varying bioavailability among brands.
Mephenytoin	Mesantoin*	ORAL: *Adults*—200 to 600 mg daily. *Children*—100 to 400 mg daily.	

cont'd. next page

*Available in U.S. and Canada
†Available in Canada only
‡Not available in Canada

96 Pocket Nurse Guide to Drugs

Table 7-2 Administration of anticonvulsants—cont'd.

Generic Name	Trade Name	Dosage and Administration	Comments
Ethotoin	Peganone‡	ORAL: *Adults*—1000 mg daily increased gradually to 2000 to 3000 mg in 4 to 6 divided doses. *Children*—500 to 1000 mg in divided doses.	
Succinimides			
Ethosuximide	Zarontin*	ORAL: *Adults*—500 mg daily increased gradually every 4 to 7 days to control seizures. *Children*—over 6 yr, as for adults; 3 to 6 yr, 250 mg daily increased gradually to control seizures.	Effective serum concentration, 40 to 80 $\mu g/ml$.
Methsuximide	Celontin*	ORAL: 300 mg daily for 1 wk, increased weekly by 300 mg to control seizures to a maximum dose of 1200 mg daily.	
Phensuximide	Milontin*	ORAL: 500 to 1000 mg 2 to 3 times daily.	

Oxazolidinediones

Trimethadione Paramethadione	Tridione Trimedone† Paradione	ORAL: *Adults*—900 mg daily divided into 3 to 4 doses, can increase by 300 mg daily every 7 days to control seizures; maximum, 2400 mg daily. *Children*—300 to 900 mg/day daily divided into 3 to 4 doses.	No longer widely used because of serious side effects and high teratogenic potential. Effective serum concentration of dimethadione (active metabolite), 700 μg/ml or higher.

Benzodiazepines

Diazepam	Valium*	INTRAVENOUSLY, to terminate status epilepticus: *Adults*—5 to 10 mg (no faster than 5 mg/min, use a large vein). Can repeat every 10 to 15 min to a maximum dose of 30 mg. *Children*—30 days to 5 yr, 0.2 to 0.5 mg slowly every 2 to 5 min, maximum 5 mg; over 5 yr, 1 mg slowly every 2 to 5 min, maximum 10 mg.	Rarely used orally as an anticonvulsant agent. Do not mix or dilute into intravenous fluids.

cont'd. next page

*Available in U.S. and Canada
†Available in Canada only
‡Not available in Canada

Table 7-2 Administration of anticonvulsants—cont'd.

Generic Name	Trade Name	Dosage and Administration	Comments
Clonazepam	Clonopin Rivotril†	ORAL: *Adults*—1.5 mg daily in 3 doses, increase every 3 days by 0.5 to 1 mg to control seizures; maximum total dose, 20 mg daily. *Children*—Infants to 10 yr, 0.01 to 0.03 mg/kg, increased by 0.25 to 0.5 mg every 3 days to control seizures to a maximum of 0.2 mg/kg daily.	Effective therapeutic plasma concentrations, 5 to 70 ng/ml.
Miscellaneous			
Acetazolamide	Diamox* Acetazolan†	ORAL: *Adults and children*—8 to 30 mg/kg in divided doses.	A weak diuretic. Tolerance usually develops.
Adrenocorticotropic hormone (ACTH)		INTRAMUSCULAR: *Infants*—10 units daily, increase by 5 units every 5 days up to 60 units for 6 to 7 wk.	If ACTH is ineffective, diazepam, 3 mg/lb, is added. If ACTH is ineffective in 2 wk, may switch to cortisone, 3 mg/lb, as an alternative to increasing ACTH. Cortisone is brought down by 1 mg/lb over 3 wk.

Anticonvulsants 99

Carbamazepine	Apo-Carbamazepine† Mazepine† Tegretol*	ORAL: *Adults and children over 12 yr,*—200 mg twice on day 1, increase by 200 mg daily to control seizures; maximum dose, 1000 mg (less than 15 yr) or 1200 mg (over 15 yr). Doses are taken every 6 to 8 hr.	Effective therapeutic plasma concentrations, 4 to 12 $\mu g/ml$.
Lidocaine hydrochloride	Xylocaine* Xylocard Hydrochloride*	INTRAVENOUS: *Adults*—to terminate status epilepticus: Infuse 1 to 3 mg/min to terminate seizures.	A last resort for terminating status epilepticus. If given in excess, lidocaine itself can induce convulsion.
Chlorazepate dipotassium	Tranxene‡	*Adults*—7.5 mg 3 times daily up to 90 mg per day *Children*—9 to 12 years: 7.5 mg twice daily up to 60 mg per day.	

cont'd. next page

---

* Available in U.S. and Canada

† Available in Canada only

‡ Not available in Canada

Table 7-2 Administration of anticonvulsants—cont'd.

Generic Name	Trade Name	Dosage and Administration	Comments
Paraldehyde		INTRAMUSCULAR, INTRAVENOUS, to terminate status epilepticus: *Adults or children*—usual dose 5 ml. Solution must be diluted. RECTAL: *Children*—0.3 ml/kg diluted 1:1 in olive oil or milk.	A last resort for terminating status epilepticus.
Valproic acid	Depakene*	ORAL: *Adults and children*—15 mg/kg daily in divided doses. Can be increased by 5 to 10 mg/kg daily every 7 days to control seizures, up to 60 mg/kg daily.	The newest anticonvulsant in the United States. Clinical potential still to be explored, but drug effective in controlling myoclonic epilepsy refractory to most other anticonvulsant drugs. Effective serum concentrations reported to be 50 to 100 μg/ml.

*Available in U.S. and Canada
†Available in Canada only
‡Not available in Canada

Anticonvulsants

ciated with an 80% incidence of spontaneous abortions or birth defects.

- Sudden withdrawal from barbiturates can precipitate convulsions; withdrawal should be gradual.
- Barbiturates are contraindicated for patients with porphyria, or who are depressed or possibly suicidal.
- Paraldehyde is contraindicated in patients with bronchopulmonary disease or liver disease.
- Patients taking anticonvulsants should avoid the use of alcohol, which can alter the seizure threshold and causes CNS depression.
- With barbiturates and primidone, observe patients for respiratory depression for 30 to 60 minutes after intramuscular injection.
- Because most anticonvulsants cause drowsiness, caution patients to avoid activities requiring mental alertness until individual effects are established.
- Central nervous system depressants should be avoided by patients taking clonazepam.
- Phenytoin should not be given intramuscularly or subcutaneously because it is highly irritating, can precipitate in tissue, and has erratic tissue absorption.

Parenteral Administration of Phenobarbital

If using powder, dilute as instructed. Desired dose of solution should be further diluted to a volume of 10 ml for IV use. Administer slowly, 60 mg per minute. In patients with status epilepticus or grand mal seizures, it may not be possible to monitor the blood pressure. Be alert for hypotension and respiratory depression.

Parenteral Administration of Phenytoin

The drug should be reconstituted only with the diluent provided by the manufacturer. The drug is incompatible with other drugs and intravenous fluids, so it should not be mixed. The drug is administered by slow intravenous push (bolus) at a rate not exceeding 50 mg per minute. Given via this route, the drug can cause hypotension and cardiac arrest. If at all

102 Pocket Nurse Guide to Drugs

possible, the patient should be attached to a cardiac monitor during intravenous administration.

Parenteral Administration of Diazepam

For intravenous use in status epilepticus:

a. The drug should not be mixed. It has limited compatibility with infusion fluids. Check with the pharmacy before mixing in an IV solution.

b. Administer at a rate not exceeding 5 mg per minute and even more slowly in children.

c. Hypotension, respiratory depression, apnea, and bradycardia may occur. Monitor vital signs.

d. It may be appropriate to have the patient attached to a cardiac monitor if large doses are being used, although this may be impossible or of limited value during a seizure.

e. Resuscitation equipment should be available.

Parenteral Administration of Paraldehyde

Intravenous paraldehyde can be extremely dangerous. Dilute as instructed in the manufacturer's literature and administer slowly, 1 ml of diluted medication per minute. Monitor vital signs.

Side Effects of Anticonvulsants

Phenobarbital can cause profound respiratory depression, and sedation, drowsiness, and paradoxical excitement in children and the elderly. The side effects of the long-acting *barbiturates* and *primidone* include rashes, gastrointestinal upset, nausea, and vomiting; intoxication or overdose may cause slurred speech, ataxia, and vertigo. Most side effects of *phenytoin* occur at higher than effective serum levels, including nystagmus, ataxia, tremors and nervousness or drowsiness and fatigue, insomnia, headache, gingival hyperplasia, folic acid or vitamin D deficiency, allergic rashes, acne, hirsutism, and congenital fetal malformations when taken in pregnancy. Toxicity and overdose with the *hydantoins* may produce ataxia, nystagmus, and slurred speech. The *succinimides* may cause dizziness, drowsiness, gastrointestinal irritation, anorexia, nausea, vomiting, diarrhea, rashes,

Anticonvulsants 103

gum hypertrophy, hirsutism, and occasionally agranulocytosis; psychiatric disturbances may occur in patients with a history of psychological problems. *Trimethadione* can cause serious allergic dermatitis, kidney and liver damage, agranulocytosis, aplastic anemia, photophobia, and spontaneous abortion or congenital anomalies when taken in pregnancy. *Diazepam* and *chlorazepate* may cause drowsiness, dizziness, ataxia, and respiratory depression (see also Chapter 1). *Clonazepam* commonly causes drowsiness, ataxia, and personality changes and may cause slurred speech, tremors, abnormal eye movements, dizziness, vertigo, confusion, and increased salivation and bronchial secretions; children may become hyperactive, irritable, aggressive, or violent; psychiatric problems may include confusion, depression, hallucinations, hysteria, psychoses, increased libido, and suicidal tendencies. *Acetazolamide* has weak diuretic effects and may cause loss of appetite, drowsiness, confusion, a tingling sensation, and metabolic acidosis. *Carbamazepine* causes increased alertness but may also cause drowsiness, dizziness, ataxia, visual disturbances, gastrointestinal upset, and infrequently rashes, liver damage, and bone marrow depression. *Lidocaine* may itself induce convulsions at high doses and can depress the heart. *Paraldehyde,* if administered too quickly intravenously, may cause bronchopulmonary irritation and severe coughing, and vein irritation and thrombophlebitis. *Valprioc acid* may cause gastrointestinal distress, sedation, CNS stimulation, excitement, tremor, alopecia, and possibly liver damage.

Nursing Implications for Anticonvulsants

General

- Women of childbearing age may wish to consider using birth control measures while on anticonvulsant therapy. If a woman desires to conceive, she should discuss her plans with her physician so that she can obtain current information about the risks associated with each drug.
- Instruct patients to continue taking anticonvulsants as ordered, even after they have been seizure free for a period of time. Suddenly discontinuing anticonvulsants increases the chances of having more seizures.

104   Pocket Nurse Guide to Drugs

- Patients on long-term anticonvulsant therapy should be encouraged to wear a medical identification tag or bracelet. In addition, suggest that they carry in their wallets a card listing current drugs and dosages and keep this listing current.
- Encourage patients to return for follow-up visits, at which time discussion and evaluation of any side effects can occur, and routine blood work to monitor for hepatic, renal, or hematopoietic effects can be done.
- Remind patients to keep all health care providers informed of all medications being taken.
- Referral to appropriate agencies for assistance and follow-up should be done.

Barbiturates

- The barbiturates may lower the blood levels of oral anticoagulants, resulting in insufficient anticoagulation and perhaps a need for an increase in dosage.

Phenytoin

- The preferred route of administration for phenytoin is the oral route. The capsule preparation manufactured by Parke-Davis has been approved for once-a-day dosing if desired instead of divided doses. Once-a-day administration may result in better patient compliance; consult the physician.
- It is important that patients continue to take the same brand of phenytoin. Switching brands may result in alterations in absorption and metabolism.
- An oral suspension of phenytoin is available. Instruct patients and parents of children to shake the bottle vigorously before preparing each dose. Without adequate resuspension the patient may be underdosed with the liquid near the top of the bottle and overdosed as the contents of the bottle near the bottom are used.
- Patients should be taught to use meticulous oral hygiene while taking hydantoins, including regular brushing and flossing, to avoid developing gingival hyperplasia. Regular

Anticonvulsants **105**

dental care should be stressed and patients instructed to tell the dentist that phenytoin is being used.

- Remember that even if phenytoin is being used for its anticonvulsant effects, it still has cardiac effects (Chapter 17).
- Phenytoin is best taken with meals, a snack, or milk to reduce gastric irritation.
- Phenytoin may cause hyperglycemia. Diabetics should monitor urine glucose levels carefully; an increase in insulin dosage may be necessary.
- Megaloblastic anemia may occur as a result of a folic acid deficiency caused by long-term phenytoin use. Symptoms develop slowly and include easy fatigability, weakness, fainting, and headache, although the first sign may be alteration in routine blood work. Treatment is with folic acid therapy.
- Symptoms of other blood dyscrasias that may be caused by hydantoins (thrombocytopenia, agranulocytosis, pancytopenia) include fatigue, pallor, easy bruising or bleeding, fever, and sore throat.

Succinimides

- Symptoms of agranulocytosis that may result from succinimides include fatigue, pallor, fever, and sore throat. Instruct the patient to report these or any unusual symptoms immediately.
- Patients taking succinimides should be instructed to use meticulous oral hygiene, including brushing and flossing, and to continue regular dental checkups. Taking the medications with meals may reduce gastric irritation.

Benzodiazepines

- Diazepam is discussed at length in Chapter 1.
- Because clonazepam may cause an increase in salivation and hypersecretion in the upper respiratory passages and depresses respiration, it should be used with caution in patients with chronic respiratory disease or in small children.

106   Pocket Nurse Guide to Drugs

- Instruct the patient to report any rash, fever, sore throat, bruising, or bleeding because these signs may indicate hematopoietic reactions related to carbamazepine.
- Patients should take carbamazepine with meals because it may improve absorption and reduce gastrointestinal side effects.
- Propoxyphene napsylate (Darvon-N) should be avoided by patients taking carbamazepine.
- Because of the wide variety of side effects of carbamazepine, patients should be monitored frequently with blood work and appropriate investigation of specific complaints. Serum drug concentrations should be monitored to assist in determining the correct dose for a patient. Therapeutic levels for adults should fall between 4 and 12 μg/ml.

Paraldehyde

- Paraldehyde decomposes readily. Use only fresh, previously unopened containers, and always check the expiration date before using.
- Paraldehyde reacts with some plastics, so glass syringes and containers should be used.
- Paraldehyde can be given via the intramuscular route but it should be well diluted with sodium chloride, and care should be taken to avoid injection into any peripheral nerves. There will be pain at the injection site.
- For rectal instillation, Paraldehyde should be diluted in 2 volumes of olive oil to prevent irritation to the mucosa. Administer as for a retention enema. It is difficult to control the amount or rate of absorption via this route.
- For oral administration, dilute the liquid form of paraldehyde in juice or milk to avoid gastrointestinal irritation. Capsules are available.
- Paraldehyde imparts a characteristic odor to the patient's breath.
- Paraldehyde is partly excreted via the lungs, and the drug may cause coughing and an increase in bronchial secretions. Especially during intravenous administration, patients should be placed on their sides, and suctioning equipment should be available.

Anticonvulsants 107

Valproic Acid

- After initiating therapy with valproic acid it is often possible to reduce the dose of or eliminate the need for some of the other drugs the patient is receiving.
- Because valproic acid is partly excreted as a ketone-containing metabolite, the urine test for ketones may be falsely positive. Patients with diabetes mellitus should be warned of this side effect.
- Valproic acid may prolong the bleeding time, although this seems to be a greater problem when the patient is taking other drugs affecting coagulation. Instruct patients to report any bleeding, bruising, or petechiae. Patients should avoid the use of aspirin unless it is cleared by the physician.
- Because of the possibility of drug interactions, it will often be necessary to monitor the serum concentrations of all the drugs the patient is receiving for several weeks after the initiation of therapy with valproic acid. Blood tests to evaluate liver function should be performed routinely.
- Taking valproic acid with meals may reduce gastric irritation.
- Valproic acid-containing capsules should be swallowed whole and not chewed to avoid irritation to the mouth and throat. There is a liquid preparation available.

Drugs for Central Motor Control: Parkinsonism and Spasm

8

Drugs for parkinsonism
  Anticholinergics
    Benztropine mesylate
    Biperiden
    Cycrimine hydrochloride
    Ethopropazine
    Procyclidine hydrochloride
    Trihexphenidyl
      hydrochloride
  Antihistamines
    Diphenhydramine
      hydrochloride
    Orphenadrine
  Other drugs
    Amantadine
    Levodopa
    Carbidopa-levadopa

Centrally acting skeletal muscle relaxants
  Drugs to treat spasticity
    Baclofen
    Dantrolene
    Diazepam
  Drugs to treat muscle spasms
    Carisoprodol
    Chlorphenesin
    Chlorzoxazone
    Cyclobenzaprine
    Diazepam
    Methocarbamol
    Orphenadrine

Drugs for Parkinsonism

Actions of Drugs for Parkinsonism

Drugs for parkinsonism lessen the severity of symptoms by blocking the excessive action of acetylcholine, or by increasing the concentration of dopamine, to return the balance of excitatory acetylcholine action and inhibitory dopamine action toward normal.

Indications for Drugs for Parkinsonism

Anticholinergic drugs are used to treat parkinsonism as well as the extrapyramidal reactions arising from use of antipsychotic drugs (Chapter 2). *Benztropine* is particularly used to reverse acute dystonic reactions to antipsychotic drugs. The *antihistamines* are less potent but are also used to treat parkinsonism. *Amantadine* is often used to control symptoms. *Levodopa* is used when the other drugs cannot adequately relieve symptoms; the combination drug *carbidopa-levodopa* causes less severe gastrointestinal side effects than levodopa alone, since lower doses of the levodopa component are possible.

Nurse Alert for Drugs for Parkinsonism

- Anticholinergic drugs are more likely to cause mental problems in older patients with preexisting mental imbalance.
- Anticholinergic drugs are contraindicated, or should be used cautiously, in patients with glaucoma, urinary or intestinal obstruction, or tachycardia.
- Because these drugs can cause drowsiness, caution the patient to avoid activities requiring alertness until effects are established.
- Levodopa should be used cautiously in patients with heart disease, asthma, emphysema, peptic ulcer, or glaucoma.

Parenteral Administration of Anticholinergic Drugs

The anticholinergic drugs are supplied in solution. Administer as ordered for intramuscular use. For intravenous use, administer slowly over several minutes, monitoring pulse and blood pressure.

Side Effects of Drugs for Parkinsonism

Common side effects of the *anticholinergic* drugs include dry mouth, constipation, urinary retention, blurred vision, impaired recent memory, confusion, insomnia, restlessness, agitation, delirium, paranoid reactions, or hallucinations.

Table 8-1 Administration of drugs for parkinsonism

Generic Name	Trade Name	Dosage and Administration
Anticholinergics		
Benztropine mesylate	Cogentin*	ORAL: *Adults*—0.5 to 1 mg at bedtime initially. Increased gradually to 4 to 6 mg if required. For drug-induced extrapyramidal reactions: ORAL, INTRAMUSCULAR, INTRAVENOUS: *Adults*—1 to 4 mg, 1 to 2 times daily. For an acute dystonic reaction: ORAL, INTRAVENOUS: *Adults*—2 mg IV, then 1 to 2 mg orally twice daily.
Biperiden	Akineton*	ORAL: *Adults*—2 mg, 3 times daily. May increase dose up to 20 mg daily if required. For drug-induced extrapyramidal reactions: ORAL: *Adults*—2 mg, 1 to 3 times daily. INTRAMUSCULAR: *Adults*—2 mg repeated as often as every 30 min but no more than 4 doses in 24 hours. *Children*—0.04 mg/kg as often as every 30 min but no more than 4 doses in 24 hours.
Cycrimine hydrochloride	Pagitane Hydrochloride	ORAL: *Adults*—1.25 mg, 3 times daily. May be increased to 12.5 to 20 mg daily if required.

Drugs for Central Motor Control: Parkinsonism and Spasm

Drug	Trade Names	Dosage
Ethopropazine	Parsidol, Parsitant	ORAL: *Adults*—50 mg, 1 to 2 times daily initially. Mild to moderate cases require 100 to 400 mg daily. Severe cases may require 500 to 600 mg daily.
Procyclidine hydrochloride	Kemadrin*, Procyclid†	ORAL: *Adults*—5 mg twice daily. Up to 20 to 30 mg daily if required. For drug-induced extrapyramidal reactions: ORAL: *Adults*—2 to 2.5 mg, 3 times daily. Increased to 10 to 20 mg daily if required.
Trihexyphenidyl hydrochloride	Artane*, Pipanol HCl, Trihexy†	ORAL: *Adults*—2 mg, 2 to 3 times daily. Increased to 15 to 20 mg daily (usually). For drug-induced parkinsonism: ORAL: *Adults*—1 mg initially. Subsequent doses are increased if symptoms do not decrease. Usual daily dose is 5 to 15 mg.

Antihistamines

Drug	Trade Names	Dosage
Diphenhydramine hydrochloride	Benadryl*	ORAL: *Adults*—25 mg 3 times daily. Increased to 50 mg 4 times daily if required. For drug-induced extrapyramidal reactions: INTRAMUSCULAR, INTRAVENOUS: *Adults*—10 to 50 mg with maximum daily dose of 400 mg. *Children*—intramuscular 5 mg/kg daily. Maximum, 300 mg in 24 hr.

cont'd. next page

*Available in U.S. and Canada
† Available in Canada only

Table 8-1   Administration of drugs for parkinsonism—cont'd.

Generic Name	Trade Name	Dosage and Administration
Orphenadrine	Disipal*	ORAL: *Adults*—50 mg 3 times daily; up to 250 mg if required.

Other Drugs to Treat Parkinsonism

Generic Name	Trade Name	Dosage and Administration
Amantadine	Symmetrel*	ORAL: *Adults*—100 mg daily after breakfast for 5 to 7 days. An additional 100 mg may be added after lunch.
Levodopa	Dopar Larodopa*	ORAL: *Adults*—initially 300 to 1000 mg daily in 3 to 7 doses during waking hours with food. Increase dosage 100 to 500 mg every 2 to 3 days or more until desired control is achieved. Usually requires 4 to 6 Gm and 6 to 8 weeks to achieve control. After several months to 1 year the dosage may be lowered.
Carbidopa-levodopa	Sinemet	ORAL: *Adults*—Initial daily dose is ¼ of the levodopa daily dose. Administer 8 hours after the last levodopa dose; given in 3 to 4 doses daily. Patients not previously receiving levodopa are started with 10:100 mg (carbidopa: levodopa) 3 times daily, gradually increase as required.

* Available in U.S. and Canada
† Available in Canada only

Drugs for Central Motor Control: Parkinsonism and Spasm 113

Antihistamines can cause drowsiness and sedation (see also Chapter 23). *Amantadine* can cause dizziness, nervousness, inability to concentrate, ataxia, slurred speech, insomnia, lethargy, blurred vision, dry mouth, gastrointestinal upset, and rash, but these side effects are less severe than with the anticholinergics. *Levodopa* can cause nausea, vomiting, anorexia, orthostatic hypotension, increased heart rate and force of contraction, cardiac arrhythmias, gastrointestinal bleeding, cough, disturbed breathing, urinary retention, increased alertness, increased sex drive, euphoria, anxiety, irritability, hyperactivity, insomnia, paranoid or psychotic episodes, and dyskinesia after prolonged therapy. *Carbidopa-levodopa* has similar effects with reduced emetic effects.

Nursing Implications for Drugs for Parkinsonism

- Patients should not suddenly discontinue their drugs for Parkinson's disease.
- Parkinson's disease is usually a disease of older adults. If, however, a premenopausal woman should have Parkinson's disease, she should consider the use of birth control measures during therapy with the antiparkinsonism drugs.
- Patients and family members should be taught about the side effects of these drugs because it may often be the family who notices side effects before the patient does.
- Monitor the blood pressure and pulse every 4 hours when patients are being started on anticholinergic drug therapy, when dosages are being changed, or when other medications are added. It may take several days for the effects of the drug to be fully manifested.
- Because of possible drowsiness and hypotension associated with anticholinergic drugs, patients should be cautioned to rise slowly and to call for assistance as needed. At night, hospitalized patients should be assisted when up.
- Instruct patients taking anticholinergic drugs to report any gastrointestinal problem such as constipation or abdominal pain. Although rare, fatal paralytic ileus has occured. If constipation is a chronic problem, encourage the patient to increase the fluid intake to 2500 to 3000 ml per day, to increase the bulk intake, to modify the diet to include foods

114   Pocket Nurse Guide to Drugs

that may have a laxative effect (e.g., prunes, juices, coffee, hot chocolate), and to increase exercise and ambulation. It may be necessary to prescribe stool softeners on a regular basis.

- Anticholinergic drugs may produce anhidrosis (inability to sweat), resulting in intolerance to heat and rarely, hyperthermia. Caution patients to limit strenuous activities, especially in hot weather, and to take frequent rest periods to cool off.
- Nausea and dry mouth can be a problem. When severe it may be necessary to reduce the dosage. Sometimes altering the times the medications are given can help decrease these side effects. Taking the medications just before meals may help with the dry mouth, unless this produces nausea. Taking the drug after meals may prevent nausea, in which case giving some mints, hard candies, or chewing gum may help to make the dry mouth more tolerable. Some patients may find the use of a commercially prepared saliva substitute to be helpful.
- Psychiatric problems (e.g., confusion, euphoria, disturbed behavior, agitation) related to anticholinergics may occur. If severe, the drug should be stopped for a few days and resumed at a lower dosage.
- Patients with a known history of cardiac arrhythmias should be watched carefully because the anticholinergics may aggravate the cardiac problems.
- Patients with a history of seizures taking amantadine should be observed closely for increased seizure activity.
- Patients with a history of congestive heart failure should be observed carefully when being started on amantadine. Weigh daily, monitor the blood pressure, check for increasing fluid retention in dependent areas, auscultate the lungs for fluid, and observe the neck veins for venous distention.
- Because amantadine can cause drowsiness and blurred vision, patients should be cautioned to avoid activities requiring mental alertness (e.g., driving, operating machinery).
- During periods of dosage adjustment or when new drugs are added to the medical regimen, patients taking amantadine

Drugs for Central Motor Control: Parkinsonism and Spasm   **115**

should have their blood pressure checked every 4 hours; hypotension is a known side effect. Caution patients to rise slowly. If dizziness or lightheadedness occurs, the patient should sit down. It may be necessary to supervise ambulation, especially at night.

- Nursing implications related to the antihistamines are described in Chapter 23.
- Nursing implications related to phenothiazines are described in Chapter 2.
- Levodopa and antidepressants that are monoamine oxidase (MAO) inhibitors should not be given concurrently; MAO inhibitors should be discontinued at least 2 weeks before administering levodopa. Levodopa is contraindicated for patients with closed-angle glaucoma, with a history of melanoma, or for patients with suspicious undiagnosed skin lesions.
- Patients on levodopa with a history of cardiovascular disease, myocardial infarction, or arrhythmia should be observed carefully for signs of cardiac irregularity or arrhythmia.
- Observe patients on levodopa with a history of peptic ulcer disease for signs of reactivation of the disease such as abdominal pain or occult blood in the stools.
- Because levodopa can cause hypotension, the blood pressure should be monitored every 4 hours during periods of dosage adjustment or when other drugs are added to the regimen. Caution patients to move slowly from supine to sitting or standing positions, to sit down if dizziness or lightheadedness occurs, and to call for assistance if needed. Supervise ambulation, especially at night. Wearing elastic stockings may be helpful.
- A variety of personality changes can occur with levodopa: confusion, hallucinations, delusions, agitation, euphoria, depression, and suicidal tendencies. Observe patients carefully for signs of personality or behavior change, and ask the patient and family to report any symptoms.
- Pyridoxine hydrochloride (vitamin B_6) reverses the effects of levodopa; therefore vitamin mixtures containing this vitamin should be avoided. Caution patients not to take

Pocket Nurse Guide to Drugs

over-the-counter vitamin preparations without first checking with the physician.

- Warn patients taking levodopa that several weeks of therapy may be necessary before full results can be seen.
- The urine, saliva, and perspiration may become darker while patients are receiving levodopa therapy. Other effects of the drug that are rare but that may cause concern are a bitter taste in the mouth, hot flashes, and foul body odor.
- Gastrointestinal side effects may be decreased by taking levodopa with meals or milk. If nausea is severe, it may be necessary for the patient to take an antiemetic. Gastrointestinal symptoms often diminish with prolonged therapy. Because of the disease and the drug side effects, the patient with Parkinson's disease may be poorly nourished. Allow the patient plenty of time to eat and weigh the patient weekly.
- Patients receiving levodopa need individualized titration of the dose and careful evaluation. Any patient complaint or unusual signs or symptoms should be carefully assessed.
- If levodopa therapy must be interrupted for prolonged periods, it may be necessary to resume the drug at a lower dose and progressively increase the dose until the desired dose is again reached.
- When starting the carbidopa-levodopa combination, levodopa alone should have been discontinued at least 8 hours previously.

Centrally Acting Skeletal Muscle Relaxants

Drugs to treat spasticity
    Baclofen
    Dantrolene
    Diazepam

Drugs to treat muscle spasms
    Carisoprodol
    Chlorphenesin
    Chlorzoxazone
    Cyclobenzaprine
    Diazepam
    Methocarbamol
    Orphenadrine

Actions of Centrally Acting Skeletal Muscle Relaxants

Diazepam and baclofen are thought to act within the spinal cord to restore some inhibitory tone. Dantrolene affects muscle directly by interfering with the intracellular release of calcium necessary to initiate contraction. Centrally acting muscle relaxants to treat spasm depress the polysynaptic pathways in the spinal cord, modulating muscle tone, and reduce anxiety that worsens muscle spasms.

Indications for Centrally Acting Skeletal Muscle Relaxants

Diazepam is used to treat spasticity associated with spinal cord injury, multiple sclerosis, and cerebral injury, and to treat muscle spasms. *Baclofen* is used to treat spasticity related to spinal cord injury and multiple sclerosis, but less for spasticity related to brain damage. *Dantrolene* is used to treat spasticity that causes pain or discomfort or limits functional rehabilitation; it may be effective for the spasticity of stroke, cerebral palsy, or multiple sclerosis. The *drugs to treat muscle spasms* are used when analgesics and other measures do not achieve relief.

Nurse Alert for Centrally Acting Skeletal Muscle Relaxants

- Dantrolene causes muscular weakness and may worsen the patient's overall condition if strength is marginal.
- Methocarbamol is not recommended for patients with epilepsy, and should not be administered parenterally to patients with impaired renal function.
- Orphenadrine is contraindicated in patients with glaucoma, myasthenia gravis, tachycardia, or urinary retention.
- These drugs should not be combined with alcohol or other CNS depressants.
- Because these drugs may cause drowsiness, patients should be cautioned to avoid activities requiring alertness until effects are determined.

Table 8-2   Administration of centrally acting muscle relaxants

Generic Name	Trade Name	Dosage and Administration
Drugs to Treat Spasticity		
Baclofen	Lioresal*	ORAL: *Adults*—Begin with 5 mg 3 times daily. Increase by 5 mg 3 times daily every 3 days as required. Maximum daily dose is 80 mg.
Dantrolene	Dantrium*	ORAL: *Adults*—25 mg 1 to 2 times daily. Increase to 25 mg 3 to 4 times daily, then 50 to 100 mg 4 times daily as required. Increments are made every 4 to 7 days.
Diazepam	Valium*	ORAL: *Adults*—2 to 10 mg 4 times daily. *Children*—0.12 to 0.8 mg/kg body weight daily divided into 3 or 4 doses.
		INTRAVENOUS: *Adults*—2 to 10 mg injected no faster than 5 mg (1 ml) per min. Do not mix or dilute with other solutions, drugs, or intravenous fluids. *Children*—0.04 to 0.2 mg/kg body weight with a maximum of 0.6 mg/kg in an 8 hr period.
Drugs to Treat Muscle Spasms		
Carisoprodol	Rela Soma*	ORAL: *Adults*—350 mg 4 times daily.
Chlorphenesin	Maolate	ORAL: *Adults*—800 mg 3 times daily. Can decrease to 400 mg 4 times daily as improvement is noted.

Drugs for Central Motor Control: Parkinsonism and Spasm

Chlorzoxazone	Paraflex	ORAL: *Adults*—250 to 750 mg 3 or 4 times daily. *Children*—20 mg/kg body weight in 3 to 4 divided doses.
Cyclobenzaprine	Flexeril*	ORAL: *Adults*—10 mg 3 times daily up to a maximum total dose of 60 mg.
Diazepam	Valium*	See Drugs to treat spasticity
Methocarbamol	Delaxin	ORAL: *Adults*—1.5 to 2 Gm 4 times daily for 2 to 3 days.
	Robamol	Decrease to 1 Gm 4 times daily for maintenance.
	Robaxin*	INTRAMUSCULAR: *Adults*—500 mg every 8 hr, alternating
	Romethocarb	between the gluteal muscles.
	Spenaxin	INTRAVENOUS: *Adults*—1 to 3 Gm daily for a maximum of 3 days. Inject no faster than 300 mg (3 ml) per min.
Orphenadrine	Flexon	ORAL: *Adults*—100 mg twice daily.
	Neocyten	INTRAMUSCULAR, INTRAVENOUS: *Adults*—60 mg twice
	Norflex*	daily.
	Tega-Flex	
	X-Otag	

*Available in U.S. and Canada

- Baclofen, dantrolene, and the other drugs for muscle spasm are not generally recommended for use in pregnancy and lactation.
- Orphenadrine is contraindicated in patients with glaucoma, intestinal obstruction, prostatic hypertrophy, obstruction of bladder neck, or myasthenia gravis.

Parenteral Administration of Dantrolene

To administer intravenous dantrolene sodium, reconstitute each vial by adding 60 ml of sterile water for injection (without bacteriostatic agent) and shake vigorously to reconstitute the powder. For treatment of malignant hyperthermia, administer via rapid intravenous injection a dose of 1 mg/kg. The dose may be repeated to a maximum accumulated dose of 10 mg/kg. Dantrolene sodium should be used in conjunction with other recognized methods of supportive care for malignant hyperthermia. Protect the reconstituted solution from direct light and use within 6 hours.

Parenteral Administration of Muscle Spasm Drugs

Intravenous doses should be given with the patient lying down. Instruct the patient to remain in a recumbent position for 15 minutes to decrease the incidence of postural hypotension. Monitor the vital signs. Side rails should be up. Caution the patient to move slowly from lying to sitting or standing positions. If dizziness, lightheadedness, or vertigo should occur on rising, the patient should sit down. Supervise ambulation until the patient is steady when walking.

Side Effects of Centrally Acting Muscle Relaxants

Diazepam may have prominent side effects of drowsiness and incoordination (see also Chapter 1). *Baclofen* may cause drowsiness, incoordination, and occasional gastrointestinal upset. *Dantrolene* can cause muscle weakness, photosensitivity, and liver damage. All the *centrally acting skeletal muscle relaxants* can cause drowsiness and dizziness, vertigo, tremor, agitation, irritability, headache, nausea, tachycardia, malaise, and confusion. *Chlorzoxazone* and *cyclobenzaprine* may cause liver changes or damage.

Nursing Implications for Centrally Acting Skeletal Muscle Relaxants

- Baclofen should be administered cautiously to patients with a history of seizures because a loss of seizure control has been reported.
- The use of baclofen may cause the following alterations in blood tests: increased SGOT, increased alkaline phosphatase, and elevated blood sugar levels. Caution diabetic patients receiving baclofen to monitor their urine sugar concentration carefully.
- Abrupt withdrawal of baclofen may cause hallucinations. Caution patients to discontinue use of this drug only on the advice of the physician.
- Because of the risk of serious hepatitis, patients receiving dantrolene sodium should be cautioned to report any jaundice, yellowing of sclera, right upper quadrant abdominal pain, nausea, or fever. In addition, blood tests, including SGOT, SGPT, alkaline phosphatase, and total bilirubin, should be monitored at regular intervals.
- Patients receiving dantrolene sodium for the first time need thorough and systematic evaluation of their spasticity on a daily basis until it can be determined whether the drug is helping. Information from direct examination of the patient should be correlated with subjective data from the patient and observations by those who care for the patient daily.
- Caution patients taking dantrolene that several days or weeks of therapy may be needed before improvement is seen.
- Additional nursing implications related to diazepam are described in Chapter 1.

Neuromuscular Drugs

Acetylcholinesterase inhibitors
for myasthenia gravis
    Ambenonium chloride
    Edrophonium chloride
    Neostigmine bromide
    Neostigmine methylsulfate
    Pyridostigmine bromide

Neuromuscular blocking drugs
    Nondepolarizing drugs
        Atracurium
        Gallamine triethiodide
        Metocurine
        Pancuronium bromide
        Tubocurarine (curare)
        Vecuronium
    Depolarizing drugs
        Succinylcholine
    Cholinesterase inhibitor
        Hexafluorenium

Acetylcholinesterase Inhibitors

Actions of Acetylcholinesterase Inhibitors

Acetylcholinesterase inhibitors allow the accumulation of acetylcholine at the neuromuscular junction and postganglionic parasympathetic synapses; this increase in the concentration of acetylcholine at the neuromuscular junction ensures that available receptors are activated.

Indications for Acetylcholinesterase Inhibitors

These drugs are used to diagnose or treat myasthenia gravis by making available more acetylcholine for receptors at the neuromuscular junction. The same drugs are used to reverse the effects of the competitive neuromuscular blocking drugs used in surgery. When *neostigmine* is used in an injectable form, muscular improvement is diagnostic of myasthenia gravis. *Pyridostigmine* is the drug of choice for the treatment of myasthenia gravis; *ambenonium* is the drug of choice for patients with bromide allergies. *Edrophonium* is used only for diagnostic purposes to determine whether muscular weakness is due to worsening of the disease (myasthenic crisis) or to overmedication (cholinergic crisis).

Nurse Alert for Acetylcholinesterase Inhibitors

- If *edrophonium* is used to differentiate between myasthenia gravis and cholinergic crisis, a patient determined to be in cholinergic crisis may require ventilatory assistance after injection.
- *All the anticholinesterase drugs* are contraindicated for patients with obstruction of the intestinal or urinary tract; they should be used cautiously in patients with bronchial asthma.

Administration of Acetylcholinesterase Inhibitors for Myasthenia Gravis

The anticholinesterase drugs used to treat myasthenia gravis are positively charged compounds of low lipid solubility. These drugs are therefore not readily absorbed orally, and the oral dose is thirty times the parenteral dose. The anticholinesterases are metabolized by plasma esterases and by hepatic enzymes to inactive compounds. The drugs and their metabolites are excreted in the urine. The effective dose must be individualized for each patient. In a given patient, stress and infection can increase the effective dose. Women in the premenstrual part of their cycle may require higher doses. Very ill patients may become unresponsive to their medication, but temporary reduction or withdrawal of the dose over a three-day period may restore their responsiveness. Parenteral administration may be required.

Side Effects of Acetylcholinesterase Inhibitors

All these drugs may produce muscle cramps, muscle fasciculations, and weakness because of overstimulation of neuromuscular receptors; parasympathetic stimulation effects may include excessive salivation, perspiration, abdominal distress, and nausea and vomiting. *Neostigmine* has a high incidence of

124   Pocket Nurse Guide to Drugs

Table 9-1   Administration of acetylcholinesterase inhibitors for myasthenia gravis

Generic Name	Trade Name	Dosage and Administration
Ambenonium chloride	Mytelase*	ORAL: *Adults* — 5 mg 3 or 4 times daily increased every 1 to 2 days as required. *Children* — 0.3 mg/kg body weight daily in divided doses, increased gradually if necessary to a maximum of 1.5 mg/kg daily.
Edrophonium chloride	Tensilon*	To differentiate a myasthenic from a cholinergic crisis: 1 to 2 mg. A cholinergic crisis if muscle strength decreases (lower medication dose). Diagnosis of myasthenia gravis is positive if muscle strength increases within 3 min (duration, 5 to 10 min). INTRAVENOUS: *Adults* — 2 mg injected over 15 to 30 sec. If no response, 8 mg is given. May repeat test after 1 hr. *Children* — 2 mg initially as above followed by 5 mg (under 75 lb) or up to 10 mg (over 75 lb).
Neostigmine bromide	Prostigmin* Bromide	ORAL: *Adults* — 15 mg every 3 to 4 hr initially,

*Available in U.S. and Canada

Neuromuscular Drugs **125**

Table 9-1 Administration of acetylcholinesterase inhibitors for myasthenia gravis—cont'd.

Generic Name	Trade Name	Dosage and Administration
Neostigmine bromide— cont'd.	Prostigmin* Bromide	then adjust upward as required. *Children* — begin with 2 mg/kg body weight daily in divided doses.
Neostigmine methylsulfate	Prostigmin* Methysulfate	INTRAMUSCULAR: *Adults* — 0.022 mg/kg body weight (atropine, IM, 0.011 mg/kg may be given to control muscarinic side effects). *Children* — 0.01 to 0.04 mg/kg (with 0.01 mg/kg atropine, IM)
Pyridostigmine bromide	Mestinon*	ORAL: *Adults* — 60 to 120 mg every 3 or 4 hr initially, increased as necessary. *Children* — 7 mg/kg in divided doses as required.
	Regonol*	INTRAMUSCULAR: INTRAVENOUS: *Adults* — 1/30 of oral dose. *Newborn infants of myasthenic mothers* — 0.05 to 0.15 mg/kg body weight.

*Available in U.S. and Canada

side effects, including cramps and diarrhea. Side effects of *pyridostigmine* are less common: miosis, sweating, salivation, gastrointestinal distress, and bradycardia. *Ambenonium* may also produce side effects such as jitteriness, headache, confusion, and dizziness. *Edrophonium* may cause hypotension, faintness, dizziness, and flushing.

Nursing Implications for Acetylcholinesterase Inhibitors

- Health care professionals should be well-versed in the difference between a myasthenic crisis and a cholinergic crisis before attempting to care for the patient with myasthenia gravis.
- The symptoms of a *myasthenic crisis* include a positive Tensilon test, increased blood pressure and pulse, difficulty chewing, swallowing and coughing, bladder and bowel incontinence, increasing ptosis, difficulty breathing and cyanosis, and decreased urinary output. Symptoms of *cholinergic crisis* include a negative Tensilon test, abdominal cramps, diarrhea, fasciculations, nausea, vomiting, and blurred vision (these symptoms can be produced by overdose with acetylcholinesterase inhibitors). Finally, note that generalized weakness, increased salivation, tearing, bronchial secretions, general feelings of apprehension, restlessness, and difficulty breathing may be seen in either kind of crisis.
- Edrophonium (Tensilon), pyridostigmine (Mestinon), atropine, neostigmine, and syringes should be kept at the patient's bedside or together in a convenient place on the hospital unit for rapid treatment of a myasthenic or cholinergic crisis.
- If the ability of the myasthenic patient to swallow is deteriorating, it may be necessary to administer a parenteral dose of medication rather than an oral dose. Ideally, the physician will have written orders for both oral and parenteral doses of anticholinesterases.
- In the hospital setting, careful scheduling of diagnostic studies and x-ray studies should be done for the patient with myasthenia because the administration of anticholinesterase medications cannot be delayed while waiting for the patient to return to the unit. If the patient is not on the unit when a medication is due, the medication should be taken to the patient.
- Appropriate parameters to assess in managing the patient with myasthenia include blood pressure, pulse, vital capac-

Neuromuscular Drugs   127

ity, the presence or degree of ptosis, muscle strength, and ability to swallow. These assessments should be made before each dose of medication is given and whenever the patient's condition seems to be changing.

- In planning for discharge of a patient with myasthenia gravis, it is important to emphasize the following points to the patient:

  a. Anticholinesterases must be taken as ordered. In all but the mildest cases of the disease, forgetting a dose of medication, taking a dose too early or too late, or omitting an inconvenient dose may cause the disease to go out of control.

  b. No medications, whether prescription or over-the-counter, should ever be taken without first checking with the physician.

  c. Patient should also be taught about and given a list of drugs known to cause weakness.

- Patients with myasthenia gravis may find it helpful to plan to take their anticholinesterase 30 to 60 minutes before meals to increase strength for chewing and swallowing.

- Taking anticholinesterases with milk or crackers will help to reduce gastric irritation.

- If the patient at home is required to take a dose of medication during the night, a reliable, nonelectric alarm clock should be used to awaken the patient.

- The patient should be reminded to keep a careful watch on the supply of medication on hand and to refill prescriptions before they run out.

- Family members need to be taught about the disease and signs and symptoms of myasthenic and cholinergic crises. If the family feels that a patient is not responding appropriately, the patient should be brought to the emergency room.

- Patients with myasthenia gravis should be encouraged to wear a medical identification tag or bracelet and to carry with them the names and doses of medications being taken.

- If neostigmine is being used, the prior or concomitant use of atropine sulfate may be appropriate to decrease muscarinic side effects. Neostigmine and atropine should never be mixed in the same syringe. When used as an antidote for tubocurarine, neostigmine is administered via slow intravenous push. Appropriate ventilatory support should be continued until the patient is breathing well unassisted. If the pulse is less than 80 beats/minute, atropine should be administered prior to the neostigmine.

- In any situation in which an anticholinesterase is being administered via continuous infusion, a volume control device and an infusion monitoring device are recommended to control the dilution and rate of administration. Monitor carefully and frequently the respiratory and cardiovascular status.

Neuromuscular Blocking Drugs

Actions of Neuromuscular Blocking Drugs

Neuromuscular blocking drugs produce complete muscle relaxation by binding to the receptor for acetylcholine at the neuromuscular junction, with or without causing depolarization of the muscle membrane.

Indications for Neuromuscular Blocking Drugs

These drugs are used primarily to provide muscle relaxation during surgery without using deep general anesthesia, and are used with light anesthesia for endotracheal entubation, for spasm of the larynx, to prevent convulsive spasms during electroconvulsive therapy, and to allow breathing to be totally controlled by a respirator during surgery.

Tubocurarine is used for muscle relaxation for surgery or electroconvulsive therapy, muscle spasm in tetanus, controlled ventilation, and in small doses for diagnosis of myasthenia gravis. *Succinylcholine* has the shortest duration of action and is a drug of choice for endoscopy, laryngospasm, endotracheal entubation, orthopedic procedures, and electroconvulsive therapy. *Hexafluorenium* is used to prolong the neuromuscular blockade of succinylcholine and reduce its effects on muscle fasciculation. *Gallamine, metocurine,* and *pancuronium* have uses similar to tubocurarine.

Nurse Alert for Neuromuscular Blocking Drugs

- Endotracheal intubation, a suction machine, oxygen, a mechanical ventilator or resuscitation bag, and resuscitation equipment and drugs should be available when neuromuscular blocking drugs are administered.
- *Tubocurarine* and *pancuronium* should be used in smaller doses in patients with renal failure or acidosis. *Metocurine* and *gallamine* should not be used in patients with renal failure.
- During therapy, the reversing agent or antagonist should be readily available. All of the nondepolarizing agents and succinylcholine can be reversed by neostigmine. In addition, tubocurarine can be reversed by edrophonium or pyridostigmine, and vecuronium by pyridostigmine. Atropine is used only in special circumstances.

Side Effects of Neuromuscular Drugs

Tubocurarine and *metocurine* may cause hypotension or bronchospasm. *Gallamine* may cause tachycardia for a few minutes after injection. *Pancuronium* increases heart rate, cardiac output, and atrial pressure. At usual doses, *atracurium* does not cause cardiac side effects. *Vecuronium* may cause only minimal side effects, like those of tubocurarine. *Succinylcholine* may cause cardiac arrythmias and bradycardia, particularly in children, muscle fasciculations, and transient rise in intraocular pressure. Patients who receive any depolarizing agent may have pain or discomfort in the back, neck, trunk, lower intercostal region, or abdominal wall when first walking.

Nursing Implications for Neuromuscular Blocking Drugs

- Monitor the blood pressure, pulse, respirations, and overall respiratory status at frequent, regular intervals. It may be appropriate to also monitor the electrocardiogram.
- Neuromuscular blocking agents are not anesthetics. Patients, unless also anesthetized, can still hear, feel sensa-

Table 9-2 Administration of neuromuscular blocking drugs

Generic Name	Trade Name	Dosage and Administration‡
Nondepolarizing (Competitive) Drugs		
Atracurium besylate	Tracrium	INTRAVENOUS: *Adults*—0.3 to 0.6 mg/kg; subsequent doses, 0.05 to 0.1 mg/kg.
Gallamine triethiodide	Flaxedil* Triethiodide	INTRAVENOUS: *Adults*—1 to 1.5 mg/kg body weight. Supplemental doses, 0.3 to 1.2 mg/kg. *Children*—2.5 mg/kg initially with 0.3 to 1.2 mg/kg supplemental doses. *Newborns*—to 1 ml, 1.5 mg/kg initially, with 1 mg/kg supplemental doses.
Metocurine iodide	Metubine*	INTRAVENOUS: *Adults*—0.1 to 0.3 mg/kg body weight. Supplemental doses, 0.02 to 0.03 mg/kg.
Pancuronium bromide	Pavulon*	INTRAVENOUS: *Adults and children*—0.04 to 0.1 mg/kg body weight initially with 0.01 to 0.02 mg/kg supplemental doses. Newborns may be very sensitive; use a test dose of 0.02 mg.
Tubocurarine chloride (curare)	Tubarine†	INTRAVENOUS: *Adults and children*—0.2 to 0.4 mg/kg body weight initially. Supplemental doses, 0.04 to 0.2 mg/kg. Diagnosis of myasthenia gravis: ⅟₁₅ to ⅓ of above dose. Intravenous injection should be slow (1 to 1½ min). Do not combine with the alkaline intravenous barbiturate solutions.
Vecuronium	Norcuron	INTRAVENOUS: *Adults*—0.07 to 0.14 mg/kg for intubation; 0.04 to 0.1 mg/kg initially, followed by 0.015 to 0.02 mg/kg as needed for surgery.

Depolarizing Drugs

Succinylcholine chloride	Anectine* Quelicin Sucostrin Sux-Cert	INTRAVENOUS: *Adults*—0.6 to 1.1 mg/kg body weight initially. Continuous infusion, 0.1% or 0.2% solution at a rate of 0.5 to 10 mg/min. *Children*—1.1 mg/kg body weight initially with 0.3 to 0.6 mg/kg supplemental doses. *Newborns*—2 mg/kg. Continuous infusion is not recommended for children and newborns. Duration is only 5 min because of hydrolysis by plasma cholinesterase. This enzyme is missing genetically in some patients, and a prolonged action is seen.

Cholinesterase Inhibitor

Hexafluorenium	Mylaxene	INTRAVENOUS: *Adults*—0.1 to 0.3 mg/kg, followed in two to three min by 0.3 to 0.5 mg/kg succinylcholine. Muscle relaxation lasts 20 to 30 min. For longer procedures, additional succinylcholine, 0.25 mg/kg, is given at 15 to 30 min intervals.

*Available in U.S. and Canada
†Available in Canada only
‡The dosages given are for use with nitrous oxide. Other inhalation anesthetics may require smaller doses.

132 **Pocket Nurse Guide to Drugs**

tions, and see, if the eyelids are opened. Avoid inappropriate discussions in the presence of the patient. Orient the patient to time and day, tell the patient what activities are going on in the environment, and arrange for periods of time during which the patient can sleep uninterrupted.

- Because the patient can still experience pain (if not anesthetized), it may be appropriate to medicate the patient with analgesics at regular intervals. Careful positioning of the patient should be done, care should be taken that equipment, instruments, and linens are not placed so as to cause discomfort to the patient, who would be unable to communicate discomfort.

- When therapy with a neuromuscular blocking agent is being discontinued, the patient should not be left unattended until enough muscle tone has returned that the patient can breathe, handle secretions, and if not intubated, call for assistance if needed. In infants, assess for the ability to hold the eyelids open or to hold up the legs.

- A variety of factors may prolong the effects of neuromuscular blockade, including hypothermia; renal or hepatic insufficiency; alterations in pH or electrolytes (especially hypokalemia or hypocalcemia); dehydration; reduced circulation time, as might be seen in congestive heart failure or shock; age (the very young or the elderly); myasthenia gravis; the concomitant use of inhalation anesthetics; many antibiotics (including aminoglycosides, polymyxins, tetracyclines, bacitracin, lincomycin, clindamycin); or other pathologic conditions such as amyotrophic lateral sclerosis or Eaton-Lambert syndrome. Quinidine, trimethaphan, and magnesium sulfate may potentiate tubocurarine. Patients with abnormalities in plasma cholinesterase activity may have prolonged apnea in response to succinylcholine. These patients include those with genetic problems with plasma cholinesterase, patients exposed to organophosphorus pesticides, or topical use of long-acting anticholinesterases (e.g., for open-angle glaucoma).

- The use of a peripheral nerve stimulator to monitor the response to a neuromuscular blockade agent is helpful.

Neuromuscular Drugs 133

- When these drugs are administered via continuous infusion, an infusion monitoring device should be used to control the rate of infusion.
- Consult the manufacturer's literature for specific guidelines regarding calculation of dosage. In most institutions, induction with a neuromuscular blockade agent must be done by the anesthesiologist or nurse anesthetist; consult institution policies for guidance.

SENSORY SYSTEM DRUGS

PART II

Drugs Affecting the Eye

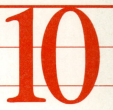

Drugs for mydriasis and cycloplegia
    Anticholinergic drugs
        Atropine sulfate
        Cyclopentolate hydrochloride
        Homatropine hydrobromide
        Scopolamine hydrobromide
        Tropicamide
        Eucatropine hydrochloride
    Adrenergic drugs
        Hydroxyamphetamine hydrobromide
        Phenylephrine hydrochloride

Drugs to treat glaucoma
    Cholinomimetic drugs
        Carbachol
        Physostigmine sulfate
        Physostigmine salicylate
        Pilocarpine nitrate
        Demecarium bromide
        Echothiophate iodide
        Isoflurophate
    Adrenergic drugs
        Epinephrine bitartrate
        Epinephryl borate
        Epinephrine hydrochloride
        Dipivefrin
        Timolol maleate
    Carbonic anhydrase inhibitors
        Acetazolamide
        Acetazolamide sodium
        Dichlorphenamide
        Methazolamide
    Osmotic agents
        Glycerin
        Isosorbide
        Mannitol
        Urea

Drugs for Mydriasis and Cycloplegia

Actions of Drugs Producing Mydriasis and Cycloplegia

Mydriasis (dilated pupil) is achieved by drugs that either block the muscarinic receptors of the sphincter muscles or stimulate the alpha receptors of the dilator muscles. Cycloplegia (paralysis of ciliary muscles with blurring of vision) results from drug actions that block muscarinic receptors. *Anticholinergic* drugs relax the sphincter and ciliary muscles and produce both conditions; *adrenergic* drugs act on the alpha receptors to produce mydriasis only.

Indications for Drugs Producing Mydriasis and Cycloplegia

Atropine sulfate (the drug of choice for children), *cyclopentolate*, *homatropine*, *scopolamine*, and *tropicamide* are used to relax eye muscles to aid in measuring refraction. *Atropine sulfate*, *cyclopentolate hydrochloride*, *homatropine hydrobromide*, and *scopolamine hydrobromide* are used in addition to treat eye inflammation. *Atropine sulfate* is also used to relax eye muscles for surgery. *Eucatropine hydrochloride* is used to dilate the eye for examination with little cycloplegia and to test for intraocular pressure rise when acute glaucoma is suspected. *Hydroxyamphetamine hydrobromide* and *phenylephrine hydrochloride* are used when only mydriasis is required for examination of internal structures of the eye.

Nurse Alert for Anticholinergic Drugs

- *Atropine* and the *belladonna alkaloids* may precipitate an attack of acute glaucoma in elderly patients or those predisposed to angle closure; thus they should be given cautiously to these patients.

Side Effects of Drugs Producing Mydriasis and Cycloplegia

Atropine has been reported to cause contact dermatitis of the eyelids. Systemic reactions of anticholinergic drugs may include dry mouth and dry skin, fever, thirst, confusion, and hyperactivity; children are most prone.

Nursing Implications for Drugs Causing Mydriasis and Cycloplegia

- Patients receiving mydriatics should be warned that their vision will be temporarily impaired. Wearing sunglasses may lessen the photophobia.

Table 10-1   Administration of drugs for producing mydriasis and cycloplegia

Drug	Trade Name	Dosage and Administration
Anticholinergic Drugs for Mydriasis and Cycloplegia		
Atropine sulfate	Atropine Sulfate Atropisol Isopto Atropine*	Topical solutions, 0.5% to 3%. *Adults*—1 drop of 1% to 3% solution to each eye. Frequency of administration depends on the condition being treated. *Children*—1 drop of 0.125 to 0.5% solution (under 8 yr) or 0.25 to 1% solution (over 8 yr) 3 times daily for 3 days before and once on the morning of the day refraction is measured. Duration: 6 days.
Cyclopentolate hydrochloride	Cyclogyl* Opto-Pentolate†	Topical solutions, 0.5%, 1%, and 2%. *Adults*—1 drop of solution in each eye, repeated after 5 min. Darker irises of children require the stronger solutions. *Children*—1 drop of solution in each eye, repeated after 10 min. Onset: 25 to 75 min. Duration: 6 to 24 hr.
Homatropine hydrobromide	Isopto Homatropine*	Topical solutions, 2% and 5%. *Adults*—for refraction 1 drop of 5% solution every 10 min 2 or 3 times. Duration: 2 days.

Drugs Affecting the Eye 139

Scopolamine hydrobromide	Isopto Hyoscine	Topical solutions, 0.2% to 0.3%. *Adults*—1 drop of solution or ointment to each eye, 1 or more times daily depending on the condition being treated. *Children*—1 drop of 0.2% to 0.25% solution or ointment twice daily for 2 days before refraction measurement. Duration: 3 days.
Tropicamide	Mydriacyl*	Topical solutions, 0.5% and 1%. 1 drop in each eye, repeated in 5 min. Onset: 20 to 35 min. Duration: 2 to 6 hr

Anticholinergic Drugs for Mydriasis Only

Eucatropine hydrochloride	Eucatropine Hydrochloride	Topical solutions, 5% and 10%. 1 drop in each eye repeated in 10 to 15 min for dilation. 2 drops in one eye to test for acute glaucoma. Onset: 30 min. Duration: 2 to 4 hr.

cont'd. next page

*Available in U.S. and Canada
†Available in Canada only

Table 10-1   Administration of drugs for producing mydriasis and cycloplegia—cont'd.

Drug	Trade Name	Dosage and Administration
Adrenergic Drugs for Mydriasis Only		
Hydroxyamphetamine hydrobromide	Paredrine	Topical use, 1 drop of a 1% solution. Maximal mydriasis in 45 to 60 min. Recovery in 6 hr.
Phenylephrine hydrochloride	AR-Nefrin Mydfrin* Neo-Synephrine Hydrochloride*	Topical solutions 0.08% to 10% Topical use, 1 drop of a 2.5% solution. Maximal mydriasis in 60 to 90 min. Recovery in 6 hr.

*Available in U.S. and Canada
†Available in Canada only

Drugs Affecting the Eye **141**

- Review with patients and parents of children receiving atropine the possible systemic side effects that can occur (Chapter 17 and 21). Instruct patients to report any unusual signs or symptoms.
- Patients receiving drugs causing cycloplegia should be cautioned to avoid activities requiring visual acuity, such as driving or operating machinery, until the paralysis of the ciliary muscles disappears and visual acuity returns to normal.
- Review with patients the anticipated duration of action of the specific eye medication being used so that the patient can anticipate how long vision may be reduced.

Drugs Used to Treat Glaucoma

Actions of Drugs for Glaucoma

The weak cholinomimetic drugs spread the trabecular spaces of the anterior chamber when the sphincter muscles contract, allowing improved uptake of aqueous humor, and relieving of intraocular pressure. Epinephrine stimulates the alpha and beta receptors to reduce resistance to the outflow of aqueous humor and decreases production of aqueous humor. Adrenergic beta blockers decrease intraocular pressure by an unclear mechanism. Carbonic anhydrase inhibitors decrease the production of aqueous humor. Osmotic agents reduce intraocular pressure short-term by drawing fluid from the eye to the hyperosmotic blood.

Indications for Drugs for Glaucoma

The weak cholinomimetics are used to treat chronic (open-angle) glaucoma. *Pilocarpine* is the drug of choice for both chronic and acute glaucoma. The strong cholinomimetics *demecarium, echothiophate,* and *isoflurophate* are used for resistant chronic glaucoma. *Epinephrine* is used in the initial treatment of glaucoma in young patients and in elderly patients with cataracts. *Timolol* may be used in the initial treatment of chronic glaucoma, or used with miotic drugs and epinephrine. *Carbonic anhydrase inhibitors* may be used in resistant cases of chronic glaucoma. *Osmotic agents* are used

Table 10-2 Administration of drugs for glaucoma

Generic Name	Trade Name	Dosage and Administration
Cholinomimetic Drugs (Weak Miotics)		
Carbachol	Carbacel Isopto Carbachol*	TOPICAL: 1 drop 0.75% to 3% solution every 8 hr. Onset: 15 to 30 min.
Physostigmine sulfate	Eserine Sulfate	TOPICAL: 1 drop of 0.25% to 1% every 4 to 6 hr. Ointment or night use primarily. Onset: 30 min.
Physostigmine salicylate	Isopto Eserine	
Pilocarpine hydrochloride	Isopto Carpine* Pilocar Various others	TOPICAL: 1 drop, 0.25% to 10% every 6 to 8 hr. Onset: 15 to 30 min.
Pilocarpine nitrate	P.V. Carpine Liquifilm*	TOPICAL: 1 drop, 0.5% to 6% every 6 to 8 hr. Onset: 15 to 30 min.
Cholinomimetic Drugs (Strong Miotics)		
Demecarium bromide	Humorsol	TOPICAL: 1 drop 0.125% to 0.25% solution every 12 to 48 hr. Onset: 12 hr.
Echothiophate iodide	Phospholine Iodide*	TOPICAL: 1 drop 0.03% to 0.06% every 12 to 48 hr. Onset: 12 hr.

Isoflurophate	Floropryl	TOPICAL: ¼ in strip of 0.025% ointment every 12 to 72 hr. Onset: 12 hr.

Adrenergic Drugs

Epinephrine bitartrate	Epitrate* Murocel Mytrate	TOPICAL: 1 drop of a 0.25% to 2.0% solution one or two times daily.
Epinephryl borate	Epinal* Eppy*	Same.
Epinephrine hydrochloride	Epifrin* Glaucon*	Same.
Dipivefrin	Propine*	TOPICAL: One drop into the conjunctival sac every 12 hrs. for glaucoma.
Timolol maleate	Timoptic*	TOPICAL: 1 drop of 0.25% solution twice daily. If not sufficient, a 0.5% solution is used.

Carbonic Anhydrase Inhibitors

Acetazolamide	Acetazolam† Diamox*	ORAL: *Adults*—250 mg every 6 hr. *Children*—10 to 15 mg/kg body weight daily in divided doses. Timed-release capsules are taken every 12 to 24 hr but may not be as effective.

cont'd. next page

*Available in U.S. and Canada
†Available in Canada only

Table 10-2 Administration of drugs for glaucoma—cont'd.

Generic Name	Trade Name	Dosage and Administration
Acetazolamide sodium	Diamox, Parenteral*	INTRAVENOUS, INTRAMUSCULAR: *Adults*—500 mg repeated in 2 to 4 hr if necessary. *Children:* 5 to 10 mg/kg body weight every 6 hr.
Dichlorphenamide	Daranide Oratrol	ORAL: *Adults*—50 to 200 mg every 6 to 8 hr.
Methazolamide	Neptazane*	ORAL: *Adults*—25 to 100 mg every 8 hr.
Osmotic Agents		
Glycerin	Glyrol Osmoglyn	ORAL: *Adults and children*—1 to 1.5 Gm/kg body weight as a 50% or 75% solution once or twice daily.
Isosorbide	Ismotic	ORAL: *Adults*—1.5 Gm/kg body weight up to 4 times daily.
Mannitol	Osmitrol*	INTRAVENOUS: *Adults and children*—0.5 to 2 Gm/kg body weight as a 20% solution infused over 30 to 60 min.
Urea	Ureaphil Urevert	INTRAVENOUS: *Adults*—0.5 to 2 Gm/kg body weight as a 30% solution infused at 60 drops/min. *Children*—0.5 to 1.5 Gm/kg body weight of a 30% solution infused over 30 min.

*Available in U.S. and Canada
†Available in Canada only

in short-term treatment to lower intraocular pressure of glaucoma prior to surgery. Emergency treatment for acute (closed-angle) glaucoma consists of a cholinomimetic, carbonic anhydrase inhibitor, epinephrine, and an osmotic diuretic prior to surgery.

Nurse Alert for Drugs for Glaucoma

- Patients with hereditary fructose intolerance should not be given urea made up in invert sugar. Timolol should be used cautiously with patients who have asthma, heart block, or heart failure, because of its systemic side effects. Carbonic anhydrase inhibitors should be used with caution in patients on digitalis because hypokalemia may be produced.

Side Effects of Drugs for Glaucoma

Cataracts may develop with the long-term administration of *demecarium, echothiophate* and *isoflurophate,* as well as muscles spasms in the eye, ocular pain, and headache. *Physostigmine* may cause depigmentation of the eyelids in blacks or conjunctivitis and allergic reactions with prolonged use. *Epinephrine* can cause browache and eye irritation, and with prolonged use, swelling of the eyelids and bloodshot eyes; side effects of systemic absorption include tachycardia, hypertension, headache, sweating, and tremors, which are rare and occur usually only with eye damage, or if the epithelium comes in contact with the drug. *Timolol* may produce systemic effects including bradycardia, hypotension, and bronchospasm. *Carbonic anhydrase inhibitors* may cause loss of appetite, gastrointestinal upset, lethargy, depression, paresthesia, and, early in treatment, a slight hypokalemia. *Glycerin* may cause hyperglycemia in diabetics, headache, nauseas, and vomiting. *Isosorbide* produces diuresis. *Mannitol* produces pronounced diuresis and commonly causes headache, nausea, and vomiting. *Urea* produces irritation on injection.

Nursing Implications for Drugs for Glaucoma

- Glycerin and isosorbide may be flavored or chilled with chipped ice to increase palatability.

146   Pocket Nurse Guide to Drugs

- Review with patients the prescribed concentration of eye preparations, and caution patients to read labels carefully, especially when prescriptions are refilled, to ensure the correct dose is being used.
- To prevent overflow of medications into the nasal and pharyngeal passages and to reduce the incidence of systemic side effects with some preparations, the patient may be instructed to occlude the nasolacrimal duct with one finger for 1 to 2 minutes after the medication has been applied and before the patient closes the eyelid. Check with the physician.
- Patients receiving miotic drugs should be warned not to drive immediately after administration of the drug. The pain and blurred vision commonly experienced at the beginning of treatment will usually diminish with repeated usage. Painful eye spasms can be relieved by application of cold compresses.
- Patients with glaucoma should be instructed that their eye medications are as important to their well-being as any other medications and should not be discontinued without prior consultation with the physician.
- One drop of a 1% to 2% epinephrine solution reverses the redness caused by the potent acetylcholinesterase inhibitors.
- Pralidoxime (PAM), 0.1 to 0.2 ml of a 5% solution, reverses the action of the irreversible acetylcholinesterase inhibitors. PAM must be injected subconjunctivally to be effective in the eye.
- Acetylcholinesterase inhibitors should be discontinued 2 weeks before surgery because of possible interactions with anesthetic agents.
- The carbonic anhydrase inhibitors and osmotic agents are discussed in chapter 14.
- Monitor the pulse of patients receiving timolol and teach the patients to check their pulse regularly, if appropriate. Because this drug causes bradycardia, it should not be administered if the pulse is below 50 or 60 beats/minute; check with the physician.
- Help patients to understand that glaucoma can be controlled with proper use of medications, but that glaucoma cannot

be cured. Drugs will have to be used on a regular, ongoing basis.

- The Ocusert Pilo-20 and Pilo-40 Systems are sustained release forms of pilocarpine. While more expensive than simple drops, the Ocusert System can be very helpful to patients who have a history of poor compliance or have conditions which make accurate instillation of eye drops difficult, such as poor vision or arthritis. The Ocusert System is inserted into the upper or lower cul-de-sac, and the medication is released slowly. Patients should be instructed to make sure that the unit is in place every morning since it may fall out at night. The unit is designed to be replaced weekly, but occasionally a unit will only be effective for a few days before needing replacement. Miosis and spasm may be a problem after the unit is inserted, so it is suggested that the unit be inserted at bedtime.
- Because glycerin can cause hyperglycemia, it may necessitate an increase in insulin dosage in diabetics. Lying down immediately after taking glycerin may reduce the headache which occasionally accompanies its use.

Local Anesthetics 11

Topical application
Benoxinate hydrochloride
Benzocaine
Butamben picrate
Cocaine hydrochloride
Cyclomethycaine sulfate
Dibucaine hydrochloride
Dyclonine hydrochloride
Hexylcaine hydrochloride
Lidocaine
Lidocaine hydrochloride
Pramoxine hydrochloride
Proparacaine hydrochloride
Tetracaine hydrochloride

Injection application
(infiltration, nerve or epidural
block, or spinal block)
Bupivacaine hydrochloride
Chloroprocaine hydrochloride
Dibucaine
Etidocaine hydrochloride
Lidocaine
Mepivacaine
Prilocaine
Procaine hydrochloride
Tetracaine

Actions of Local Anesthetics

Local anesthetics inhibit nerve conduction in the area of administration and affect all neurons, including sensory, motor, and autonomic neurons.

Indications for Local Anesthetics

For Topical Anesthesia:

Benoxinate hydrochloride is applied topically to anesthetize the cornea and conjunctiva. *Benzocaine* is used for relief of sunburn, itching, and mild burns. *Butamben picrate* is nonprescription drug used for relief of itching and burning. *Cocaine hydrochloride* is used in ear, nose, and throat procedures for shrinking of mucous membranes and vasoconstriction as well as for local anesthesia, and is used to anesthetize the cornea and conjunctiva. *Cyclomethycaine sulfate* and *dibucaine hydrochloride* are nonprescription drugs used for skin anesthesia. *Dyclonine* is used to suppress the gag reflex and for genitourinary endoscopy. *Hexylcaine* is used in

148

bronchoscopy, endotracheal intubation, gastroscopy, and genitourinary procedures. *Lidocaine* is used for topical anesthesia in ear, nose, and throat procedures, upper digestive tract procedures, and genitourinary procedures. *Proparacaine* is used topically to anesthetize the cornea and conjunctiva. *Tetracaine* is used topically for anesthesia and in ophthalmic instillations.

For Injection:

Bupivacaine and *chloroprocaine* are used for epidural anesthesia in labor. *Dibucaine* is the most potent and toxic of the local anesthetics. *Etidocaine* is used for epidural block for abdominal surgery and other anesthetic purposes, but not for labor. *Lidocaine* and *mepivacaine* are used for local anesthesia for many purposes. *Prilocaine* is often used for outpatient surgery because of fewer side effects. *Procaine* is unreliable for epidural block. *Tetracaine* is most commonly used for spinal anesthesia. (See also "Administration of Local Anesthetics" section.)

Nurse Alert for Local Anesthetics

- With topical applications to mucous membranes, use the lowest concentration of the drug to avoid systemic toxicity and side effects.
- With administration by injection, aspirate syringe to ensure blood vessel has not been entered.
- Spinal anesthesia is hazardous for abdominal surgery in poor-risk patients because of potential for sudden vasodilation and hypotension.
- Because allergic reactions may occur with any local anesthetic, epinephrine and resuscitation equipment should be available.

Side Effects of Local Anesthetics

All local anesthetics act as CNS stimulants if absorbed systemically, producing anxiety, paresthesia, tremors, tinnitus, and even convulsions. Cocaine is unique among local anesthetics in causing euphoria and vasoconstriction. A high

150   Pocket Nurse Guide to Drugs

Table 11-1   Administration of local anesthetics

Generic Name	Trade Name	Surface Applications			Maximum Dosage
		Eye**	Mucous Membranes†	Skin	
Benoxinate hydrochloride	Dorsacaine	+	0	0	—
Benzocaine	Americaine	0	0	+	—
Butamben picrate	Butesin Picrate	0	0	+	—
Cocaine hydrochloride		+	+	0	—
Cyclomethycaine sulfate	Surfacaine	0	+‡	+	—
Dibucaine hydrochloride	Nupercaine Hydrochloride	0	0	+	—
Dyclonine hydrochloride	Dyclone	0	+	+	—
Hexylcaine hydrochloride	Cyclaine	0	+	0	—
Lidocaine	Xylocaine*	0	+	+	—
Lidocaine hydrochloride	Xylocaine Hydrochloride*	0	+	+	—

Local Anesthetics 151

Generic Name	Trade Name				Maximum Dosage
Pramoxine hydrochloride	Tronothane Hydrochloride*	0	+‡	+	—
Proparacaine hydrochloride	Ophthaine Hydrochloride*	+	0	0	—
Tetracaine hydrochloride	Pontocaine Hydrochloride*	+	+	+	20-50 mg

*Available in U.S. and Canada

**+ indicates suitable site for application; 0 indicates site not suitable for application.

†Mucous membranes include the bronchotracheal mucosa and the mucosa of the urethra, rectum, and vagina.

‡Not for application to the bronchotracheal mucosa.

Administration by Injection

Generic Name	Trade Name	Local Infiltration or Nerve Block or Epidural Block**	Spinal Block (Sub-Arachnoid)	Duration†	Maximum Dosage
Bupivacaine	Marcaine*	+	Investigational	Long‡	200 mg
Chloroprocaine hydrochloride	Nesacaine	+	Investigational	Short	800 mg

cont'd. next page

*Available in U.S. and Canada

**+ indicates suitable use; 0 indicates use not suitable.

†Duration without epinephrine: short, 1 hr; intermediate, 2 hr; long, 3 hr (approximations).

‡Duration of bupivacaine in nerve block is 6 to 13 hr.

Table 11-1 Administration of local anesthetics—cont.

Generic Name	Trade Name	Administration by Injection		Duration†	Maximum Dosage
		Local Infiltration or Nerve Block or Epidural Block**	Spinal Block (Sub-Arachnoid)		
Dibucaine	Nupercaine	0	+	Long	2.5-10 mg
Etidocaine	Duranest	+	0	Long	—
Lidocaine	Xylocaine*	+	+	Intermediate	300 mg (4.5 mg/kg)
Mepivacaine	Carbocaine*	+	0	Intermediate	400 mg (7 mg/kg)
Prilocaine hydrochloride	Citanest Hydrochloride*	+	0	Intermediate	600 mg (8 mg/kg)
Procaine hydrochloride	Novocain*	+	+	Short	600 mg (10 mg/kg)
Tetracaine	Pontocaine Hydrochloride*	0	+	Long	2-5 mg

*Available in U.S. and Canada

** + indicates suitable use; 0 indicates use not suitable.

†Duration without epinephrine: short, 1 hr; intermediate, 2 hr; long, 3 hr (approximations).

‡Duration of bupivacaine in nerve block is 6 to 13 hr.

plasma concentration of local anesthetics may cause CNS depression, including hypotension, respiratory depression, and coma. Vasodilation and cardiac depression may occur. Allergic responses may occur, although anaphylaxis is rare. Lidocaine may cause drowsiness, fatigue, and amnesia. Vasodilation frequently occurs with spinal anesthesia. Some local anesthetic solutions contain epinephrine to retard distribution of the anesthetic away from the injection site. Absorption of the epinephrine may cause cardiac stimulation, hypertension, and central nervous system stimulation.

Nursing Implications for Local Anesthetics

- Patients should be questioned about possible allergies to local anesthetics. Remember, to many people "Novocain" is the term applied to all local anesthetics, regardless of the actual preparation.
- Following spinal anesthesia, the patient should be kept flat for the specified number of hours (usually 12).
- If the patient has not voided within 8 to 12 hours after surgery, notify the physician.
- Patients who have received spinal anesthesia should be assisted when getting up the first time.
- Keep the siderail up for all patients who have received any form of spinal anesthesia until it is clear that the patient's sensation has returned in the lower extremities.
- Position the patient carefully in the bed because there will be no sensation in the lower extremities to warn the patient of wrinkles, tight sheets, or other irritations to the skin.
- Application of heat or cold to areas numb from local or spinal anesthesia should be done with extreme caution as the patient will be unable to indicate if there is skin irritation or burning.
- If some form of local anesthesia is being used for delivery, be certain to monitor not only the mother but also the baby. Monitor fetal heart tones every 5 to 15 minutes. The mother's sensation of uterine contractions may be absent or altered, and she may need additional instructions to assist with the delivery.

Pocket Nurse Guide to Drugs

- Conversation and noise should be kept to a minimum as some patients find excessive conversation overstimulating. Care should be taken to avoid discussing other patients, pathology reports, or complications as these topics might alarm the patient.
- Patients should be cautioned to use surface anesthetics as instructed and not to increase the frequency of application or to use the preparation on surfaces for which it was not designed.
- After a local anesthetic has been used, the body is not able to perceive pain in the anesthetized area, and injury may occur. For this reason it is important to instruct patients carefully about the extent to which they may use an anesthetized area until the effects of the local anesthesia wear off.

CARDIOVASCULAR SYSTEM DRUGS

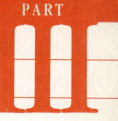

PART III

Drugs to Improve Circulation 12

Sympathomimetics for
hypotension and shock
  Dobutamine hydrochloride
  Dopamine hydrochloride
  Epinephrine hydrochloride
  Isoproterenol hydrochloride
  Levarterenol bitartrate
  (norepinephrine)
  Mephentermine sulfate
  Metaraminol bitartrate
  Methoxamine hydrochloride
  Phenylephrine hydrochloride
Antianginal drugs
  Beta-adrenergic receptor
  antagonists (see Ch. 13)
  Calcium channel blockers
  (see Ch. 13)
  Direct acting vasodilators
    Amyl nitrite
    Erythrityl tetranitrate
    Isosorbide dinitrate
    Nitroglycerin
    Pentaerythritol tetranitrate

Vasodilators for peripheral
vascular disease
  Cyclandelate
  Dihydrogenated ergot
  alkaloids
  Isoxsuprine
  Nicotinyl alcohol
  Nylidrin hydrochloride
  Papaverine hydrochloride
  Pentoxifylline
  Tolazoline hydrochloride

Sympathomimetics for Hypotension and Shock

Actions of Sympathomimetics for Hypotension and Shock

Levarterenol is an agonist of alpha-1 and beta-1 adrenergic receptors and produces potent peripheral vasoconstriction and inotropic actions, dramatically raising blood pressure with small change in heart rate but stronger contractions of the heart. *Epinephrine* is an agonist of alpha-1, beta-1 and beta-2 receptors, increasing heart rate and force of contraction, with vasoconstriction but little or no increase in blood pressure. *Isoproterenol* stimulates beta-1 and beta-2 adrenergic receptors, increasing heart rate and cardiac output, decreasing peripheral resistance, and stimulating smooth muscle. *Dopamine* stimulates alpha and beta adrenergic receptors and dopaminergic receptors to increase cardiac output while heart rate and mean blood pressure are generally unchanged. *Dobutamine* at low doses increases contractility of the heart without increasing heart rate. *Methoxamine* and *phenylephrine* stimulate alpha adrenergic receptors and increase blood pressure. *Metaraminol* is both a direct alpha adrenergic agonist and an indirect sympathomimetic, increasing diastolic and systolic blood pressure with increased contractility; heart rate usually falls as a result of reflex bradycardia.

Indications for Sympathomimetics for Hypotension and Shock

Levarterenol is used to restore blood pressure in acute hypotensive states after blood volume has been restored. *Epinephrine* is the drug of choice for anaphylactic shock; it may be used for bronchospasm from asthma or allergic reactions, and it is occasionally used for cardiac arrest. *Isoproterenol* is used principally as a bronchodilator (see Chapter 27) but also to stimulate cardiac contractility in heart block or cardiogenic shock secondary to myocardial infarction or septicemia. *Dopamine* is used most commonly for shock. *Dobutamine* is used to improve cardiac output in cardiogenic shock or congestive heart failure. *Methoxamine* and *phenylephrine* are used to treat hypotension of anesthesia, primarily for spinal and general anesthesia, and to terminate paroxysmal supraventricular tachycardia. *Metaraminol* and *mephentermine* are used to maintain blood pressure during spinal, epidural, or general anesthesia.

Nurse Alert for Sympathomimetics for Hypotension and Shock

- Levarterenol is contraindicated in cases of vascular thrombosis and patients anesthetized with a drug that sensitizes

Table 12-1 Administration of sympathomimetics for hypotension and shock

Generic Name	Trade Name	Dosage and Administration
Dobutamine hydrochloride	Dobutrex*	INTRAVENOUS: *Adults*—2.5 to 10 μg/kg/min.
Dopamine hydrochloride	Intropin* Revimine†	INTRAVENOUS: *Adults*—1 ampule (40 mg of the chloride salt in 5 ml) is diluted in 250 ml (800 μg/ml) or 500 ml (400 μg/ml of solution. Initial intravenous infusion is 2 to 5 μg/kg/min. Onset: 5 min. Duration: 10 min.
Epinephrine hydrochloride	Adrenalin Chloride	INTRAMUSCULAR, SUBCUTANEOUS, INTRAVENOUS: *Adults*—0.5 ml of 1:1000 solution IM or SC followed by 0.25 to 0.5 ml of a 1:10,000 solution IV every 5 to 15 min. *Children*—0.3 ml of a 1:1000 solution IM. May be repeated every 15 min for 1 hr if necessary. Onset: minutes. Duration: 1 to 4 hr.
Isoproterenol hydrochloride	Isuprel Hydrochloride*	INTRAVENOUS: *Adults*—1 to 2 mg (5 to 10 ml) diluted in 5% dextrose and infused at a rate of 1 to 10 μg/min. Onset: minutes. Duration: 1 to 2 hr.
Levarterenol (norepinephrine) bitartrate	Levophed Bitartrate*	INTRAVENOUS: *Adults*—2 to 8 ml in 500 ml 5% dextrose and given by continuous infusion for desired response. 8 to 12 mg/min initially, then 2 to 4 mg/min. Onset: immediate. Duration: minutes.

Mephentermine sulfate	Wyamine Sulfate*	INTRAVENOUS: *Adults*—600 mg to 1 Gm is diluted in 1 L 5% dextrose and given by continuous infusion to maintain pressure, usually 1 to 5 mg/min. Onset: immediate. Duration: 30 to 45 min.
Metaraminol bitartrate	Aramine	INTRAMUSCULAR, INTRAVENOUS: *Adults*—2 to 5 mg as a single intravenous injection or 200 to 500 mg diluted in 1 L 5% dextrose given by continuous infusion to maintain pressure. Alternatively, 5 to 10 mg given IM. Onset: 1 to 2 min. Duration: 20 to 60 min.
Methoxamine hydrochloride	Vasoxyl*	INTRAMUSCULAR, INTRAVENOUS: *Adults*—5 to 20 mg in a single intramuscular dose or 2 to 5 mg given slowly IV. Onset: immediate. Duration: 60 min.
Phenylephrine hydrochloride	Neo-Synephrine Hydrochloride* Isophrin	ORAL, INTRAMUSCULAR, SUBCUTANEOUS, INTRAVENOUS: *Adults*—1 to 10 mg IM or SC; 0.25 to 0.5 mg given IV or 10 mg in 500 ml 5% dextrose infused slowly 40-180 mg/min; 20 mg 3 times per day orally for orthostatic hypotension. Onset: minutes. Duration: 1 to 2 hr.

*Available in U.S. and Canada
†Available in Canada only

160 **Pocket Nurse Guide to Drugs**

the heart to catecholamine-induced arrhythmias and with patients taking an antidepressant drug.

- Epinephrine is contraindicated for patients taking a drug that sensitizes the heart to catecholamines, for patients with narrow-angle glaucoma, and for women in labor; it should be used cautiously in patients with cardiac arrhythmias, cardiovascular disease, hypertension, or hypotension; it should not be administered simultaneously with isoproterenol.
- Isoproterenol is contraindicated for patients taking digitalis or epinephrine or patients disposed to cardiac arrhythmias.
- Dopamine is contraindicated for patients disposed to cardiac arrhythmias, women in labor receiving oxytocic drugs, and patients receiving general anesthetics that sensitize the heart to catecholamines.
- Methoxamine, phenylephrine, mephentermine, and metaraminol have contraindications similar to those of other sympathomimetic vasopressors.
- All adrenergic drugs should be used cautiously with patients receiving monoamine oxidase inhibitors or tricyclic antidepressants because a hypertensive crisis may be precipitated.
- Propranolol may interfere with the actions of levarterenol, epinephrine, dopamine, isoproterenol, and dobutamine.

Side Effects of Sympathomimetics for Hypotension and Shock

Levarterenol may cause anxiety, a slow forceful heartbeat, and transient hypertension causing a severe headache. *Epinephrine* may cause fear and anxiety, a throbbing headache, dizziness, pallor, tremor and weakness, and palpitations; serious reactions include cerebral hemorrhage and cardiac arrhythmias. *Isoproterenol* may cause palpitations, tachycardia, headache, flushing, sweating, mild tremors, nervousness, dizziness, and nausea. *Dopamine* may cause tachycardia, palpitations, nausea and vomiting, angina, headache, hypertension, and vasoconstriction. *Dobutamine* commonly causes increased heart rate and blood pressure and more rarely palpitations, shortness of breath, angina, nausea, and headache. *Methoxamine* may cause sustained hypertension, severe headache, pilomotor erection, desire to urinate, and vomiting. *Metaraminol* may cause headache, palpitations, nausea and vomiting and difficulty in voiding. *Mephentermine* may cause drowsiness, weeping, incoherence, and occasionally convulsions.

Nursing Implications for Sympathomimetics for Hypotension and Shock

- Safe care of the patient receiving intravenous sympathomimetic drugs for the treatment of shock or hypotension includes the following:
  a. A microdrip intravenous administration set should be used to regulate the dose being administered more accurately.
  b. The patient's blood pressure and pulse should be monitored every 2 to 5 minutes until the blood pressure and rate of drug administration are stable, then every 15 minutes. The patient should not be left unattended.
  c. An electronic IV monitor or regulator should be used to accurately control the rate of IV fluid and drug administration.
  d. If possible, the central venous pressure should be monitored as frequently as the blood pressure is monitored.
  e. Monitor the fluid intake and output. Urinary output should be monitored and recorded every 30 to 60 minutes.
  f. Read the labels of the drug ampules carefully, since not all forms of a drug may be administered intravenously. Some forms of epinephrine and ephedrine solutions are safe for IV administration, whereas others are not. Do not use any solution or medication if discolored or sediment is present.
  g. Most adrenergic drugs are incompatible with many other drugs. For this reason, they are not added to IV solutions containing other medications, including sodium bicarbonate, and they are not added to blood. If in doubt, consult the pharmacist.

162 Pocket Nurse Guide to Drugs

h. All patients should be observed for hypertensive crisis. If this does occur, the adrenergic drug should be slowed or discontinued, the physician notified, and the specific drug antidote administered as ordered. Phentolamine, an adrenergic blocking agent, may be ordered, if necessary.

i. If available, cardiac monitoring should be done while the patient is receiving intravenous adrenergic drugs.

j. Data such as the pulmonary capillary wedge pressure, cardiac output, and other hemodynamic parameters that can be measured via a balloon flotation catheter should be obtained, when possible, on a regular basis during administration of adrenergic drugs. These data will assist in evaluating the success of the drug therapy.

- Extravasation of intravenous levarterenol, dopamine, or methoxamine may cause tissue necrosis and sloughing. For this reason, it is preferable to administer these drugs in a large central vein if possible. The intravenous insertion site should be inspected frequently. In the event of extravasation, the physician may order the site of injury infiltrated with a solution of 5 to 10 mg of phentolamine, an adrenergic blocker, diluted in 10 to 15 ml of normal saline solution.

- Solutions of dopamine, dobutamine, or metaraminol should be discarded if over 24 hours old.

- Patients who are markedly hypotensive or in shock may be anxious as a response to inadequate oxygenation of the brain and have a sense of "impending doom," symptoms that can accompany circulatory failure. Administration of adrenergic medications may cause palpitations and tachycardia. Provide calm reassurance to patients being treated with these drugs.

Epinephrine and Isoproterenol

- The usual dose of epinephrine used for treating anaphylactic shock is 0.1 to 1 ml (0.1 to 1 mg) of 1:1000 solution given subcutaneously.

- Epinephrine and isoproterenol are both strong cardiac stimulants and should not be administered simultaneously; they may be used alternately.

Drugs to Improve Circulation   **163**

- Epinephrine causes hyperglycemia, which may result in an increased insulin requirement in patients with diabetes mellitus.
- Some forms of epinephrine solutions are safe for IV administration, whereas others are not. Do not use any solution or medication if discolored or sediment is present.

Dopamine

- Dopamine may be diluted in any of the following solutions: sodium chloride injection, dextrose 5% injection, dextrose 5% and socium chloride 0.9%, dextrose 5% and 0.45% sodium chloride solution, dextrose 5% in lactated Ringer's solution, sodium lactate (1/6 Molar) injection, or lactated Ringer's injection. Do NOT add this drug to 5% sodium bicarbonate or other alkaline solution. The addition of 400 mg of drug to 250 ml of solution, or 800 mg of drug to 500 ml of solution, will create a concentration of 1600 μg per ml.

Dobutamine

- This drug comes as a powder, and must be reconstituted with sterile water for injection or 5% dextrose injection. Once reconstituted, the drug may be stored for 6 hours at room temperature, or 48 hours refrigerated. After being reconstituted, the drug must be further diluted to at least 50 ml prior to administration, in 5% dextrose injection, 0.9% sodium chloride injection, or sodium lactate injection. Intravenous solutions should be used within 24 hours. See the manufacturer's literature.
- Solutions of this drug may exhibit a slight color, which will increase with time. There is no loss of potency if used within time periods stated above.

Levarterenol (Norepinephrine) Bitartrate

- This drug should be administered in 5% dextrose in water or 5% dextrose in sodium chloride; administration in saline solution alone is not recommended. In the usual dilution, 4 mg of drug is added to 500 ml of solution (2 mg of drug to 250 ml of solution) to obtain a dilution of 8 μg per ml.

Metaraminol

- This drug may be diluted for intravenous administration in sodium chloride injection or 5% dextrose injection; for other solutions, check the manufacturer's directions or the pharmacy.

Antianginal Drugs

    Amyl nitrite
    Erythrityl tetranitrate
    Isosorbide dinitrate
    Nitroglycerin
    Pentaerythritol tetranitrate
    Beta adrenergic receptor antagonists (see Chapter 13)
    Calcium-channel blocker (see Chapter 13)

Actions of Antianginal Drugs

The antianginal nitrites and nitrates dilate coronary arterioles, increasing myocardial oxygen supply and they dilate peripheral arteries and veins, reducing blood pressure and cardiac work (oxygen demand).

    Beta adrenergic blockers and calcium channel inhibitors decrease cardiac work and are used as prophylactic antianginal agents. These drugs are also used as antihypertensive drugs and are discussed in Chapter 13.

Indications for Antianginal Drugs

Amyl nitrite is used for relief of acute angina attacks. *Erythrityl tetranitrate* is used prophylactically to prevent angina attacks. *Isosorbide dinitrate* is to relieve acute angina attacks and is possibly effective prophylactically. *Nitroglycerin* is the drug of choice for treatment of acute anginal episodes or prophylactically in expectation of an episode; oral sustained-release and ointment forms are for prophylactic therapy. *Pentaerythritol tetranitrate* is possibly effective as prophylactic treatment for angina pectoris.

Nurse Alert for Antianginal Drugs

- After treatment is initiated for angina pectoris, the patient should be monitored and observed for additional attacks.

Side Effects of Antianginal Drugs

The antianginal drugs may cause flushing, dizziness, headache, generalized or orthostatic hypotension, and a reflex increase in heart rate.

Nursing Implications for Antianginal Drugs

- In addition to the proper use of antianginal agents, patients will often find additional relief by losing weight until the desired weight for their height is achieved, ceasing smoking, and becoming involved in a therapeutic exercise program if one is available and if the physician feels it is appropriate.
- If possible, the patient should identify and learn to avoid angina-producing situations or learn how to regulate the medications to prevent pain.
- It may be helpful for patients with high serum levels of cholesterol or triglycerides to modify their diets; consultation with a dietitian will be helpful.
- Encourage the patient to report to the physician any pain that differs from the patient's characteristic anginal attack. Differences might occur in duration, location, intensity, response to medication, or precipitating event.
- Assessment of complaints of chest pain would include evaluation of blood pressure and pulse; auscultation of lungs and heart; intensity, duration, location, and quality of pain; response to medication; presence of diaphoresis; electrocardiogram changes; precipitating factors; patient's objective degree of distress; patient history; and subjective patient complaints.
- Alcohol should be avoided because it potentiates the hypotensive effects of the antianginal agents.
- Hypotension may be potentiated in patients receiving antianginal medications who are also receiving other drugs

Table 12-2   Administration of antianginal drugs

Generic Name	Trade Name	Dosage and Administration
Amyl nitrite	Amyl Nitrite Vaporole	INHALATION: 0.18 to 0.3 ml Onset: immediate. Duration: 5 min.
Erythrityl tentranitrate	Cardilate*	SUBLINGUAL: 5 mg 3 times daily. ORAL, CHEWABLE: 10 mg 3 times daily. If required, the dose may be increased every 2 to 3 days up to 30 mg 3 times daily. Onset: 5 min for sublingual or chewable; 30 min for oral. Duration: 4 hr.
Isosorbide dinitrate	Angidil Iso-Bid Isordil* Isotrate Sorbide Sorbitrate	SUBLINGUAL: 2.5 to 5 mg every 4 to 6 hours CHEWABLE: 5 to 10 mg every 2 to 3 hours Onset: 2 to 5 min. Duration: 1 to 2 hr. ORAL: 5 to 30 mg 4 times daily. Timed-release forms, 40 mg 2 to 4 times daily. Onset: 15 to 30 min. Duration: 4 to 6 hr.
Nitroglycerin	Nitroglycerin Nitrostat*	SUBLINGUAL: tablets of 0.15 to 0.3 mg initially, up to 0.6 mg as required in individual patients. Individual dosages may be repeated at 5 min intervals, up to 3 tablets in 15 min. Peak action: 3 min. Duration: 10 min.
	Many trade names	ORAL, SUSTAINED-RELEASE: 2.5 to 6.5 mg every 8 to 12 hrs. Onset: slow variable. Duration: 8 to 12 hours.

Drugs to Improve Circulation   167

	Susadrin	BUCCAL: 1 mg 3 times daily. May increase to 2 mg. Kept in mouth for several hours. May increase to 4 times daily or add extra for acute prophylaxis, but no more than every 2 hours.
	Nitrodisc Nitro-Dur Transderm-Nitro	TRANSDERMAL: apply patch to a site free of hair. Do not apply to hands or feet. Change daily to a new site.
Nitroglycerin ointment, 2%	Nitro-Bid* Nitrol*	TOPICAL: initially 1 inch to 2 inches every 8 hours is spread over an area of skin. This is increased by ½-inch increments as required. Absorption is improved by covering the area with plastic. Onset: 30 to 60 min. Duration: up to 3 hr.
Pentaerythritol tetranitrate	PETN Plus* Peritrate* Many others	ORAL: Initially 10 to 20 mg 4 times daily. If required dosage may be adjusted up to 40 mg 4 times daily. Onset: 30 min. Duration: 4 to 5 hr. SUSTAINED RELEASE: 30 to 80 mg twice a day. Onset: 30 to 60 min. Duration: 12 hr.

*Available in U.S. and Canada

168   Pocket Nurse Guide to Drugs

that can cause hypotension, such as diuretics, antihypertensives, central nervous system depressants, narcotics, and sedatives. Instruct the patient to keep all health care practitioners informed of all medications being taken.

- Antianginal drugs used on a regular basis, that is, *not* on a prn basis, should be discontinued slowly to decrease the possibility of a withdrawal reaction in the form of more anginal attacks.
- The presence of a severe headache in response to antianginal drugs may indicate too high a dosage; notify the physician.

Sublingual (Rapidly Acting) Antianginal Agents

- The standard guideline for the use of sublingual antianginal agents is to have the patient use 1 tablet. If relief is not obtained, the dose may be repeated at 5-minute intervals until a total of 3 tablets has been taken. If the pain persists, the patient should call the physician or seek medical care. Ascertain that the patient clearly understands how to use the medication.
- Instruct the patient not to remove sublingual nitroglycerin tablets from the original glass container and to obtain refills before the medication loses its potency.
- There are very few medications taken via the sublingual route. Make certain that the patient knows to let the tablet completely dissolve under the tongue before swallowing; otherwise it will not be effective.
- The patient who experiences syncope (fainting) or hypotension characterized by dizziness, light-headedness, or weakness, should be instructed to lie down before taking one of these agents.
- Because nitroglycerin decomposes rapidly, it is usually dispensed in small quantities (e.g., 25 tablets) and in light-resistant containers. Instruct the patient to obtain a new supply when the pills have lost their potency. Fresh (nondecomposed) nitroglycerin will cause a tingling sensation when used; old tablets will not. A bottle opened and carried on the body should probably be replaced in 6 weeks. An unopened bottle should be stored in the refrigerator.

Drugs to Improve Circulation   **169**

- The patient's family should know the need for and how to place a tablet under the patient's tongue if the patient is unable to do so.
- When the patient with angina pectoris is in the hospital, it is often customary to keep a small supply (e.g., 10 tablets) of sublingual tablets at the bedside for the patient to use as necessary. The patient should be instructed to notify the staff as each tablet is used. In addition, the bedside supply should be counted and restocked every 8 hours. The frequency of tablet use, in addition to a brief patient assessment, should be recorded in the patient's record.

Oral Antianginal Agents

- Taking oral antianginal preparations with meals may reduce gastric irritation.
- Note that there are several dosage forms for the oral agents. The physician's orders should be checked carefully to avoid error. The patient should be instructed clearly on how to take the prescribed medication. Make certain the patient knows the difference between the sublingual and oral preparations if both have been prescribed.

Amyl Nitrite

- Amyl nitrite is packaged in glass ampules wrapped in a protective covering. Instruct the patient to wrap the ampule in a cloth or handkerchief (to protect the fingers) and to crush the ampule to use. The medication is very strong smelling, but the patient should take a few deep inhalations.
- Family members should be instructed how to break and use the ampules if the patient is unable to do so.

Antianginal Ointment

- These ointments are usually ordered in inches. Small sheets of paper with one-half inch markings supplied by the manufacturer are provided for measuring the correct dose.
- Sites of application should be rotated. The rate of absorption does vary slightly depending on the site used, but there is no reason to limit application to one spot. The drug is usually applied to the chest or upper extremities. Markedly

170   Pocket Nurse Guide to Drugs

hairy areas, scars, and the lower extremities should be avoided as absorption is diminished. On the other hand, hairy areas should not be shaved because it may increase the chance of skin irritation.

- Although the ointment should cover a large surface area (several inches by several inches) the goal of application is not to rub in or to massage the ointment. Spreading the correct dose onto the plastic wrap before applying it to the skin will help prevent this.
- The ointments do discolor clothing; choice of site should take this into account.
- To protect the clothing and bed linens, plastic wrap is usually placed over the ointment and taped or wrapped in place.
- To avoid absorption through the fingertips, the practitioner should apply the ointment with the measuring guide or the plastic wrap.
- Skin irritation or contact dermatitis should be reported to the physician. If it is severe enough, it may be necessary to discontinue the medication.
- This is an unusual route of administration; make certain that the patient can perform it correctly before discharge.

Unit Dose Adhesive Bandages

- There are several unit dose adhesive bandages available for use. These units are all made differently, each with different advantages and disadvantages. Patients should be instructed not to interchange products without notifying the physician.
- Ciba's *Transdermal Therapeutic System* (TTS) is a flat unit designed to provide controlled release of nitroglycerin through a semipermeable membrane over a 24-hour period. It comes as a self-adhesive patch, which should be applied over a non-hairy site. There is an illustrated patient instruction sheet which should be reviewed with the patient. The membrane should not be torn, as it may result in uncontrolled drug release. This system may be worn during swimming and other water activities.
- Key's *Transdermal Infusion System* (TIS) has nitroglycerin in a gel-like matrix. The disc has a ring of adhesive around the edge to secure the patch to the skin. There is an

Drugs to Improve Circulation **171**

illustrated patient instruction sheet which should be reviewed with the patient.

- Searle's form is the *Microseal Drug Delivery system* (MDD), consisting of a solid polymer containing the drug bonded to an adhesive bandage. There is an illustrated patient instruction sheet which should be reviewed with the patient.
- If the patch loosens or comes off, it should be replaced. Application sites should be rotated to avoid irritation. Side effects are the same as with other nitrate preparations.
- Beware of mistakes confusing *Transderm-Nitro* (a long-acting nitroglycerin patch) with *Transderm-V* (a long-acting scopalamine preparation for treating motion sickness). Transderm-V has been reported to have been confused with the 5 mg dosage patch of Transderm-Nitro.
- This is an unusual route of administration. Make certain that the patient can perform the prescribed dosage administration correctly before discharge.

Vasodilators for Peripheral Vascular Disease

Cyclandelate
Dihydrogenated ergot alkaloids
Isoxsuprine
Nicotinyl alcohol
Nylidrin hydrochloride
Papaverine hydrochloride
Pentoxifylline
Tolaxoline hydrochloride

Actions of Vasodilators for Peripheral Vascular Disease

Cyclandelate relaxes vascular smooth muscle. *Dihydrogenated ergot alkaloids* block alpha adrenergic receptors in the periphery and brain to reduce vascular tone and slow the heart rate. *Nylidrin* stimulates blood flow in muscle and is believed to directly relax smooth muscle. *Papaverine* relaxes smooth muscle. *Pentoxifylline* improves blood flow by decreasing blood viscosity and improving red blood cell flexibility. *Tolazoline* is an alpha adrenergic antagonist with an additional direct vasodilating effect.

Indications for Vasodilators for Peripheral Vascular Disease

Cyclandelate is used in vasospastic disorders. *Dihydrogenated ergot alkaloids* are used to treat symptoms of hypertensive brain disease by lowering blood pressure. *Isoxsuprine* has no proven clinical use for peripheral vascular disease. *Nicotinyl alcohol* has not been proven effective for vasospastic disorders. *Nylidrin* may be used in treating vasospastic disorders. *Papaverine* is used to relieve smooth muscle spasm in vascular disease or colic. *Pentoxifylline* improves blood flow in intermittent claudication secondary to occlusive arterial disease of the limbs. *Tolazoline* is used to relieve vasospastic disorders.

Nurse Alert for Vasodilators for Peripheral Vascular Disease

- Vasodilators are of little value if peripheral vessel narrowing results from arteriosclerosis, and vasodilators may even worsen this condition.
- Vasodilators should be used cautiously in patients with glaucoma.
- Caution patients to avoid the use of alcohol, which potentiates the hypotensive effects of vasodilators.

Parenteral Administration of Vasodilators for Peripheral Vascular Disease

Papaverine

- Papaverine may be given intramuscularly or intravenously.
- For intravenous administration, it may be given undiluted or mixed with equal parts of sterile water for injection. Do not add to intravenous solutions. It is compatible with lactated Ringer's solution and protein hydrolysate. Before mixing with other medications, consult with the pharmacy.

Drugs to Improve Circulation 173

Table 12-3 Administration of vasodilators for peripheral vascular disease

Generic Name	Trade Name	Dosage and Administration
Cyclandelate	Cyclospasmol* Cyclanfor Cydel	ORAL: 300 to 400 mg 4 times daily. Can be decreased gradually to 100 to 200 mg 4 times daily.
Dihydrogenated ergot alkaloids	Hydergine*	SUBLINGUAL, ORAL: 1 mg 3 times daily.
Isoxsuprine	Vasodilan* Isolait Vasoprine	ORAL: 10 to 20 mg 3 to 4 times daily. INTRAMUSCULAR: 5 to 10 mg 2 to 3 times daily.
Nicotinyl alcohol	Roniacol*	TIMED-RELEASE: 300 to 400 mg every 12 hr. TABLET: 50-100 mg 3 times daily.
Nylidrin hydrochloride	Arlidin* Circlidrin Rolidrin	ORAL: 3 to 12 mg 3 to 4 times daily.
Papaverine hydrochloride	Many trade names	ORAL: 100 to 300 mg, 3 to 5 times daily. TIMED-RELEASE: 150 mg every 12 hr. Can give up to 150 mg every 8 hr or 300 mg every 12 hr. INTRAVENOUS: 30 to 120 mg, over 1 to 2 min. INTRAMUSCULAR: 30 to 120 mg.
Pentoxifylline	Trental	ORAL: 400 mg, 3 times daily with meals.
Tolazoline hydrochloride	Priscoline* Tolzol	TIMED-RELEASE: 80 mg every 12 hr. INTRAMUSCULAR, SUBCUTANEOUS, INTRAVENOUS: 10 to 50 mg 4 times daily.

*Available in U.S. and Canada

174   Pocket Nurse Guide to Drugs

- Administer slowly intravenously—1 ml (30 mg) over a period of 2 minutes.
- If possible, monitor the electrocardiogram during administration because the drug can produce ectopic ventricular rhythms (usually transient).
- Monitor the pulse, respirations, and blood pressure during administration and for an hour afterwards.

Tolazoline Hydrochloride

- Tolazoline hydrochloride may be given intravenously, intramuscularly, subcutaneously, and, in rare instances, intraarterially (by a physician).
- In the event of overdose or severe hypotension, place the patient in the Trendelenburg position, administer fluids, and administer a vasopressor such as ephedrine; avoid epinephrine or norepinephrine.
- Marked hypertension has been reported in rare instances. Monitor the blood pressure for at least an hour after parenteral administration.

Side Effects of Vasodilators for Peripheral Vascular Disease

Cyclandelate may cause belching and heartburn, headache, weakness, and increased heart rate. *Dihydrogenated ergot alkaloids* may cause sublingual irritation, nausea, gastrointestinal upset, and reduced heart rate. *Isoxsuprine* may cause flushing, dizziness, hypotension, increased heart rate, and rashes. *Nicotinyl alcohol* may cause pronounced flushing, orthostatic hypotension, gastrointestinal upset, and rashes. *Nylidrin* may cause trembling, nervousness, weakness, dizziness, palpitations, and nausea and vomiting. *Papaverine* may cause flushing, malaise, gastrointestinal upset, headache, perspiration, appetite loss, increased heart rate, increased depth of respiration, and rarely a hypersensitivity reaction with liver symptoms. *Pentoxifylline* may cause gastrointestinal upset, dizziness, headache and tremor. *Tolazoline* commonly causes headache, nausea, chills, flushing, skin tingling, and gastrointestinal upset, and occasionally arrhythmias or a pounding heart.

Nursing Implications for Vasodilators for Peripheral Vascular Disease

- Because vasodilators can cause hypotension, patients should be monitored carefully when first beginning a vasodilator or when dosages are changed. Symptoms of hypotension include vertigo, dizziness, light-headedness, syncope, increased heart rate, and decreased blood pressure. If postural hypotension occurs, instruct patients to move slowly from lying to sitting to standing. If a dose of medication is missed, patients should not "double up" on the next dose to catch up.
- Hypotension may be potentiated in patients receiving vasodilators who are also receiving other drugs that can cause hypotension, such as diuretics, antihypertensives, central nervous system depressants, narcotics, and sedatives. Instruct the patient to keep all health care practitioners informed of all medications being taken.
- The sublingual route of administration may be unfamiliar to patients taking dihydrogenated ergot alkaloids. Teach patients to let the tablet dissolve completely before swallowing.
- Taking oral preparations with meals will reduce gastric irritation.
- The safety of the vasodilators during pregnancy and lactation has not been established. Women of childbearing age may wish to use birth control measures during vasodilator therapy, or at least discuss with their physicians the benefits versus risks of taking these preparations.
- Isoxsuprine has been used to relax the uterus in cases of premature labor. Because of the undesirable side effects (maternal hypotension, maternal and fetal tachycardia) patients should be monitored carefully with frequent determinations of blood pressure and pulse and supervised ambulation. Fetal heart tones should be measured frequently.
- Most of the vasodilators can cause flushing; forewarn patients that this is an expected effect of therapy.

Antihypertensive Drugs

13

Beta-adrenergic receptor antagonists
  Acebutolol
  Atenolol
  Metoprolol
  Nadolol
  Pindolol
  Propranolol
  Timolol maleate
Alpha-adrenergic receptor antagonists
  Phentolamine hydrochloride or mesylate
  Phenoxybenzamine hydrochloride
  Prazosin hydrochloride
Alpha- and beta-adrenergic receptor antagonist
  Labetalol hydrochloride
Drugs interfering with norepinephrine storage or release
  Reserpine
  Rauwolfia
  Alseroxylon
  Deserpine
  Rescinnamine
  Guanadrel
  Guanethidine sulfate

Diuretics (see Ch. 14)
Centrally acting sympathetic nervous system inhibitory drugs
  Clonidine hydrochloride
  Guanabenz acetate
  Methyldopa
Vasodilators
  Hydralazine hydrochloride
  Minoxidil
Vasodilators—Calcium channel blockers
  Diltiazem
  Nifedipine
  Verapamil
Vasodilator—angiotensin converting enzyme inhibitor
  Captopril
  Enalapril
Drugs for hypertensive emergencies
  Diazoxide
  Sodium nitroprusside
  Trimethaphan camsylate

Actions of Antihypertensive Drugs

Table 13-1 summarizes and compares the antihypertensive actions of the categories of antihypertensive drugs.

176

Table 13-1 Categories of antihypertensive drugs

Category	Type	Drugs	Antihypertensive Action
Diuretics	Thiazide-type Loop Potassium-sparing	See Ch. 14	Reduce body salt and water which decreases arterial blood pressure. May reduce plasma volume. Counteract the fluid retention caused by certain antihypertensive drugs: methyldopa, reserpine, guanethidine, guandrel, prazosin, hydralyzine, minoxidil, and diazoxide. Enhance the action of most antihypertensive drugs given chronically.
Sympathetic Depressant Drugs	Beta-Adrenergic Receptor Antagonist	Acebutolol Atenolol Metoprolol Nadolol Pindolol Propranolol Timolol	Reduce cardiac output. Reduce renin release from the kidney. May have a central antihypertensive action. Preferred for individuals with high renin levels, typically young Caucasians. Shown to decrease the incidence of sudden death in patients with a recent heart attack. The cardioselective (beta-1 adrenergic receptors) drugs are acebutolol, atenolol, and metoprolol.
	Alpha-Adrenergic Receptor Antagonist	Prazosin Phenoxybenzamine Phentolamine	Block the vasoconstrictive action of norepinephrine, thereby decreasing peripheral resistance.

cont'd. next page

Table 13-1 Categories of antihypertensive drugs—cont'd.

Category	Type	Drugs	Antihypertensive Action
Sympathetic Depressant Drugs—cont'd.	Alpha- and Beta-Adrenergic Receptor Antagonist	Labetalol	Both alpha and beta receptor antagonistic actions (above) apply. Alpha receptor antagonist actions predominate. New drug class.
	Centrally Acting Drugs	Clonidine Methyldopa Guanabenz	Inhibit sympathetic outflow from the brain by stimulating alpha receptors in the vasomotor center of the medulla. The result is a decrease in peripheral resistance.
	Centrally & Peripherally Acting Drug	Reserpine	Depletes norepinephrine stores peripherally and centrally resulting in a decrease in peripheral resistance.
	Ganglionic Blocking Drugs	Trimethaphan Mecamylamine	Block the nicotinic receptors of the autonomic ganglia to inhibit both sympathetic and parasympathetic function. Peripheral resistance is decreased.
	Drugs Blocking Norepinephrine Release	Guanethidine Guanadrel	Loss of peripheral sympathetic tone decreases peripheral resistance by reducing both cardiac output and peripheral resistance. Used for severe hypertension.

Vasodilators	Drug Blocking Norepinephrine Synthesis	Metyrosine	Decreases peripheral resistance, particularly when there is a norepinephrine-producing tumor (pheochromocytoma). Rarely used.
	Monamine Oxidase Inhibitor	Pargyline	Decreases peripheral resistance. Rarely used because of serious drug and food interactions.
	Arterial Vasodilator	Hydralazine, Minoxidil, Diazoxide	Relax arterial smooth muscle to lower peripheral resistance. Used alone, cause rebound tachycardia (increased heart rate) and edema.
	Arterial and Venous Vasodilator	Nitroprusside	Generalized vasodilation. Useful in hypertensive emergencies.
	Calcium Channel Blockers	Diltiazem, Nifedipine, Verapamil	Reduce the tone of blood vessels by reducing intracellular calcium, thereby causing arteriolar dilation and decreased total peripheral resistance. New drug class.
Angiotensin Antagonists	Inhibitors of Angiotensin II Formation	Captopril, Enalapril	Reduces peripheral resistance in individuals with high plasma renin levels. New drug class.
	Angiotensin II Antagonist	Saralasin	Reduces peripheral resistance by blocking angiotensin II, a potent vasoconstrictive agent, from its receptors. Useful in diagnosing hypertensive patients with high renin levels. New drug class.

Indications for Antihypertensive Drugs

Current antihypertensive drug therapy is based on *stepped-care* approach in which drugs are added by class until blood pressure is brought under control. *Step one* is usually an oral diuretic (see Ch. 14) or a beta-adrenergic receptor antagonist (particularly with individuals with high plasma renin levels or coronary artery disease). *Step two* adds a sympathetic depressant drug: a beta-adrenergic receptor antagonist, methyldopa, clonidine, prazosin, reserpine, guanabenz, or guanadrel. *Step three* adds a vasodilator, most commonly hydralazine, minoxidil, or prazosin. *Step four* drugs, usually only for severe hypertension, include substituting guanethedine for the step two depressant or substituting captopril for the beta adrenergic antagonist. The role of calcium channel blockers is not fully clear but they may be used in selected cases to depress cardiac activity (diltiazem and verapamil) or to decrease vascular tone (diltiazem and nifedipine). The alpha-adrenergic receptor antagonists are used to treat hypertension caused by pheochromocytoma or selected other conditions. In *hypertensive emergencies* in which end-organs are threatened, particularly the brain, eyes, or heart, diazoxide, sodium nitroprusside, or trimethaphan camsylate may be used to rapidly lower blood pressure.

Nurse Alert for Antihypertensive Drugs

- The use of antihypertensives during pregnancy or lactation is warranted only if the benefits outweigh the risks; the patient should consult her physician.
- Dosages of beta-adrenergic blockers and other antihypertensives must be individualized for each patient.
- Beta-adrenergic blockers should be reduced gradually rather than discontinued suddenly, or angina, myocardial infarction, or ventricular dysrhythmias may be precipitated.
- Beta-adrenergic blockers must be used cautiously in patients with poor cardiac function, asthma, peripheral vascular disease, and diabetes.
- The beta-adrenergic blockers are contraindicated in patients with borderline cardiac reserve, bradycardia, bronchospas-

Text continued on p. 187

Antihypertensive Drugs **181**

Table 13-2 Administration of antihypertensive drugs

Generic Name	Trade Name	Dosage and Administration
Diuretics (Chap. 14)		
Beta-Adrenergic Receptor Antagonists		
Acebutolol	Sectral	ORAL: 400 mg once a day initially. Range for maintenance dose: 200-1200 mg daily. Do not exceed 800 mg daily in elderly patients. Reduce dose 50-75% for patients with renal failure.
Atenolol	Tenormin*	ORAL: 50 mg daily, increase to 100 mg if needed. Reduce dose to 50 mg on alternative days for renal failure.
Metoprolol	Betaloc* Lopresor† Lopressor	ORAL: 50 mg 2 times daily. Dosage may be increased to 200 mg daily to control hypertension, maximum 450 mg.
Nadolol	Corgard*	ORAL: *Adults*—40 mg once daily to start. Dosages are increased by 40 to 80 mg every 3 to 7 days until optimal blood pressure control is achieved. The dose range for maintenance is 80 to 320 mg daily.
Pindolol	Visken*	ORAL: 10 mg twice daily or 5 mg 3 times daily. Dose may be increased in increments of 10 mg/day every 2-3 weeks to achieve a satisfactory response. Maximum dose, 60 mg daily.

cont'd. next page

*Available in U.S. and Canada
†Available in Canada only

Table 13-2   Administration of antihypertensive drugs—cont'd.

Generic Name	Trade Name	Dosage and Administration
Propranolol hydrochloride	Inderal*	For hypertension: ORAL: 20 mg 3 times daily with a diuretic. Dosage may be increased to 640 mg daily to control hypertension. For angina: ORAL: 10 mg 3 or 4 times daily, initially; increase to control symptoms. Usual range is 160 to 240 mg daily. For pheochromocytoma: ORAL: 20 mg three times daily with an alpha-adrenergic blocking drug to control symptoms from pheochromocytoma. Dosage is increased to 60 mg daily for 3 days prior to surgery to remove pheochromocytoma. For arrhythmias: ORAL: 10 to 80 mg 3 to 4 times daily. INTRAVENOUS: 0.5 to 3 mg every 1 to 2 min.
Timolol maleate	Blocadren*	ORAL: 10 mg daily initially. Maintenance is 20-40 mg daily. Maximum, 60 mg daily in 2 doses.

Alpha-Adrenergic Receptor Antagonists

Phentolamine hydrochloride; phentolamine mesylate	Regitine Hydrochloride;	ORAL: *Adults*—50 mg every 4 to 6 hr. *Children*—25 mg every 4 to 6 hr.

	Regitine Mesylate	INTRAMUSCULAR, INTRAVENOUS: *Adults*—5 mg. *Children*—1 mg.
Phenoxybenzamine hydrochloride	Dibenzyline	ORAL: 10 mg daily. May be increased by 10 mg/day to a maximum dose of 60 mg daily.
Prazosin hydrochloride	Minipress*	ORAL: initial dosage 2 to 3 mg in divided doses. Dosage may be increased gradually to 20 to 30 mg/day.

Alpha- and Beta-Adrenergic Receptor Antagonist

Labetalol hydrochloride	Trandate Vescal	ORAL: 100 mg twice daily, initially. Maintenance doses are 200- 800 mg daily for mild to moderate hypertension; 600-1200 mg daily for moderately severe hypertension; 1200-1400 mg daily for severe hypertension.

Drugs Interfering with the Storage and/or Release of Norepinephrine

Reserpine	Lemiserp Rau-Sed Reserpoid Sandril Serpasil*	ORAL: *Adults*—initial dosage 0.25 to 0.5 mg daily; maintenance dosage 0.1 to 0.25 mg daily. *Children*—0.25 to 0.5 mg daily.
Rauwolfia	Raudixin*	ORAL: initial dosage 50 to 400 mg daily in 1 or 2 doses; maintenance dosage 50 to 300 mg daily in 1 or 2 doses.

cont'd. next page

*Available in U.S. and Canada
†Available in Canada only

Table 13-2   Administration of antihypertensive drugs—cont'd.

Generic Name	Trade Name	Dosage and Administration
Alseroxylon	Rauwiloid	ORAL: initial dosage 2 to 4 mg daily; maintenance dosage 2 mg daily.
Deserpidine	Harmonyl	ORAL: initial dosage 0.75 to 1 mg daily; maintenance dosage 0.25 mg daily.
Rescinnamine	Moderil	ORAL: initial dosage 0.5 mg 2 times daily; maintenance dosage 0.25 to 2 mg daily.
Guanadrel	Hylorel	ORAL: 10 mg daily initially, increased daily or less often until desired response is obtained. Maintenance dose is usually 25-75 mg daily. May divide the daily dosage.
Guanethidine sulfate	Ismelin*	ORAL: *Adults*—initial dosage 10 mg daily. Dosage may be increased every 7 days by increments of 10 mg to a maximum daily dosage of 100 mg. Further increments of 25 mg to the daily dosage may then be made every week to a maximum of 300 mg daily. *Children*—initial dosage 0.2 mg/kg of body weight daily. Increments of 0.2 mg/kg may then be made of the daily dosage every 7 to 10 days.

Centrally Acting Antihypertensive Drugs that Inhibit the Activity of the Sympathetic Nervous System

Clonidine hydrochloride	Catapres*	ORAL: 0.1 mg to 2 or 3 times daily. Dosage may be increased daily in increments of 0.1 to 0.2 mg. Maintenance doses are commonly 0.2 to 0.8 mg daily and are seldom larger than 2.4 mg daily. Withdrawal symptoms will occur when doses are larger than 1.2 mg daily unless doses are reduced gradually.
Guanabenz acetate	Wytensin	ORAL: 4 mg twice daily. May increase gradually to 32 mg twice daily or 64 mg once a day.
Methyldopa	Aldomet*	ORAL: *Adults*—initial dose 250 mg in the morning. After 1 week, the dose may be doubled, giving the second 250 mg at bedtime. Dosage may then be increased to a maximum of 2 Gm daily. *Children*—initial dosage 10 mg/kg body weight divided into 2 to 4 doses. Dosage may be increased gradually after 2 days in increments to a maximum dosage of 65 mg/kg daily.

Vasodilators

Hydralazine hydrochloride	Apresoline*	ORAL: *Adults*—initial dosage 10 to 25 mg 2 or 3 times daily. Dosage may be increased by 10 to 25 mg daily. Maximum dosage, 400 mg in 4 divided doses. *Children*—initial dosage 0.75 mg/kg in 4 divided doses. Dosage may be increased over 3 to 4 weeks to a maximum dosage of 7.5 mg/kg daily.

cont'd. next page

*Available in U.S. and Canada
†Available in Canada only

Table 13-2   Administration of antihypertensive drugs—cont'd.

Generic Name	Trade Name	Dosage and Administration
Minoxidil	Loniten*	ORAL: *Adults*—initial dosage 2.5 mg twice daily, increased to 5 mg twice daily after 1 week if needed. Up to 40 mg daily may be given. *Children*—initial dosage 0.1 to 0.2 mg/kg body weight daily in 2 doses. Increase gradually to 1.4 mg/kg of body weight daily if required.

Vasodilators—Calcium Channel Blocker

Nifedipine	Procardia Adalat†	ORAL: *Adults*—10 mg three times daily. May increase to 20 mg three times daily.
Diltiazem	Cardiazem*	ORAL: *Adults*—180-270 mg. daily.
Verapamil	Calan Isoptin	ORAL: *Adults*—240 to 480 mg daily in 3 or 4 doses. Primarily used to treat angina, arrhythmias.

Vasodilators—Angiotensin Converting Enzyme Inhibitor

Captopril	Capoten	ORAL: *Adults*—25 mg three times daily. May increase up to 50 mg three times daily in 1-2 weeks.
Enalapril	Vasotec	ORAL: *Adults*—10 to 20 mg. daily, up to 80 mg. daily.

*Available in U.S. and Canada
†Available in Canada only

Antihypertensive Drugs **187**

Table 13-3 Drugs for hypertensive emergencies

Generic Name	Trade Name	Dosage and Administration
Diazoxide	Hyperstat*	INTRAVENOUS: *Adults*—150 mg or 1 to 5 mg/kg body weight. *Children*—5 mg/kg body weight. The drug is injected within 30 sec. The injection may be repeated after 30 min.
Sodium nitroprusside	Nipride*	INTRAVENOUS: dissolve 50 mg in 500 to 1000 ml of 5% dextrose. Infuse 0.5 to 8 μg/kg/min. Solution must be protected from light and discarded after 4 hr.
Trimethaphan camsylate	Arfonad*	INTRAVENOUS: administered as a 0.1% (1 mg/ml) infusion in 5% dextrose. The rate of infusion is begun at 0.5 to 1 mg/min and increased gradually until the blood pressure falls by 20 mm Hg. After several minutes, the rate is again increased until the blood pressure reaches the desired level.

*Available in U.S. and Canada

tic disease, greater than first-degree heart block, and chronic occlusive peripheral vascular disease.

- Reserpine or methyldopa may cause serious depression and should be used cautiously in patients who may become suicidal.
- Guanethidine is contraindicated in patients with angina, cerebral insufficiency, or coronary artery disease.
- Clonidine must not be suddenly discontinued, or sympathetic rebound may occur with restlessness, insomnia, tremors, tachycardia, headache, abdominal pain, nausea, and hypertensive crisis.

188 **Pocket Nurse Guide to Drugs**

- Clonidine may cause depression; monitor patients for changes in mood or affect.
- Hydralazine patients should be monitored for the appearance of anti-DNA antibodies and lupus erythematosus cells.
- Rebound hypertension may occur if guanabenz is discontinued suddenly.
- With patients receiving sodium nitroprusside or trimethaphan for hypertensive emergency, monitor the blood pressure constantly.

Side Effects of Antihypertensives

Beta-adrenergic blockers. Side effects include bronchospasm, prolongation of insulin-induced hypoglycemia, aggravation of peripheral vascular insufficiency, cardiac depression, dizziness, fatigue, insomnia, sedation, rashes, nasal stuffiness, agranulocytosis, reduced exercise tolerance, tingling in fingers or toes, gastrointestinal upset, depression, sexual dysfunction (impotence in men), and more serious effects in patients with abnormal cardiovascular function: pulmonary edema, hypotension, cardiac failure, and AV atrioventricular nodal block.

Alpha-adrenergic blockers. Phentolamine and *phenoxybenzamine* may cause postural hypotension, reflex tachycardia, nasal congestion, and gastrointestinal upset; with intravenous administration, anginal pain and arrhythmias may occur. *Prazosin* may cause faintness, dizziness, palpitation, headache, drowsiness, dry mouth, fluid retention, depression, rashes, difficulty in urination, and arthralgia.

Alpha-and beta-adrenergic antagonist. Labetalol may cause orthostatic hypotension, gastrointestinal upset, fatigue, nervousness, dry mouth, tingling of the scalp, and the side effects of other beta-adrenergic antagonists.

Drugs interfering with norepinephrine storage or release. Reserpine may cause sedation or depression, lethargy, increased appetite, increased dreaming and nightmares, vasodilation, a flushed warm feeling, nasal congestion, salivation, stomach cramps, and diarrhea. *Guanethidine* may cause postural hypotension, bradycardia, diarrhea, sodium retention, and in men, failure of erection or ejaculation.

Centrally acting sympathetic nervous system inhibitory drugs. *Clonidine* commonly causes drowsiness, dry mouth, and constipation. *Guanabenz* commonly causes drowsiness, dry mouth, dizziness, weakness, and headache. *Methyldopa* causes drowsiness, sedation, depression, nightmares, fatigue, bradycardia, diarrhea, dry mouth, and occasional ejaculatory failure in men.

Vasodilators. *Hydralazine* commonly causes headache, palpitation, loss of appetite, nausea, vomiting, diarrhea, tachycardia, angina in susceptible individuals, and with long-term therapy, the appearance of a lupus-like syndrome. *Minoxidil* may cause excessive hairiness, transient nausea, headache, tachycardia, and fatigue.

Calcium channel blockers. *Nifedipine* and *diltiazem* may cause headache, tachycardia, dizziness, fatigue, nausea, edema, flushing, orthostatic hypotension, tinnitus, leg cramps, and skin rash.

Angiotensin converting enzyme inhibitors. *Captopril* and *enalapril* have a small but significant risk of severe side effects: skin rash that may be accompanied by fever, loss of sense of taste, anorexia, nausea and gastrointestinal disturbances, progression of renal disease in affected individuals, proteinuria, neutropenia, and hyperkalemia.

Drugs for hypertensive emergencies. *Diazoxide* may cause retention of sodium and water, and hyperglycemia. *Nitroprusside* used for several days may cause tinnitus, blurred vision, and hypothyroidism. *Trimethaphan* may cause loss of parasympathetic tone and pupillary dilation, loss of accommodation, drying of mucous surfaces, constipation, and urinary retention.

Nursing Implications for Antihypertensive Drugs

General Guidelines for Patients Receiving Antihypertensive Drugs

- Losing weight and adhering to a low sodium diet decreases the need for antihypertensive drugs.
- The poor compliance frequently seen in drug therapy for

Pocket Nurse Guide to Drugs

hypertension results in part from the fact that patients do not feel any better while on antihypertensives and may in fact feel worse.

- Hypotension is a common side effect of antihypertensive therapy, especially when the patient moves rapidly from a supine to a sitting or upright position (postural hypotension). Symptoms include dizziness, light-headedness, weakness, and syncope (fainting). If symptoms occur, instruct the patient to sit or lie down until symptoms pass, then to rise slowly. Postural hypotension is often worse in the mornings, and it may be aggravated by long periods of standing, hot weather, hot showers or baths, ingestion of alcohol, and exercise, especially if the exercise is followed by immobility. Hypotension is also worse when patients are begun on therapy and during periods of dosage adjustment.
- When beginning a patient on antihypertensive therapy, during periods of dosage adjustment, or when other medications are being added to the regimen, the blood pressure should be monitored frequently, at least every 4 hours in the ambulatory hospitalized patient, and whenever a patient complains of the symptoms of hypotension. In some instances the patient or family can be taught to measure the blood pressure at home.
- Supervise the ambulation of hospitalized patients to guard against injury should the patient become dizzy or faint.
- The elderly are more sensitive to the antihypertensives and find hypotension to be more of a problem.
- When antihypertensives are given to patients taking other drugs that also cause hypotension, the incidence of hypotensive episodes may be increased. Such drugs might include other antihypertensives, diuretics, central nervous system depressants, and barbiturates. For the same reason, patients should be instructed not to take over-the-counter medications without clearance from their physicians.
- When used alone, the antihypertensives often contribute to fluid retention and weight gain. Weigh patients daily under standard conditions. Other signs of fluid retention are pitting edema. A daily weight gain of 2 pounds or more should be reported to the physician.

Antihypertensive Drugs **191**

- Adherence to a low sodium diet may reduce the possibility of fluid retention.
- Measure the fluid intake and output of hospitalized patients.
- Help the patient find a creative way to remember to take the medications as ordered.
- If a dose of antihypertensive drug is missed, the patient should be instructed not to "double up" to make up for the missed dose but to resume the prescribed schedule the next time the medication is due.
- There are preparations available containing a combination of an antihypertensive with a diuretic (one example is Aldoril, containing methyldopa and hydrochlorothiazide). Patients taking combination products are potentially at risk for side effects resulting from any of the component drugs and should be taught about them.
- Many of the antihypertensives cause drowsiness or sedation, especially when first being used or when dosages are increased. Warn patients about this side effect, and caution them to avoid or to at least perform carefully any activity that requires mental alertness, such as driving, operating dangerous equipment, or engaging in any potentially dangerous activity. Concomitant use of other drugs that produce central nervous system depression may enhance the drowsiness (examples include alcohol, barbiturates, and sedatives).
- Intravenous administration
  a. Measure the blood pressure frequently (every 3 to 5 minutes) until stable, then every 15 to 30 minutes.
  b. An electronic infusion monitoring device should be used when constant infusion is required.
  c. A microdrip infusion set should be used for constant infusions.
  d. Monitor the pulse.
  e. Depending on the patient's general medical condition, it may be appropriate to attach the patient to a cardiac monitor.
  f. Patients should remain in bed for up to 3 hours after the drug has been administered.

192   Pocket Nurse Guide to Drugs

- Many antihypertensives cause tachycardia or bradycardia. Monitor the pulse when the blood pressure is monitored.
- If possible, antihypertensives should be discontinued before the patient has surgery.
- Careful and sympathetic questioning of patients taking antihypertensive medication, particularly those patients exhibiting poor compliance, may help health care personnel to develop a more individualized plan for reducing the patient's blood pressure.

Beta-Adrenergic Receptor Antagonists

- Prior to administering these drugs, take the apical pulse for a full minute. The usual guideline states that when the apical pulse is less than 60 beats per minute in an adult or 90 to 110 beats per minute in a child, the dose should be withheld, and the physician notified. Be especially sensitive to possible bradycardia if the patient is also receiving a cardiac glycoside.
- These drugs should not be discontinued suddenly. Patients should be instructed to consult with their physicians before changing the dose or discontinuing the drug. Caution patients to check their supply of medications regularly to avoid running out. In patients with a history of angina, sudden withdrawal or cessation of these medications may precipitate recurrence of angina, arrhythmias, even myocardial infarction.
- These drugs may cause a slight increase in serum potassium levels, but when potassium-losing diuretics are being used concomitantly, hypokalemia may still be a problem.
- The maximal effects of these drugs may not be seen for several weeks, and the dosage of the individual drug must be carefully and individually titrated.
- Beta blockers may cause, prolong or mask the symptoms of hypoglycemia, (increased pulse rate and blood pressure changes). This may be less of a problem with the cardioselective drugs. Caution diabetic patients to be aware of this problem.
- These drugs may be taken with or without food. Taking with food may decrease gastrointestinal distress, and

Antihypertensive Drugs 193

absorption may be improved. Patients should be encouraged to be consistent in the way the medications are taken, either with or without food.

- Long term therapy with these drugs may mask developing thyrotoxicosis, and sudden withdrawal of the drugs has precipitated thyroid storm. These drugs should be discontinued slowly, with the dosage reduced gradually over a one-to two-week period.
- Many of these drugs cross the placenta, and also accumulate in breast milk. They should be used in pregnancy only when the benefits clearly outweigh the risks. Women of childbearing age may with to consider the use of some form of birth control while taking these drugs. Consult the physician.
- Plasma levels of the beta blockers do not correlate well with dosage, and are not a useful guide to therapy. Decisions about dosage must be based on clinical evaluation of the patient.
- All of the beta blockers seem to be effective in classic angina, but should generally be avoided in variant angina (see chapter 12).
- Indomethacin may counteract the antihypertensive effects of propranolol. Cimetidine may increase the bioavailability of propranolol and metoprolol, necessitating a reduction in dosage of the beta blocker. Beta blockers may potentiate the effects of neuromuscular blocking agents. Enzyme-inducing agents (e.g., phenobarbital, pentobarbital, and phenytoin) enhance the metabolism of propranolol and metoprolol, and may do the same with pindolol and timolol, although less is known about the latter two.
- Propranolol is used for prophylactic treatment of common migraine headaches. It does not seem to help once the migraine is in progress.
- Propranolol may interfere with the glaucoma screening test, and cessation of the drug may increase intraocular pressure.
- Propranolol is the only beta blocker which is given parenterally. Do not mix it with any other medication. During IV administration, the ECG and central venous pressure should be carefully monitored. The drug should be

administered no faster than 1 mg per minute. The dose of propranolol must be checked carefully. Usual oral doses are in the range of 20 to 40 mg; IV doses are in the range of 0.5 to 3 mg.
- Treatment of overdose with the beta blockers is symptomatic. Bradycardia may be treated with atropine, cardiac failure with digitalization and diuretics, hypotension with vasopressors, and bronchospasm with isoproterenol and aminophylline.
- The beta blockers may reduce HDL cholesterol, and increase serum triglyceride levels.

Phentolamine and Phenoxybenzamine

- In treatment of overdose of phenoxybenzamine, discontinue the drug, and place the patient in a recumbent position. In severe cases, institute measure to counteract shock. Epinephrine is countraindicated; levarterenol should be used.
- Intravenous phentolamine: Monitor the blood pressure, pulse, central venous pressure, and cardiac rhythm every 2 to 5 minutes until the patient stabilizes, then every 15 minutes. The patient should not be left unattended.
- The treatment of shock caused by hypotension is intravenous leverterenol.
- An electronic IV monitor or regulator should be used to accurately control the rate of intravenous infusion.
- Urinary output should be monitored and recorded every 30 to 60 minutes.
- Phentolomine can be mixed with most IV solutions but should probably not be mixed with other drugs. Solutions are stable for 48 hours but should then be discarded. If in doubt, consult the pharmacist.

Prazosin

- Patients beginning therapy, adding a diuretic to the drug regimen, or increasing the dose of prazosin are susceptible to the "first dose" syndrome. Although characterized by hypotension, this syndrome can be severe enough to result in syncope and loss of consciousness. This hypotensive response usually occurs 30 to 90 minutes after taking the dose; it is more common with a first dose of 2 mg than 1 mg, so patients are usually started on the lower dose. Treatment is to lay the patient flat; the condition is self-limiting. In rare cases the episode is preceded by a tachycardia in which rates of heartbeat up to 180 beats per minute are reported.

- Because first dose syndrome effects may occur for a couple of days after initiating or changing the dose of therapy, patients should be cautioned to avoid activities in which a syncopal episode might be dangerous.
- To minimize the possibility of the first dose syndrome, patients may be instructed to take their first dose at bedtime and to remain lying down for at least 3 hours after the dose has been taken.
- Families of patients receiving prazosin should also be instructed about the hypotensive effects, both to allay anxiety should it occur and also to ensure that the patient will receive correct treatment of the problem.

Labetolol

- Labetolol has side effects, and associated patient care implications, similar to the beta blockers (see above).
- The hypotensive effects of this drug are most pronounced when the patient is upright, and during exercise.
- This drug accumulates in the choroid. No adverse effects have been reported, but periodic eye examinations are recommended.
- When administering this drug intravenously, the supine blood pressure should be measured immediately before administration, and 5 to 10 minutes afterwards to evaluate the effectiveness. Administer at a rate of 20 mg over at least two minutes.

Guanethidine and Guanadrel

- Although orthostatic hypotension can affect patients taking any of the antihypertensives, it is a common problem with guanethidine.
- Postural blood pressure determinations (blood pressure taken with the patient in lying, sitting, and standing

196   Pocket Nurse Guide to Drugs

positions) should be obtained with these drugs, since the maintenance dose is partially determined by the standing blood pressure. The standing blood pressure should be measured after the patient has been standing for at least 10 minutes.

- These drugs cause bradycardia. Monitor the pulse, and be especially careful when the patient is also taking a cardiac glycoside.
- Monoamine oxidase (MAO) inhibitors should be stopped for at least a week before initiating therapy with these drugs.
- If diarrhea is severe enough, it may be necessary to treat it. Also be alert to electrolyte imbalances in patients with severe chronic diarrhea.
- These drugs should not be used in patients with pheochromocytoma.

Reserpine and Related Drugs

- Patients may find this group of drugs convenient to take because once-a-day therapy is usually sufficient.
- Reserpine has a delayed onset of action and may require 4 to 6 weeks of therapy before its full effect can be seen. When discontinued, effects may persist for several weeks.
- Taking reserpine with meals may reduce gastric irritation. Reserpine should not be used by patients with a history of ulcer disease or ulcerative colitis.
- Reserpine can cause bradycardia; this may be a problem in patients who also receive digitalis or other drugs causing bradycardia.
- Cardiac arrhythmias have occurred in patients receiving the rauwolfia preparations; use cautiously in patients taking digitalis or quinidine.
- Reserpine is available in a form suitable for intramuscular injection, but this is rarely used.
- Parenteral reserpine, if given to treat eclampsia, crosses the placental barrier, causing drowsiness, nasal congestion, cyanosis, and anorexia in the newborn infant.
- In an overdose serious enough to require vasopressor therapy, phenylephrine, levarterenol, or metaraminol should be used.

Methyldopa

- If sedation is a problem, suggest that the patient add any increases in dosage in the evening rather than the morning.
- Urine may darken when left exposed to the air.
- Although most patients who develop a positive Coombs' test while on methyldopa therapy are exhibiting a false positive result, it cannot be assumed that this is so. Evaluation for possible hemolytic anemia includes blood counts done before initiating therapy and at regular intervals during therapy. Liver function tests should also be performed at regular intervals.
- Intravenous administration
  a. Intramuscular or subcutaneous administration is not recommended because of the erratic absorption that occurs.
  b. Methyldopa is not the drug of choice for intravenous antihypertensive control.
  c. Dilute the medication with enough 5% dextrose in water to make 100 ml.
  d. Administer the ordered dose over 30 to 60 minutes. See general guidelines.
  e. The patient should be switched to oral doses as soon as possible.

Clonidine and Guanabenz Acetate

- The side effects of dry mouth, drowsiness and sedation often diminish with continued therapy. Orthostatic hypotension may occur occasionally.
- Impress on patients that stopping the drug suddenly can be dangerous.
- Patients taking clonidine should have regular eye examinations; in animal studies the drug has produced retinal degeneration.

Hydralazine

- Hydralazine seems to be better tolerated when used in combination with other drugs than when used alone.
- This drug does not cause sedation or other central nervous system effects as commonly as do other antihypertensives.

198 Pocket Nurse Guide to Drugs

- There are parenteral forms available for intravenous and intramuscular use, but these are rarely used. Consult the pharmacy with questions.
- Some brands of hydralazine contain FD&C coloring number 5 (tartrazine), which may cause an allergic response in some individuals. Although rare, this response is more common in individuals with aspirin hypersensitivity.

Minoxidil

- This drug can cause hypertrichosis (excessive hairiness) after several weeks of therapy. Instruct patients to report this side effect. Caution patients not to discontinue the medications without contacting their physician.
- Observe patients for pericardial effusion, a rare side effect. The patient may complain of chest pain or pain in the shoulder or arm. There may be dyspnea, tachycardia, distended jugular veins, and changes in heart sounds.
- Fluid retention can be a serious problem, but may not result in loss of blood pressure control. Observe patients for edema.
- ECG changes are frequently seen. These changes include flattening or inversion of T waves, or increased QRS voltage. They may disappear with time, are usually asymptomatic, and reversible following discontinuation of therapy.

Calcium Channel Blockers

- Side effects of these drugs include hypotension, headache, bradyarrhythmias, nausea, swelling, edema, arrhythmias, constipation, rashes, uticaria, and others. As these drugs are used more, additional side effects may become recognized. Instruct the patient to report any unusual findings.
- When initiating therapy or changing dosages, monitor the blood pressure and pulse.
- If hypotension occurs, instruct the patient to move slowly from sitting or lying to standing. Some patients may find wearing elastic stockings to be helpful.
- These drugs should be used during pregnancy only when the benefits clearly outweigh the risks. Women of childbear-

Antihypertensive Drugs 199

ing age may wish to consider the use of some form of contraception while taking these drugs. These drugs should be used during lactation only after consultation with a physician.

Verapamil

- Bradycardia is common. Monitor the pulse. It may be appropriate to instruct the patient to monitor and record the pulse at regular intervals at home.
- Constipation is a frequent side effect, but this can often be prevented or corrected by having the patient maintain adequate fluid intake (if not restricted by the medical problems), eat foods high in roughage and fiber, maintain a regular exercise program, and judiciously use foods known to stimulate defecation. In some patients, it may be necessary to use stool softeners.
- Severe hypotension, bradycardia, cardiac failure, and arrhythmias have been produced in patients receiving both verapamil and beta blockers.
- Verapamil should be avoided in patients with sick sinus syndrome, second or third degree A-V block, cardiogenic shock, or advanced congestive failure.
- Verapamil may increase serum digoxin levels; digoxin dosage may need to be reduced significantly during concomitant administration with verapamil.
- This drug has been reported to cause an increase in transaminase and alkaline phosphatase levels; hepatitis has also been reported.
- The intravenous form should be given slowly over at least two minutes. When administering this drug intravenously, the patient should be connected to a cardiac monitor, and resuscitation equipment should be readily available.

Nifedipine

- This drug is a more potent vasodilator than verapamil, so hypotension may be more of a problem. Instruct patients to move slowly from sitting or lying to a standing position. In the hospital, monitor the blood pressure carefully.

Pocket Nurse Guide to Drugs

- Reflex tachycardia has been reported; angina may also be exacerbated.
- This drug should be used carefully concomitantly with beta blockers.
- This drug may increase serum digoxin levels, requiring a reduction in the dose of digoxin.
- Glucose intolerance has been reported. Monitor the blood and urine sugar.

Diltiazem

- This drug is similar to verapamil.

Captopril

- This drug should be taken one hour before meals because absorption is reduced when taken with food.
- The initial dose of the drug may cause a severe drop in blood pressure. After receiving the first dose, patients should be observed carefully for several hours.
- Monitor the urine protein, serum potassium, and white blood cell counts at regular intervals during therapy.
- Agranulocytosis has been reported. Instruct patients to report any fever, sore throat, or sign of infection.

Saralasin

- Review the manufacturer's literature for information about dosage, administration, and interpretation of results.

Diazoxide

- Diazoxide can be administered undiluted and fairly rapidly. The usual adult dose (150 mg) should be administered over 30 seconds. It may also be diluted and given as a slow infusion over a period of 20 to 30 minutes, at a rate of 15 to 30 mg/min.
- Severe hypotension is uncommon, but can be treated with a sympathomimetic agent such as norepinephrine.
- As always in hypertensive emergencies, appropriate drugs and equipment should be available for treating possible side effects.

Antihypertensive Drugs **201**

- Hyperglycemia is common. Monitor the blood and urine glucose levels.
- The medication is highly alkaline and should not be given intramuscularly or subcutaneously. Extravasation should be avoided.
- Monitor the vital signs, fluid intake and output, and weight.

Sodium Nitroprusside

- This drug should not be given undiluted. Dissolve 50 mg of drug in 2 to 3 ml of 5% dextrose in water. There are reports that sterile water may be safely used, but it *must not contain a preservative* (if in doubt, consult the pharmacy). The concentrated solution should then be further diluted in 500 or 1000 ml of 5% dextrose in water to make concentrations of 100 or 50 μg/ml. The solution may have a faint brownish tint; if highly colored, the solution should be discarded. The diluted solution should be covered with foil and the infusion tubing covered to protect from light. The solution should be used immediately; discard solution over 24 hours old. Do not mix with any other medications.
- The rate of infusion should be prescribed by the physician and be based on the response of the blood pressure, but the usual rate is 0.5 to 8 μg/kg over a period of 1 minute.
- Monitor the fluid intake and output.
- This drug should only be administered in an acute care setting where appropriate equipment and drugs are available should an emergency arise.
- To treat an overdose, discontinue the infusion of nitroprusside. Administer amyl nitrite for 15 to 30 seconds each minute until a sodium nitrite solution for intravenous administration can be prepared. A 3% sodium nitrite solution should be administered intravenously at a rate of 2.5 to 5 ml per minute up to a total dose of 10 to 15 ml. After this, inject sodium thiosulfate intravenously, 12.5 Gm in 50 ml of 5% dextrose in water over a 10-minute period. Monitor the patient carefully throughout. Signs of overdose can reappear for up to several hours, and sodium nitrite and sodium thiosulfate can be repeated at half the dose listed.

Pocket Nurse Guide to Drugs

- Thiocyanate levels should be determined daily if the drug is used longer than 72 hours. If serum thiocyanate levels do not exceed 10 mg/dl, it is probably safe to continue the drug.

Trimethaphan Camsylate

- This drug *must* be diluted before administration. This is usually done by adding one ampule (500 mg or 10 ml) to 500 ml of 5% dextrose injection to make a concentration of 1 mg/ml. The use of other diluents is not recommended.
- The drug is administered via constant infusion, and the dose is titrated in response to the blood pressure, which should be measured at 2- to 3-minute intervals. The physician should determine the goal of therapy, that is, the acceptable blood pressure.
- This drug should be used in an acute care setting where equipment and drugs are available for treatment of any possible side effects.
- If the blood pressure does not come down as anticipated with the patient in the supine position, the head of the bed can be raised. Do so carefully, however, as cerebral anoxia is to be avoided.
- Note that the drug produces pupillary dilation so this parameter may not be helpful in evaluating the patient.
- Monitor the pulse and respiration frequently.
- In the event of overdose or severe hypotension requiring vasopressors, phenylephrine or mephentermine should be used, with norepinephrine reserved for refractory cases.
- Monitor the fluid intake and output. This drug may cause urinary retention; the insertion of a Foley catheter may assist in evaluating renal function.
- Trimethaphan camsylate should not be mixed with any other drugs.

Diuretics

14

Loop diuretics
  Ethacrynic acid
  Furosemide
  Bumetanide
Thiazides and related diuretics
  Chlorothiazide
  Chlorothiazide sodium
  Hydrochlorothiazide
  Benzthiazide
  Hydroflumethiazide
  Bendroflumethiazide
  Methyclothiazide
  Trichlormethiazide
  Polythiazide
  Cyclothiazide
  Metolazone
  Quinethazone
  Chlorthalidone
  Indapamide

Potassium-sparing diuretics
  Spironolactone
  Triamterene
  Amiloride
Carbonic anhydrase inhibitors
  Acetazolamide
  Methazolamide
Osmotic diuretics
  Mannitol
  Urea
Organomercurials
  Mersalyl with theophylline
  Mercaptomerin sodium

General Actions of Diuretics

Most diuretics increase water excretion by increasing sodium ion excretion. Osmotic diuretics are exceptions.

Nursing Implications

For All Diuretics (for specific classes, see later sections)

- Measure and record fluid input and urine output.
- Weigh patient daily or more often to evaluate diuretic effectiveness.
- Monitor blood pressure regularly.
- Caution patient against use of alcohol.
- Teach patient how to cope with orthostatic hypotension.

204 Pocket Nurse Guide to Drugs

Table 14-1 Summary of diuretic effects on tubular transport

	Excretion Increased					Excretion Blocked		
Loop diuretics	Na^+	H_2O	K^+	Cl^-	—	Uric acid	Li^+	—
Thiazides and related drugs	Na^+	H_2O	K^+	Cl^-	HCO_3^-	Uric acid	Li^+	—
Potassium-sparing diuretics	Na^+	H_2O	—	—	HCO_3^-	—	—	K^+,H^+
Carbonic anhydrase inhibitors	Na^+	H_2O	K^+	—	HCO_3^-	Uric acid	—	—
Osmotic diuretics	(Na^+)*	H_2O	(K^+)*	(Cl^-)*	—	—	—	—
Organomercurials	Na^+	H_2O	—	Cl^-	—	Uric acid	—	—

*Large doses.

NOTE: The effects on ion transport shown are those commonly observed in humans during chronic therapy with normal clinical doses. With prolonged therapy, those ions whose excretion is increased may become depleted from the body, whereas those whose excretion is blocked may accumulate. Lithium ion accumulation is clinically important only for those patients receiving lithium carbonate therapy for mania. Uric acid accumulation is usually important only for those patients predisposed to gout.

Table 14-2 General indications for classes of diuretics

Conditions Responding to Diuretics	Loop Diuretics	Thiazides and Related Compounds	Potassium-sparing Diuretics	Carbonic Anhydrase Inhibitors	Osmotic Diuretics
Essential hypertension	+	+	+		
Edema caused by congestive heart failure, renal disease, cirrhosis of the liver	+	+	+		
Pulmonary edema	+				
Diabetes insipidus		+			
Acute mountain sickness				+	
Open-angle glaucoma				+	
Excessive intraocular pressure				+	+
Brain edema					+

- Measure body circumferences to determine fluid retention; check dependent areas for edema.
- If potassium supplement is used, teach client about proper use.
- Maintain dietary control for patients with hypertension, cardiovascular disease, or renal disease.
- Teach clients about effects of salt and salt substitutes in diet.
- Prepare patients for effects of diuretic therapy, such as increased urination.
- Caution patient to avoid nonprescription medications or to check with physician first.
- Consult with the physician concerning increased ingestion of liquid to combat increased thirst.
- Be alert to signs of potassium depletion, especially if patient is also taking digitalis.

Loop Diuretics

Ethacrynic acid   Furosemide   Bumetanide

Actions of Loop Diuretics

Loop diuretics inhibit the active reabsorption of chloride ion in Henle's loop, causing the excretion of NaCl and water. Potassium ion is also excreted more than normally. Furosemide, in addition, may increase bicarbonate excretion.

Indications for Loop Diuretics

Loop diuretics are for control of edematous states as occur in congestive heart failure, renal disease, cirrhosis of the liver, lymphedema, nephrotic syndrome, and ascites associated with cirrhosis or malignancy. Furosemide is preferred for infants; safe doses of bumetanide or ethacrynic acid for infants have not been established.

Nurse Alert for Loop Diuretics

- Contraindicated for use with lithium or in patients with hypersensitivity or anuria.

Diuretics   **207**

- Ethacrynic acid should not be used in infants.
- Use cautiously in hepatic coma or in patients with severe electrolyte depletion.
- Use cautiously with patients on aminoglycoside antibiotics, digitalis, potassium-depleting steroids, high doses of salicylates and tubocurarine.

Parenteral Administration of Loop Diuretics

Furosemide

- Furosemide is incompatible with acidic solutions but will mix with isotonic saline solution, 5% dextrose in water, and lactated Ringer's solution. If in doubt, consult the pharmacy; flush the tubing before administering intravenously.
- Furosemide may be given intravenously undiluted. The rate should not exceed 20 mg over a period of 2 minutes.
- Do not mix with any other medication in a syringe.
- Use only fresh solutions and discard after 24 hours.
- Store at room temperature. Do not use if the solution has turned yellow.
- Intramuscular injection may produce transient pain at the injection site.

Ethacrynic Acid

- Ethacrynic acid should not be given intramuscularly or subcutaneously.
- The usual dilution is 50 mg of ethacrynic acid in 50 ml of 5% dextrose in water or sodium chloride injection. Hazy or opalescent solutions should not be used.
- A single dose should not exceed 100 mg (100 ml).
- Ethacrynic acid may be administered by direct intravenous injection or by continuous infusion. Do not mix with other medications, do not add to intravenous solutions, and do not mix with blood or its derivatives. If in doubt, consult the pharmacy.
- The rate of administration should not exceed 10 mg (10 ml) per minute.
- Check the infusion site carefully; extravasation causes pain and tissue irritation.
- Discard solutions after 24 hours.

Table 14-3   Administration of loop diuretics

Generic Name	Trade Name	Dosage and Administration	Diuretic Effect		
			Onset	Peak	Duration
Ethacrynic acid	Edecrin*	ORAL: *Adults*—50 to 100 mg initially; thereafter 50 to 200 mg daily. *Children*—25 mg initially, increasing by 25 mg to maintain.	30 min	1 to 2 hr	6 to 8 hr
		INTRAVENOUS: *Adults*—50 mg. Not recommended for children by this route.	5 to 10 min	15 to 20 min	1 to 3 hr
Furosemide	Lasix* Novosemide†	ORAL: *Adults*—20 to 80 mg once or twice daily. *Children*—2 mg/kg initially, increasing by 1 or 2 mg/kg after 6 to 8 hr; maximum dose, 6 mg/kg.	60 min	1 to 2 hr	6 to 8 hr
		INTRAVENOUS: *Adults*—20 to 40 mg once or twice daily. *Children*—1 mg/kg initially, increasing by 1 mg/kg after 2 hr; maximum dose 6 mg/kg.	5 to 10 min	15 to 20 min	1 to 3 hr

Bumetanide	Bumex	ORAL: *Adults*—1 mg each morning; if needed, a second dose may be given 6 to 8 hr later; Usual daily doses are less than 4 mg, except in severe renal failure where doses may reach 15 mg daily.	30 min	1 to 2 hr	6 to 8 hr
		INTRAVENOUS: *Adults*—Initially 0.5 to 1 mg to relieve pulmonary edema; repeat dose in 20 min if necessary.	5 to 10 min	15 to 20 min	1 to 3 hr

*Available in U.S. and Canada
†Available in Canada only

Bumetanide

- Bumetanide may be administered intravenously or intramuscularly.
- Intravenous administration should be over 1 to 2 minutes.
- Bumetanide will mix with 5% dextrose in water, 0.9% sodium chloride, and lactated Ringer's solution. Do not use if the solution contains particulate matter or is discolored.
- Discard solutions after 24 hours.

Side Effects of Loop Diuretics

All

All loop diuretics may cause some or all of the following: acute dehydration, potassium depletion, hyperuricemia, electrolyte depletion with accompanying weakness, dizziness, muscle cramps; mental confusion; vomiting, nausea, diarrhea, gout; hyperglycemia (less commonly with ethacrynic acid); agranulocytosis resulting in chills, fever, sore throat, enlarged lymph nodes; and dermatologic reactions such as photosensitivity, rashes.

Ethacrynic Acid

Ethacrynic acid may cause vascular thromboses, emboli; ototoxicity, resulting in transient or permanent deafness; excessive anticoagulation in patients on warfarin; and gastrointestinal bleeding.

Furosemide

Furosemide may cause dermatitis, blood dyscrasias, urinary bladder spasm, it may also result in impaired glucose tolerance, and may precipitate diabetes mellitus. Allergic interstitial nephritis resulting from use of furosemide may produce reversible renal failure.

Bumetanide

Side effects of bumetanide may include azotemia, impaired glucose tolerance, blood dyscrasias, rashes, gastrointestinal distress, and myalgia in patients with renal failure on large doses.

Additional Nursing Implications for Loop Diuretics

- See general nursing implications, pp. 203, 205.
- Teach patient to report diarrhea, vomiting, and anorexia because these conditions contribute to potassium loss.
- Administer oral preparations with meals to reduce gastric irritation.
- Monitor patient carefully to detect signs of any of possible side effects.

Thiazide and Related Diuretics

Chlorothiazide
Hydrochlorothiazide
Hydroflumethiazide
Methyclothiazide
Polythiazide
Metolazone
Chlorthalidone

Chlorothiazide sodium
Benzthiazide
Bendroflumethiazide
Trichlormethiazide
Cyclothiazide
Quinethazone
Indapamide

Actions of Thiazide Diuretics

Thiazide diuretics block sodium and chloride reabsorption in the distal convoluted tubule, leading to the excretion of NaCl and water. Carbonic anhydrase is inhibited in the proximal convoluted tubule, increasing the excretion of bicarbonate.

Indications for Thiazide Diuretics

Less potent than loop diuretics and more suitable for outpatients, thiazide diuretics are used to control edema associated with heart or kidney disease, corticosteroid or estrogen therapy, and hypertension.

Nurse Alert for Thiazide Diuretics

- Thiazide diuretics are contraindicated for patients on lithium.
- Use cautiously with patients on corticosteroids, digitalis, ACTH, tubocurarine, and diabetic patients on insulin control.

Table 14-4   Administration of thiazide diuretics

Generic Name	Trade Name	Dosage and Administration	Diuretic Effect		
			Onset	Peak	Duration
Chlorothiazide	Diuril* Ro-chlorozide	ORAL: *Adults*—0.5 to 1 Gm once or twice daily. *Children*—22 mg/kg daily in 2 doses. *Infants*—under 6 months of age, maximum dose of 33 mg/kg daily in 2 divided doses.	2 hr	4 hr	6 to 12 hr
Chlorothiazide sodium	Diuril [Sodium]	INTRAVENOUS: *Adults*—500 mg twice daily.	15 min	30 min	6 to 12 hr
Hydrochlorothiazide	Chlorzide Diuchlor-H† Esidrix* HydroDiuril* Novohydrazide† Oretic	ORAL: *Adults*—Initially, 25 to 200 mg daily administered in 1 or 2 doses; maintenance, 25 to 100 mg daily or less frequently. *Children*— 2 mg/kg daily in 2 doses.	2 hr	4 hr	6 to 12 hr
Benzthiazide	Aquatag Exna Proaqua Urazide	ORAL: *Adults*—50 to 200 mg; once daily for low doses, divide doses over 100 mg daily. *Children*—1 to 4 mg/kg daily in 3 doses initially; dose reduced for maintenance.	2 hr	4 to 6 hr	12 to 18 hr

Hydroflumethiazide	Diurcardin* Saluron	ORAL: *Adults*—50 to 200 mg; once daily for low doses; divide doses over 100 mg daily. *Children*—1 mg/kg daily; adjust as needed for maintenance.	1 to 2 hr	3 to 4 hr	18 to 24 hr
Bendroflumethiazide	Naturetin*	ORAL: *Adults*—Initially, 5 mg once daily; maintenance, 2.5 to 15 mg once daily or less frequently. *Children*—Maximum dosage 0.4 mg/kg daily in 2 doses; reduce dose for maintenance.	1 to 2 hr	6 to 12 hr	18 to 24 hr
Methyclothiazide	Aquatensen Duretic† Enduron	ORAL: *Adults*—2.5 to 10 mg once daily. *Children*—0.05 to 0.2 mg/kg daily.	2 hr	6 hr	24 hr
Trichlormethiazide	Diurese Metahydrin Naqua	ORAL: *Adults*—1 to 4 mg once daily. *Children*—0.07 mg/kg daily in single or divided dose.	2 hr	6 hr	24 hr
Polythiazide	Renese*	ORAL: *Adults*—1 to 4 mg once daily; maintenance, 0.5 to 8 mg daily, according to response. *Children*—0.02 to 0.08 mg/kg daily.	2 hr	6 hr	36 hr

cont'd. next page

* U.S. and Canadian trade name.
† Canadian trade name only.

214 **Pocket Nurse Guide to Drugs**

Table 14-4 Administration of thiazide diuretics—cont'd.

Generic Name	Trade Name	Dosage and Administration	Diuretic Effects		
			Onset	Peak	Duration
Cyclothiazide	Anhydron Fluidil	ORAL: *Adults*—1 to 2 mg daily; maintenance, 1 mg 2 to 4 times weekly. *Children*—initially, 0.02 to 0.04 mg/kg daily; reduce dose for maintenance.	6 hr	7 to 12 hr	18 to 24 hr
Non-thiazide Diuretics With Mechanisms Similar to Thiazides					
Metolazone	Diulo Zaroxolyn*	ORAL: *Adults*—5 to 20 mg once daily.	1 hr	2 hr	12 to 24 hr
Quinethazone	Aquamox† Hydromox	ORAL: *Adults*—50 to 100 mg once daily, or 150 to 200 mg on alternate days or 3 times weekly.	2 hr	6 hr	18 to 24 hr
Chlorthalidone	Hygroton* Novothalidone†	ORAL: *Adults*—50 to 100 mg after breakfast daily or less frequently. *Children*—2 mg/kg 3 times weekly.	2 hr or less	2 hr	48 to 72 hr
Indapamide	Lozol	ORAL: *Adults*—2.5 mg/day taken in the morning; may be increased after a few days to 5 mg/day.	1 to 2 hr	2.3 to 3.5 hr	24 to 72 hr

* U.S. and Canadian trade name.
† Canadian trade name only.

Parenteral Administration of Chlorothiazide

- Chlorothiazide is not safe for intramuscular or subcutaneous administration.
- Dilute each vial (0.5 Gm) with at least 18 ml of sterile water. Further dilution may be done with 5% dextrose in water or sodium chloride injection.
- Unused solutions should be discarded after 24 hours.
- Administer slowly (0.5 Gm over a period of 5 minutes).
- This medication is incompatible with many other drugs and with blood or its derivatives. If in doubt, consult with the pharmacy.
- Check the intravenous insertion site carefully; avoid extravasation.

Side Effects of Thiazide Diuretics

Fluid and electrolyte imbalance may cause thirst, weakness, lethargy, restlessness, muscle cramps, fatigue; metabolic alkalosis. Increased uric acid levels may precipitate gout. GI effects may include nausea, vomiting, constipation, jaundice, or pancreatitis. CNS effects include dizziness, headache, paresthesia. Blood dyscrasia, urticaria, allergic reactions or orthostatic hypotension may occur. Endocrine effects include changes in glucose tolerance or calcium metabolism.

Additional Nursing Implications for Thiazide Diuretics

- See general nursing implications, pp. 203, 205.
- Watch for signs and symptoms of hypokalemia, hypochloremic alkalosis, hyponatremia, and hypomagnesemia.
- Monitor urine sugar levels; diabetics may need to increase insulin dosage.
- Use cautiously in pregnancy (research is ongoing).
- Discontinue thiazide administration before testing parathyroid function.
- Thiazides may cause a paradoxical antidiuretic effect in patients with diabetes insipidus.
- Exacerbation of systemic lupus erythematosis has been reported with thiazide use.
- Administer oral preparations with meals to reduce gastric irritation.

- Monitor patient carefully to detect signs of any possible side effects.

Potassium-sparing Diuretics

Spironolactone   Triamterene   Amiloride

Actions of Potassium-sparing Diuretics

Potassium-sparing diuretics inhibit the pump mechanism that exchanges potassium for sodium in the distal convoluted tubule. Spironolactone blocks the action of aldosterone on this pump, leading to the excretion of sodium but not potassium. Triamterene and amiloride produce the same effects via a mechanism not dependent on aldosterone.

Indications for Potassium-sparing Diuretics

These drugs are used when a smaller increase in sodium excretion is required (control of edema in congestive heart failure, cirrhosis of the liver, nephrotic syndrome, hypertension) and for reversing potassium loss caused by various conditions. Spironolactone is more effective in cases of elevated aldosterone. Triamterene and amiloride can be used regardless of aldosterone level. Amiloride is more effective for metabolic alkalosis, and in long-term therapy results in less sodium excretion and less potassium retention than spironolactone or triamterene.

Nurse Alert for Potassium-sparing Diuretics

- May cause dangerous increases in serum potassium levels.
- Patients with impaired renal function or high potassium intake are at greatest risk, including for fatal cardiac arrhythmias.
- Avoid in diabetes because of the risk of hyperkalemia.
- Contraindicated for patients receiving potassium supplements or other potassium-sparing diuretics.
- Contraindicated in pregnancy and lactation.
- Use cautiously and adjust dosages for patients using other antihypertensives or receiving norepinephrine under local or general anesthesia.

Table 14-5 Administration of potassium-sparing diuretics

Generic Name	Trade Name	Dosage and Administration	Diuretic Effect		
			Onset	Peak	Duration
Spironolactone	Aldactone*	ORAL: *Adults*—25 to 200 mg daily in divided doses. *Children*—3.3 mg/kg daily in divided doses.	Effects build over a period of days		
Triamterene	Dyrenium*	ORAL: *Adults*—100 mg twice daily after meals; do not exceed 300 mg daily. *Children*—2 to 4 mg/kg daily in divided doses.	2 to 4 hr	6 hr (maximal effect not seen for several days)	7 to 9 hr
Amiloride	Midamor	ORAL: *Adults*—5 to 10 mg daily.	Similar to triamterene		

* Available in U.S. and Canada

Pocket Nurse Guide to Drugs

Side Effects of Potassium-sparing Diuretics

Spironolactone may cause endocrine abnormalities such as menstrual irregularities, hirsuitism, and voice deepening in females, and gynecomastia and erection difficulties in males. *Triamterene* and *amiloride* may cause reversible azotemia with increased BUN. All may cause gastrointestinal disturbances, rashes, and drug fever.

Additional Nursing Implications for Potassium-sparing Diuretics

- See general nursing implications, pp. 203, 205.
- The potassium-sparing diuretics may cause hyperkalemia or hyponatremia, although the latter may be a result of excessive water ingestion.
- Because of the likelihood of hyponatremia, a normal salt intake (sodium intake) may be permitted.
- Many combination products contain both a potassium-sparing diuretic and a potassium-losing diuretic. The goal of the combination products is to promote diuresis while maintaining normal serum potassium levels. Patients are potentially at risk for side effects resulting from any of the component drugs.
- It is theoretically possible that the potassium-sparing diuretics may alter the serum levels of lithium.

Carbonic Anhydrase Inhibitors

Acetazolamide
Methazolamide

Actions of Carbonic Anhydrase Inhibitors

Carbonic-anhydrase-inhibiting diuretics prevent the secretion of hydrogen ion into the renal tubule and the reabsorption of carbon dioxide from the renal tubule, thus increasing the excretion of bicarbonate along with sodium ion. The bicarbonate excretion is much greater; these drugs are classified as weak diuretics.

Indications for Carbonic Anhydrase Inhibitors

Primarily for the treatment of glaucoma, congestive heart failure, and convulsive disorders.

Nurse Alert for Carbonic Anhydrase Inhibitors

- Not for long-term administration because metabolic acidosis may occur, preventing the diuretic action.
- Because potassium excretion is enhanced, potassium depletion may occur, especially with corticosteroids or ACTH administration; digitalis toxicity is increased by low serum potassium.
- Increased risk of toxicity from quinidine, tricyclic antidepressants, amphetamines, erythromycin, procainamide, and salicylates.

Parenteral Administration of Carbonic Anhydrase Inhibitors

- Dilute each 500 mg of acetazolamide with at least 5 ml of sterile water for injection.
- Administer slowly via intravenous injection (500 mg over a period of 5 minutes). It may be added to intravenous solutions and administered over 4 to 8 hours. Consult with the pharmacy before mixing with other medications. It is incompatible with protein hydrolysate.
- Because of an alkaline pH, intramuscular injection is very painful; the intravenous route is preferred.

Side Effects of Carbonic Anhydrase Inhibitors

Reactions are rare, especially in short-term or intermittent therapy. Carbonic anhydrase inhibitors may cause a variety of blood dyscrasias, fever, and rash. CNS symptoms may include paresthesia, nervousness, sedation, lassitude, depression, headache, and vertigo. They may worsen the condition of patients with chronic obstructive pulmonary disease (COPD) or respiratory acidosis.

Table 14-6 Administration of carbonic anhydrase inhibitors

Generic Name	Trade Name	Dosage and Administration	Diuretic Effect		
			Onset	Peak	Duration
Acetazolamide	Acetazolam† Diamox* Hydrazol	ORAL, INTRAVENOUS: *Adults*—250 to 375 mg once daily; alternate-day therapy may be used.	About 1 hr	2 to 4 hr	6 to 12 hr
Methazolamide	Neptazane	ORAL: *Adults*—50 to 100 mg 2 or 3 times daily.	2 to 4 hr	6 to 8 hr	10 to 18 hr

*Available in U.S. and Canada
†Available in Canada only

Nursing Implications for Carbonic Anhydrase Inhibitors

- Long-term therapy with the carbonic anhydrase inhibitors is usually limited to patients with primary open-angle glaucoma and other chronic glaucomas.
- With chronic therapy, the diuretic effect of the carbonic anhydrase inhibitors subsides, probably because of the metabolic acidosis the drugs create. Signs and symptoms of this acidosis include headache, mental dullness, and increased respiratory rate with characteristic deep respirations; the arterial pH is below 7.35. In the most severe cases, disorientation, coma, and death will occur. Other side effects of these drugs, which may or may not be related to the acidosis, include anorexia, nausea, vomiting, diarrhea, weakness, decreased libido, impotence, and malaise. In infants, failure to thrive may result from acidosis. To reduce the problem with acidosis, intermittent therapy is often used. Because many of these side effects may be mild and develop insidiously, the practitioner needs to question patients carefully about their response to the drugs.
- Rarely, carbonic anhydrase inhibitors can produce drug fever, thrombocytopenia (abnormally low number of platelets), agranulocytosis (depressed production of white blood cells), and aplastic anemia. The patient should be instructed to report any unexplained fever, rash, sore throat, bruising, or bleeding.
- Renal colic (severe flank pain), hematuria (blood in the urine), and oliguria are signs and symptoms of renal calculus formation.
- The use of potassium supplements depends on the patient's response. In many patients, the serum potassium level drops initially but returns to normal within a couple of weeks unless another potassium-losing drug is also being given.
- Elevation of serum uric acid levels has been reported, but exacerbation of gout is rare.
- Hyperglycemia and glycosuria are rare but may require a change in insulin dose for diabetics.

- Because carbonic anhydrase inhibitors alter electrolyte balance, clients receiving lithium should be watched carefully for alterations in serum lithium levels.

Osmotic Diuretics

Mannitol
Urea

Actions of Osmotic Diuretics

Osmotic diuretics become highly concentrated in renal tubular fluid, reducing the reabsorption of water and increasing the production of urine. Sodium excretion increases only with high doses.

Indications for Osmotic Diuretics

Osmotic diuretics are used to prevent permanent damage during acute renal failure, and to increase the osmolality of the plasma so as to reduce osmotic pressure inside the eye and in cerebrospinal fluid.

Nurse Alert for Osmotic Diuretics

- Patients with reduced cardiac reserve are at risk because of possible acute expansion of extracellular fluid volume.
- Urea is contraindicated in patients with liver failure.

Administration of Osmotic Diuretics

Usually administered intravenously.

Administration of Mannitol

- Dilution of mannitol is not necessary. It should not be added to other intravenous solutions or medications or mixed with blood.
- The rate of administration is usually 1 to 2 Gm/kg over 30 to 90 minutes, but up to 3 Gm/kg has been given.

- Mannitol comes in several concentrations, ranging from 5% solutions to 25% solutions. If in doubt about the dosage, consult the physician and pharmacist.
- Before administering, check the bottle or ampule for crystallization, a frequent problem. If crystals are present, warm the container under running water until the crystals dissolve. Let cool to body temperature before administering. An in-line intravenous filter should be used.

Administration of Urea

- Urea must be diluted to make a 30% solution (30% solution equals 30 Gm of urea/100 ml or 300 mg/1 ml). Dilution may be done with 5% or 10% dextrose in water or with 10% invert sugar in water; some manufacturers supply the diluent. Patients with hereditary fructose intolerance (aldolase deficiency) may have a severe reaction to the invert sugar solution if it is used as diluent. Symptoms include hypoglycemia, nausea, vomiting, tremors, coma, or convulsion.
- The rate of infusion should not exceed 4 ml per minute (1200 mg per minute).
- Only fresh solution should be used; discard any unused portion.
- Do not mix urea with blood or other drugs in the same syringe. If in doubt about the dilution or the compatibility, consult the pharmacy.
- Check the intravenous insertion site frequently and avoid extravasation. Venous irritation is more common with urea than with mannitol. The use of hypothermia while urea is being administered increases the risk of venous thrombosis and hemoglobinuria (hemoglobin in the urine).

Side Effects of Osmotic Diuretics

Fluid and electrolyte imbalances may occur, particularly with renal impairment. Occasionally seen are pulmonary congestion, acidosis, thirst, blurred vision, convulsions, nausea and vomiting, diarrhea, tachycardia, fever, angina-like pain, and local irritation with thrombophlebitis.

Additional Nursing Indications for Osmotic Diuretics

- See general nursing implications, pp. 203, 205.
- Mannitol is preferred over urea in most situations because it is easier to administer, has fewer side effects, and causes less rebound in cerebral edema when discontinued.
- Assess patients frequently for signs of pulmonary or cardiac difficulty by monitoring such parameters as the pulse, blood pressure, respiratory rate, color, ECG, and subjective complaints.
- Hyponatremia is possible with mannitol.
- Diuresis occurs rapidly and copiously after administration of mannitol or urea; it is usually necessary to insert a urinary catheter (Foley). If the urine output should fall before 30 to 50 ml per hour, notify the physician.
- Deafness has been reported in patients receiving mannitol who are also receiving kanamycin. Signs of hearing difficulty include tinnitus, decreased hearing acuity, and vertigo.
- Because both mannitol and urea affect electrolyte balance, serum lithium levels may be altered.
- Urea can cause both hyponatremia and hypokalemia.
- Osmotic diuretics are often administered to patients who have a decreased level of consciousness. Patients should be monitored frequently and carefully for side effects.
- Do not confuse the drug mannitol with mannitol hexanitrate, an antianginal drug.

Organomercurials

Mersalyl with theophylline
Mercaptomerin sodium

Actions of Organomercurials

Organomercurial compounds inhibit active chloride-ion transport in ascending limb of Henle's loop, increasing chloride excretion and the excretion of sodium ion and water. The excretion of potassium, ammonium ion, calcium, and magnesium is also increased.

Diuretics 225

Table 14-7 Administration of organomercurials

Generic Name	Trade Name	Dosage and Administration	Diuretic Effect		
			Onset	Peak	Duration
Mersalyl with theophylline	Mercurasol Mersalyn Theo-Syl R	INTRAMUSCULAR, INTRAVENOUS: *Adults*—initial dose 50 mg mersalyl and 25 mg theophylline; thereafter, 100 to 200 mg mersalyl and 50 to 100 mg theophylline (1 to 2 ml of drug as supplied) once or twice weekly. *Children*—doses are half those of adults.	30 to 40 min	2 to 4 hr	About 12 hr
Mercaptomerin sodium	Thiomerin Sodium	INTRAMUSCULAR, SUBCUTANEOUS: *Adults*—25 to 250 mg daily (0.2 to 2 ml of drug as supplied).	30 to 40 min	2 to 4 hr	12 hr

Indications for Organomercurials

These drugs are seldom used in modern practice because safer agents are available.

Nurse Alert for Organomercurials

- The risk of mercury poisoning is increased in patients with renal disease.
- Mersalyl with theophylline should be given in small test doses because of possibility of side effects, or a skin test should be used to test for allergic reaction.

Parenteral Administration of Organomercurials

- The organomercurials are not recommended for intravenous administration because they may produce ventricular fibrillation. If necessary, however, mersalyl with theophylline may be given via this route.
- Dilute 0.5 ml of the medication with 5 to 10 ml of sterile water.
- Do not mix with any other medication in a syringe or add to an infusion.
- Administer each 0.5 ml of actual medication over a period of at least 2 minutes.
- Monitor the ECG while administering.
- Check the intravenous insertion site carefully because extravasation can cause tissue necrosis and sloughing.
- Mersalyl with theophylline should not be given subcutaneously.

Nursing Implications for Organomercurials

- See general nursing implications, pp. 203, 205.
- An allergic, sometimes fatal, reaction is characterized by a precipitous fall in blood pressure, dyspnea, gasping, cyanosis, and cardiac irregularities. If an allergic reaction occurs, discontinue the drug, notify the physician, and treat symptomatically.
- Mercury poisoning can also occur after prolonged use. Symptoms include cardiac arrhythmias, an ashen gray

appearance around the mouth and pharynx, a metallic taste, diarrhea, stomatitis, sore gums, foul breath, and excessive salivation. Treatment includes discontinuing the drug and administering dimercaprol (BAL).

- The organomercurials can produce hypochloremic alkalosis, hyponatremia, hypokalemia, hypocalcemia, and hypomagnesemia.

Cardiotonic Drugs: Cardiac Glycosides and Drugs for Congestive Heart Failure

Cardiac glycosides
    Digoxin
    Digitoxin
    Ouabain
    Deslanoside
    Gitalin
    Digitalis leaf

Other drugs used in congestive
heart failure
    Dobutamine (see Ch. 12)
    Dopamine (see Ch. 12)
    Ephedrine (see Ch. 28)
    Diuretics (see Ch. 14)
Vasodilators
    Sodium nitroprusside
    (see Ch. 13)
    Isosorbide dinitrate
    (see Ch. 12)
    Nitroglycerin (see Ch. 12)

Note: The drugs other than the cardiac glycosides listed above are considered in this chapter only to allow comparison of the full range of drugs used in the treatment of congestive heart failure. These others are discussed only in the section on Indications; see the chapters noted above for complete information.

Actions of Cardiac Glycosides

The cardiac glycosides, a group of complex steroid-like structures linked to sugar molecules, are used to treat congestive heart failure because they directly improve the strength of heart muscle and therefore elevate cardiac output. Contractility is increased by the accumulation of calcium in heart cells because the cardiac glycosides inhibit Na^+, K^+-ATPase. The result is increased output, improved blood flow to kidneys and periphery, lowering of venous pressure, and excretion of excess fluid.

Indications for Cardiac Glycosides and Other Drugs for Congestive Heart Failure

Indications for Cardiac Glycosides

The cardiac glycosides are used primarily in the treatment of congestive heart failure, but also for the control of cardiac arrthymias.

Indications for Other Drugs for Congestive Heart Failure

Drugs that stimulate the beta-1 adrenergic receptors in the heart increase contractility by increasing cyclic AMP. *Dobutamine* increases contractility without increasing blood pressure or heart rate and is used to increase cardiac output in severely ill patients. *Dopamine* in low doses increases renal blood flow and promotes diuresis, and in higher doses directly stimulates the heart; it is usually used only for patients with congestive heart failure complicated by hypotension. *Ephedrine* increases contractility of the heart, but also produces the usually unwanted effects of increasing heart rate and peripheral vascular resistance; it has the advantage of being an oral agent.

Diuretics, most commonly furosemide, are used in controlling the pulmonary edema accompanying severe congestive heart failure; they may also directly improve cardiac function.

Vasodilators such as sodium nitroprusside, isosorbide dinitrate, and nitroglycerine are used in late chronic congestive heart failure because they reverse the persistent vasoconstriction and thus increase cardiac output and reduce the heart's work load.

Nurse Alert for Cardiac Glycosides

- Precautions for the use of cardiac glycosides primarily involve care required in adjusting dosages (see following section on Administration) and prevention and treatment of side effects (see later section on Side Effects). Because

230   **Pocket Nurse Guide to Drugs**

toxic reactions are dose related, many hospitals have established assays to measure active cardiac glycosides in the blood as an aid to establishing safe doses. Toxicity is increased by thiazide and loop diuretics and low levels of intracellular potassium.

Administration of Cardiac Glycosides
General Note on Administration

Because of the long half-lives of the cardiac glycosides, the final therapeutic concentrations are not achieved for weeks following the start of therapy. To avoid this delay a loading dose is usually used, followed by a smaller maintenance dose on a regular schedule that is continued indefinitely or until the patient's condition warrants adjustment.

Special Notes on Administration of Cardiac Glycosides
Digitoxin

Digitoxin is usually given orally in a dose to produce and to maintain the therapeutic level in plasma of 14 to 26 ng/ml. The dose required to produce the maximum therapeutic effect varies considerably from patient to patient and must be individualized. Digitalizing, or loading, doses would be expected to range around 0.8 to 1.2 mg per day. Since 97% of this drug is reversibly bound to protein in the bloodstream and is inactive, the dose given the patient must take into account that only 3% of the dose in the bloodstream is active. Since the half-life of digitoxin is about 6 days, about 10% of the total body store of the drug is excreted each day. The routine daily dose of the drug must compensate for this drug loss. Maintenance doses should be expected in the range of 0.05 to 0.2 mg per day. Consideration of the half-life of the drug is also important when toxicity occurs; toxicity may persist for long periods because the drug is only slowly removed from the system.

Digoxin

Digoxin is usually given orally in a dose to produce and to maintain a therapeutic plasma level of 0.8 to 1.6 ng/ml.

Table 15-1 Pharmacokinetics of cardiac glycosides

	Oral Absorption	Plasma Protein Binding	Plasma Half-Life	Route of Excretion
Digoxin	60 to 100%*	23%	32 to 48 hr	Renal
Digitoxin	90 to 100%	97%	5 to 7 days	Hepatic
Ouabain	Unreliable	42%	21 hr	Renal
Deslanoside	Unreliable	25%	33 to 36 hr	Renal

*60% for the tablet form, but up to 100% with the soft gelatin capsule.

Table 15-2 Time course of action of cardiac glycosides

Drug	Route	Onset	Peak	Duration
Digoxin	oral	1 to 2 hr	1.5 to 6 hr	2 to 6 days
	intravenous	5 to 30 min	1 to 4 hr	2 to 6 days
Digitoxin	oral	1 to 4 hr	8 to 14 hr	14 days
	intravenous	30 to 120 min	4 to 12 hr	14 days
Ouabain	intravenous	3 to 10 min	30 to 120 min	1 to 3 days
Deslanoside	intravenous	10 to 30 min	1 to 3 hr	2 to 5 days
Gitalin	oral	2 to 4 hr	8 to 12 hr	12 days
Digitalis leaf	oral	2 to 4 hr	12 to 14 hr	14 days

Pocket Nurse Guide to Drugs

Dosage regimens with this drug must also be individualized for the patient. Digitalizing doses should be expected to be in the range of 1 to 1.5 mg per day. This drug is less highly bound to plasma protein than digitoxin and has a much shorter half-life. The maintenance dose of digoxin must replace the 37% of the total body store of the drug that is lost every day. Maintenance doses should be expected to be in the range of 0.125 to 0.5 mg per day.

Ouabain

Ouabain is used only in emergencies when the intravenous route of administration is required and rapid action is imperative. Ouabain has no role in long-term therapy of congestive heart failure. Maintenance doses of oral cardiac glycosides are started usually within 12 or 24 hours after initial therapy with ouabain, and after intravenous ouabain is discontinued.

Deslanoside

Deslanoside is used only in emergencies when the intravenous route of administration is required. Like ouabain, deslanoside has no role in long-term therapy of congestive heart failure, its only advantage being the rapid action when given intravenously. However, deslanoside is usually no more rapid in onset of action than digoxin given intravenously. Moreover, adjusting doses when the patient is switched to oral maintenance therapy is more problematic with deslanoside than with digoxin. For these reasons, deslanoside is not widely used.

Glycoside Mixtures

Various natural products or partially purified extracts from natural products contain a variety of cardiac glycosides, including the highly active compound digitoxin. These preparations can be used orally for maintenance therapy or long-term therapy of congestive heart failure. Some of these products contain glycosides that interfere with the assay of active cardiac glycosides.

Side Effects of Cardiac Glycosides

Side effects may result within many different body systems. Gastrointestinal effects include anorexia, nausea, vomiting, and diarrhea. Visual changes may include dimness of vision, double vision, blind spots, flashing lights, blurred vision, or altered color vision. Neurological effects may include weakness, fatigue, fainting, headache, confusion, disorientation, or restlessness. Cardiac effects may include decreased pulse rate, perceived changes in cardiac rhythm, bradycardia, and occasionally tachycardia. Psychiatric disturbances range from mood alterations to psychoses or hallucinations. The concomitant use of a cardiac glycoside with some drugs has the following effects: with cholestyramine or barbiturates, diminished effectiveness of the glycoside may result; with antacids or Kaopectate, decreased absorption of the glycoside may result; with reserpine or sympathomimetics, increased frequency of arrhythmias may result; with propranolol, excessive bradycardia may result.

Nursing Implications for Cardiac Glycosides

- Patients receiving cardiac glycosides need careful observation to validate the effectiveness of the drug and dosage and to diagnose early toxicity. Desired effects of the cardiac glycosides might include a decrease in pulse and heart rate; slower, less labored respiration; diuresis with accompanying weight reduction; less coughing; less distended neck veins; and better tolerance of exertion.
- Low serum potassium levels predispose to digitalis toxicity. The serum potassium level should be checked by the nurse whenever the measurement is obtained and prior to administration of the prescribed dose of medication. If the potassium level is excessively low, notify the physician. Signs of hypokalemia include weakness, thirst, depression, anorexia, nausea, vomiting, abdominal distention, postural hypotension, and hypoactive reflexes. Vomiting, chronic diarrhea, nasogastric suctioning, and any state of alkalosis can cause excessive potassium loss from the body. In

234 Pocket Nurse Guide to Drugs

addition, potassium loss can occur as a side effect associated with the administration of potassium-losing diuretics, chronic steroids, amphotericin B, and chronic glucose infusions.

- Increased toxicity of cardiac glycosides is also seen when there are preexisting low serum magnesium levels, elevated serum calcium levels, or with hypothyroidism.
- If digitalis toxicity occurs, the drug is withheld until the patient's condition is no longer toxic. Any arrhythmias that occur are treated with appropriate drugs (Chapter 17).
- Patients receiving cardiac glycosides must be checked frequently for extra beats or other arrhythmias.
- Take the apical pulse for 1 minute before administering a digitalis preparation. The usual rule states that if the apical pulse is less than 60 beats per minute in an adult or 90 to 110 beats per minute in a child, the dose should be omitted and the physician notified.
- If a serum digitalis level determination has been ordered, check the value before administering the drug.
- If the patient is on a cardiac monitor or is having frequent electrocardiogram (ECG) tracings done, it is possible to monitor the effects of the cardiac glycoside on the heart by checking these tracings. Digitalis preparations can cause prolongation of the P-R interval, S-T segment sagging, any degree of atrioventricular block, atrial tachycardia with or without atrioventricular block, bigeminal pulse, ventricular tachycardia, and premature ventricular contractions.
- Check carefully the name and dose of digitalis preparations because there are several different preparations that have similar spellings.
- The patient's overall response to heart disease should be monitored daily. Physical assessment should include daily weight, fluid intake and output, breath sounds, checking for edema, especially in the sacral area and lower extremities, as well as other signs, symptoms, and measurements previously discussed.
- Taking digitalis preparations with meals may reduce gastric irritation.

Cardiotonic Drugs 235

- Before discharge, the patient needs thorough teaching about the cardiac glycoside as well as any other prescribed medications. In addition to knowledge about side effects, correct dosage, and frequency for each individual medication, the patient must understand the interaction of the medications. If appropriate, the patient needs to be taught to measure and record the apical or radial pulse at regular intervals (e.g., daily, or once a week). Referral to a community-based nursing agency may be appropriate for patient follow-up.
- Intravenous digitalis preparations need to be administered slowly (usually 1 ml per minute or more slowly). They should not be mixed with infusion fluids. Check with the pharmacy if in doubt.
- Ouabain is the fastest acting cardiac glycoside. It is usually reserved for emergencies and should only be given intravenously. Administer slowly, 0.5 ml per minute, and do not mix with other infusion fluids.
- Instruct patients that if a dose of medication is missed, they should not try to "double up" the next time a dose is taken to catch up.
- Weight gain in excess of 2 to 5 pounds per week, or as determined by the health care provider, should be reported by the patient. Consult the physician.
- Elderly patients are especially prone to side effects with cardiac glycosides. Significant cardiac toxicity may develop without some of the earlier signs of toxicity, such as gastrointestinal disturbances. In addition, elderly patients may not think it is important to report anorexia or visual changes, attributing these and other symptoms to aging or other medical conditions.
- Instruct patients to report all drugs being taken and to avoid the use of over-the-counter preparations unless the drug and dose are first cleared with the physician.
- Diet therapy may also be important in the treatment of the patient's cardiac condition. Weight loss, sodium restriction, and maintaining adequate potassium intake may all be prescribed.

Fluids and Electrolytes

16

Parenteral therapy
- Isotonic saline solution
- Hypotonic saline solution
- Ringers solution
- Lactated Ringers solution
- Dextrose in water
- Potassium chloride solution
- Sodium bicarbonate solution
- Magnesium sulfate solution

Blood, blood components, and blood substitutes
- Whole blood
- Plasma
- Human albumin
- Plasma protein fraction
- Dextrans
- Hetastarch
- Hypertonic dextrose solution
- Crystalline amino acids
- Intralipid
- Travamulsion
- Liposyn

Actions of Fluids and Electrolytes

Fluids and electrolytes are used in various clinical situations to reestablish normal salt and water balances and thereby return the body to homeostasis. Fluids and electrolytes used in replacement therapy have essentially the same actions as fluids and electrolytes normally present in the body.

Indications for Fluid and Electrolyte Therapy

Fluid and electrolyte therapy is indicated for *extracellular fluid deficit* as may result from sudden hemorrhage, prolonged vomiting, excessive diarrhea, plasma loss through burns, inadequate fluid intake, or high-volume renal failure; for *fluid excess* as may result from heart failure or renal impairment or the improper administration of intravenous fluids; and for *electrolyte imbalances* such as hypernatremia, hyponatremia, hyperkalemia, hypokalemia, or acid-base imbalances from various causes.

Isotonic saline is used to replace extracellular fluid volume and to treat sodium depletion and metabolic alkalosis.

236

Hypertonic saline is used to correct severe hyponatremia. *Ringer's solution* is replacement therapy for patients with loss of fluid and electrolytes through the alimentary tract, burn patients, postoperative patients, and others. *Lactated Ringer's* is appropriate when the patient has electrolyte imbalances and is acidotic. *Isotonic dextrose in water* is used in most situations when rehydration is needed but electrolyte replacement is not required; *hypertonic dextrose solutions* are used to shift fluid from the interstitial space into the plasma. *Dextrose in saline* may be used to hydrate patients and replace sodium loss. *Potassium chloride* may be added to IV fluids to replace potassium lost from the gastrointestinal tract or kidney. *Sodium bicarbonate* is used occasionally to reverse metabolic acidosis. *Magnesium sulfate* is used to correct severe magnesium deficiencies, as maintenance during total parenteral nutrition, and to control convulsions of eclampsia.

Whole blood is used in patients who have lost more than 20% of their blood volume. *Plasma* is used for replacement when cross-matched whole blood is not available or is not required for oxygen transport. *Human albumin* and *plasma protein fraction* are used to expand plasma volume. *Plasma protein fraction* is used for hypovolemic shock in adults, for dehydration in children, and to replace plasma proteins in patients with hypoproteinemia. *Dextran* and *hetastarch* also expand plasma volume by generating osmotic forces that cause water to enter blood vessels; *dextran* is used for shock, and *hetastarch* for shock or hypervolemia.

Hypertonic dextrose is used for total parenteral nutrition. *Amino acids* are used in total parenteral nutrition to prevent negative nitrogen balance and the breakdown of protein in the body. *Fat emulsions* and *vitamin* and *mineral supplements* may be employed in addition to total parenteral nutrition fluids to prevent deficiencies.

Nurse Alert for Fluid and Electrolyte Therapy

- *Isotonic or hypertonic saline* carry the risk of circulatory overload and hypernatremia. *Hypertonic saline* solutions must be administered carefully in small volumes.

Table 16-1   Administration of fluids and electrolytes

Solution	Trade Names	Dosage for Intravenous Administration
NaCl in water (0.45%, 0.9%, 3.0%, 5.0%)	—	Isotonic (0.9%) and hypotonic (0.45%) 90-125 ml/hr but may range much higher for initial therapy; 3% solution up to 80 ml/hr; 5% solution up to 50 ml/hr.
Ringers solution (0.86% NaCl, 0.03% KCl, and 0.033% $CaCl_2$	—	90-125 ml/hr commonly employed.
Lactated Ringers (0.6% NaCl, 0.03% KCl, 0.02% $CaCl_2$, 0.31% Na lactate)	—	90-125 ml/hr commonly employed.
Dextrose in water (2.5%, 5%, 10%, 20%, 50%, 70%)	—	Isotonic (5%) 90-125 ml/hr usual but may range much higher; doses of hypertonic solutions are individualized for specific purposes.
KCl in water (11.25%, 15%, 24%)	—	Must be diluted before use and administered at rates less than 10-15 mEq/hr for minimally depleted patients or up to 40 mEq/hr for severely depleted patients.
Sodium bicarbonate, 1.4% in water	—	Doses are calculated to reverse acidosis (individualized for each patient).
Magnesium sulfate (10%, 50%)	—	The 10% solution should be infused at rates less than 1.5 ml/min. The more concentrated solution is for intramuscular administration.

Whole blood	—	One unit = 450 ± 45 ml blood + 63 ml of CPD (citrate-phosphate-dextrose) or CPDA-1 (citrate-phosphate-dextrose-adenine), administered intravenously through a 170 micron filter.
Plasma	—	Monitored by clinical response to intravenous infusion.
Human Albumin (5%, 25%)	Albuminar Albutein Buminate Plasbumin	Adjusted according to need of the patient, but should be less than 250 g/48 hr.
Plasma Protein Fraction (5%)	Plasmanate Plasma Plex Plasmatein Protenate	*Adults:* 1-1.5L of 5% solution infused at 5-8 ml/min, adjusted as necessary. *Children:* 33 ml/kg infused at 5-10 ml/min to correct dehydration.
Dextrans (Dextran 40, Dextran 70, Dextran 75)	—	Infusion rates may be rapid initially, but total daily dose should not exceed 20 mg/kg.
Hetastarch (6% in 0.9% NaCl)	Hespan	Rates of infusion for acute hemorrhagic shock are 20 ml/kg/hr or less.
Hypertonic dextrose (50% or 70%)	—	Diluted with water or amino acid solutions to concentrations initially of approx. 12.5%. Longer term therapy may ultimately require 25 to 30% solutions. Minimal adult requirements for dextrose are around 150 g daily. Initial infusion of 1000 to 1200 ml of 12.5% dextrose approximates that requirement; dosage can be gradually increased as needed to meet caloric requirements.

cont'd. next page

Table 16-1   Administration of fluids and electrolytes—cont'd.

Solution	Trade Names	Dosage for Intravenous Administration
Crystalline amino acids	Aminosyn FreAmine III Travasol TrophAmine Veinamine	May be given at about 1 g/kg body weight per day, as needed to prevent protein breakdown and negative nitrogen balance. Solutions contain mixtures of essential and non-essential amino acids. TrophAmine contains taurine, an amino acid required by neonates.
Fat emulsions	Intralipid (10%, 20%) Travamulsion (10%) Liposyn (10%, 20%)	May be given by peripheral vein 1 ml/min for 10% or 0.5 ml/min for 20% over 30 minutes initially as needed to supply calories (20% contains 2000 cal/liter) or replace essential fatty acids. This preparation should supply 60% or less of the total calories taken by a patient. Dosage should not exceed 2.5 g fat/kg body weight daily. Children and infants require lower infusion rates.

Fluids and Electrolytes **241**

- Renal function must be evaluated before using *Ringer's solution,* because the potassium in the solution may accumulate to dangerous levels if the kidney cannot eliminate it.
- *Dextrose in saline* must be used cautiously in patients with cardiac, renal, or liver disease because of the fluid shift from plasma into the interstitial space.
- Replacement with *potassium chloride* must be performed carefully to avoid causing hyperkalemia and to prevent tissue damage from extravasation.
- With *whole blood* transfusions, cross-matching to avoid reactions is mandatory.
- *Human albumin preparations* contain sodium in amounts that may cause problems for patients with cardiovascular disease.
- *Hypertonic dextrose* should be administered via a large central vein where blood flow is sufficient to dilute the strong sugar solution and prevent tissue damage.
- The parenteral form of *magnesium sulfate* is contraindicated in patients with myocardial damage or heart block; emergency resuscitation equipment must be readily available whenever parenteral magnesium sulfate is used.

Side Effects and Potential Problems with Fluid and Electrolyte Therapy

Side effects and problems with *any parenteral fluid administration* may include fluid overload (edema, distended neck veins, noisy or rapid respirations) and problems at the infusion insertion site including extravasation, phlebitis, generalized septicemia causing fever, chills, or signs of shock, or occluded infusion due to poor positioning of the extremity, the viscosity of the substance being infused, or the needle lodging against the vein wall.

Overdose of *magnesium sulfate* may cause flushing, sweating, hypotension, respiratory and circulatory collapse, and depressed deep tendon reflexes. Intramuscular *calcium replacements* cause burning and occasionally abscesses; this route should not be used for children. *Whole blood* transfusions may cause allergic reactions, including rashes, itching,

242 Pocket Nurse Guide to Drugs

bronchospasm, and angioedema, and febrile reactions including chills, headache, and malaise; circulatory overload may also occur with whole blood, especially with the elderly, small infants, and patients with cardiac disease. *Dextrans* and *hetastarch* may lead to circulatory overload or allergic or hypersensitivity reactions; dextrans may also increase bleeding time. With infusions for *total parenteral nutrition,* fluid overload may also occur; dry flaky skin, hair loss, and rashes may indicate a deficiency in essential fatty acids or zinc. *Fat emulsions* may lead to thrombophlebitis, vomiting, chest pain, and hypersensitivity reactions. Side effects of *amino acid* transfusions frequently include nausea, vomiting, flushing, and a sensation of warmth; less frequent side effects are chills, headache, abdominal pain, dizziness, rashes, hyperglycemia, and glycosuria.

Nursing Implications for Fluid and Electrolyte Therapy

General Implications for All IV Fluid Administration

- The administration of any substance directly into the vascular system has the potential for serious, sometimes rapid, consequences.
- The nurse should carefully inspect the patient receiving intravenous fluids each time the nurse sees the patient. Observe for fluid overload, reaction to the medications being administered, edema, distended neck veins, noisy or rapid respirations.
- The practicing nurse must learn the policies on intravenous infusions of the agencies or institution.
- Because intravenous injection/infusion breaks the integrity of the skin, the infusion insertion site must be maintained and monitored carefully for infection.
- Once an infusion is going, the system should not be opened except to replace an empty bag or bottle, or via needle through the injection sites.
- Master the infusion equipment prior to using it with a patient.
- Check carefully any infusion rates which must be calcu-

Fluids and Electrolytes 243

lated; double check rates supplied by the pharmacy. Some institutions require that two nurses double check any infusion rate for pediatric patients. The nurse should question any rate which does not make logical sense.

- The rate of delivery of intravenous fluids depends on the diameter of the needle or catheter, the height of the fluid reservoir above the patient, the viscosity of the fluid or solution, the length of tubing between the reservoir and the patient, and the infusion drip set; volume control devices and mechanical control or alarm devices have advantages, but they do not replace careful assessment by the nurse.
- Inspect all intravenous solutions carefully before administering. Solutions containing particulate matter should not be used. If there is a question that the IV bottle or bag is cracked, punctured, or otherwise possibly contaminated, it should not be used.
- Label all intravenous medications carefully, especially when additives have been included. Record the administration of all IV solutions carefully, just as all medications would be.
- To assess for fluid overload, weigh the patient regularly, measure intake and output. Inspect the sacral area, feet and legs for edema. Other parameters to monitor include skin turgor, urine specific gravity, pulse, blood pressure, heart sound, breath sound, central venous pressure (if available), and pulmonary artery pressure (if available).
- Check the compatibility of drugs administered IV "push" with infusing solutions prior to administration of the push drugs. It may be necessary to flush the tubing prior to administering a drug.
- If an infusion falls behind, it is not appropriate to "catch up" by doubling or increasing the rate for the next hour or two. Falling behind in the infusion rate is best prevented by frequently checking the patient. If, after all appropriate nursing measures have been tried, the rate is still too slow, it may be necessary to restart the IV infusion at another site.

Potassium

- The importance of carefully checking calculations in preparing KCl for intravenous infusions cannot be overem-

244   Pocket Nurse Guide to Drugs

phasized. Be sure to label carefully containers to which KCl has been added.

- Monitor the electrocardiogram and the serum potassium level of patients receiving KCl.
- The usual rate of administration of intravenous KCl is in concentrations of 40 mEq/L at a rate not to exceed 10 to 15 mEq/hr. The total dose per day would usually not exceed 100 to 300 mEq/24 hours. In rare situations, when the patient's serum potassium is less than 2 mEq/L, potassium may be given cautiously in concentrations as high as 60 mEq/L at a rate of 40 mEq/hr. Note that potassium is never administered undiluted.
- If hyperkalemia occurs, emergency treatment is with parenteral sodium bicarbonate, calcium gluconate (if not contraindicated because of cardiac conditions), and regular insulin for parenteral use. In extreme cases, dialysis may be necessary.
- Potassium should not be administered to patients receiving potassium-sparing diuretics (Chapter 14).
- Since potassium is well absorbed via the gastrointestinal tract, it is usually desirable to put the patient on oral potassium replacement, if needed, as soon as the patient's condition warrants it. However, oral preparations are often unpalatable or difficult to take. Effervescent preparations are often unpalatable, and patients soon stop taking them. Oral solutions work well, but often have a bitter, salty taste. These solutions can be diluted in juice or milk, but this may also be unacceptable to the patient. Enteric-coated or controlled release tablets have been implicated in small bowel ulceration caused by high local concentrations of potassium. These preparations should be reserved for use in patients who refuse other forms. Taking potassium with meals may help reduce gastric irritation. It is important to work with the patient to try to find an acceptable potassium replacement form, which the patient is willing to take on a regular basis.
- Dietary sources of potassium include citrus fruits and juices; grape, cranberry, apple, pear, and apricot juices; bananas; whole grain cereal; tea and cola beverages, peanut

Fluids and Electrolytes 245

butter, and nuts. Note, however, that many of these commercially prepared foods are also high in sodium, so may be contraindicated for a patient on that basis. Some patients may wish to augment their drug regime with dietary replacement.

- Licorice can cause potassium excretion, and should be avoided by patients with hypokalemia.
- Salt substitutes contain varying amounts of potassium and sodium. Patients should discuss the use of any specific salt substitute with the physician, nurse or dietitian prior to use.
- Instruct the patient to inform all caregivers of potassium replacements. The patient should avoid the use of over-the-counter medications without first consulting the physician or pharmacist, as many contain potassium, and may predispose to hyperkalemia.
- Some oral preparations contain FD & C coloring number 5 (tartrazine), which may cause an allergic response in some individuals. Although rare, this response is more common in individuals with aspirin hypersensitivity. Read carefully the literature supplied with potassium replacements.
- Occasionally, hyperkalemia is treated with administration of sodium polystryrene sulfonate (Kayexalate), a resin which exchanges sodium for potassium in the intestine. Its effect is not evident for up to 24 hours, after administration; it is used in non-life-threatening hyperkalemia, or after emergency treatment has already been given. Adverse effects include hypokalemia, hypocalcemia, anorexia, nausea, vomiting, and constipation. Monitor the electrolytes. Be particularly careful when the patient is also receiving a digitalis preparation, as hypokalemia enhances digitalis intoxication. The drug can be administered orally (the preferred route), or rectally as an enema. When given orally, constipation is frequently a problem, so a mild laxative (e.g., sorbitol) is usually given concomitantly. For oral administration, the drug may be diluted in water, syrup, fruit juice, or a soft drink; it may be given via stomach tube. If sorbitol is used as the laxative, it should be administered every 2 to 3 hours until a stool is passed, then once or twice a day as needed to prevent constipation.

246 Pocket Nurse Guide to Drugs

Magnesium Sulfate

- In pregnancy, the goal is to achieve a serum level which will inhibit the development of seizures, but which will not cause respiratory or cardiac paralysis. Several dosage regimens are used for this; most begin with a loading dose, which is reduced then to a maintenance dose. Assess the patient's peripheral reflexes, respiratory rate, and urinary output. If the reflexes become diminished or absent, the respiratory rate decreases, or the urinary output drops below 30 to 100 ml/hour, the dose of magnesium sulfate may need to be reduced. Monitor the vital signs, fluid intake and output, and serum magnesium levels. Newborn infants of mothers who received parenteral magnesium sulfate should be monitored carefully for the first few hours after birth for signs of hypermagnesemia.
- The drug causes pain when administered intramuscularly. To reduce the discomfort, 1 ml of 2% lidocaine may be added to the drug dose (with approval of the physician). The drug should be administered slowly.
- Magnesium sulfate 10% solution may be administered intravenously at a rate not exceeding 1.5 ml/min.

Sodium Bicarbonate

- Except during resuscitation, this drug will be diluted when given intravenously. During resuscitation, sodium bicarbonate is administered via direct intravenous push at approximately 5 minute intervals to help correct metabolic acidosis. It is usually found in prelabeled syringes in the emergency drug box or on the resuscitation cart, for use in this emergency situation.
- Signs of overdose (or when too rapid administration has occurred) are those of metabolic alkalosis and hypernatremia. Emergency treatment of overdose would be with parenteral calcium gluconate and 2.14% ammonium chloride solution.
- Because sodium bicarbonate renders the urine alkaline, it may cause the following drug interactions: the effects of amphetamines, mecamylamine, pseudoephedrine, and qui-

Fluids and Electrolytes 247

nine may be enhanced, while the effects of lithium, phenobarbital and salicylates may be reduced.

Calcium

- Patients on digitalis preparations who receive intravenous calcium preparations must be monitored very carefully, as increases in serum calcium predispose to digitalis toxicity.
- Patients receiving intravenous calcium should have their electrocardiogram monitored, as well as vital signs, serum electrolytes and pH.
- Severe hypocalcemia may manifest itself as tetany. Chvostek's sign and Trousseau's signs may be positive (see a physical assessment book for illustration of these signs). Pad the side rails. Have resuscitation equipment readily available.
- Hypercalcemia can occur as a result of abnormalities of the parathyroid, some cancers, and as a result of some medications (see treatment Chapter 38).
- There are many good dietary sources of calcium, including milk products, cheese, yogurt; dark green leafy vegetables such as spinach, kale and greens, and sardines, clams and oysters.

Whole Blood, Plasma, Albumin, Plasma Protein Fraction

- Whole blood is administered via a blood infusion tubing set, which usually contains an in-line blood filter. The tubing is primed, usually with normal saline (solutions with dextrose may hemolyze the blood, while solutions containing calcium, as in Lactated Ringer's solution, may clot the blood), and the blood is piggybacked to the priming solution. This method helps prevent the blood from clotting as the infusion nears an end, and allows for the maintenance of a patent IV access line, even if the blood infusion must be discontinued, as might happen in a severe incompatibility reaction.
- Carefully check the patient's identification, and the labeling on whole blood, prior to beginning an infusion. The administration of incompatible blood is a potentially fatal

248 Pocket Nurse Guide to Drugs

complication, and death can occur after as little as 50 to 100 ml of blood.

- After initiating a blood transfusion, the nurse should remain with the patient for 10 to 15 minutes, monitoring and recording the vital signs. Any unexpected finding should be thoroughly investigated, the infusion of blood stopped (although a patent IV line should be maintained by restarting the priming solution), and the physician notified. The nurse should know where emergency equipment is prior to administering blood.

- Febrile reactions usually begin within the first 15 minutes of infusion, but may not begin until one to two hours later. They are characterized by high fever (39.4-40° C or 103-104° F), chills headache and malaise. Again, the infusion of blood should be stopped, the physician notified, and the cause investigated.

- No medications should ever by mixed with blood. If it is necessary to administer an IV medication via the same IV access line, the infusion of blood must be interrupted, and the infusion line flushed with normal saline before and after the medication is infused.

- Because of the character and size of the blood cells, a large diameter (18g or larger) needle or catheter should be used for infusions.

- When there is a possibility of circulatory overload, red cell concentrates may be used. These provide the patient with blood of 70 - 80% hematocrit, without the fluid volume. The cells may be fresh or frozen. If frozen, they must be thawed before use, usually by putting in a cool water bath (in its protective package).

- Units of whole blood should usually be administered within 2 to 4 hours; if left hanging longer than that, they will often clot. In extreme emergencies (e.g., hypovolemic shock), pressure may be applied to the blood-containing bag to deliver the blood in 10 minutes or less. Red cell concentrates may be primed with normal saline to increase their rate of flow; because the volume is smaller, they may be administered over a shorter period of time.

Fluids and Electrolytes **249**

- Cryoprecipitated factor VIII (for hemophiliacs), and other special blood fractions are administered the same way as blood. They are usually of smaller volume, and it may be necessary to administer several units over a short period of time.
- All blood products rapidly deteriorate if not stored properly, and not used promptly. Frozen products should not be thawed unless they will be used; blood should not be obtained from the blood bank until the patient is ready for the infusion. Blood products should never be left lying around the patient care unit. Finally, check and observe all expiration dates on blood products.

Dextrans and Hetastarch

- These products are artificially produced, and are not derived directly from the blood. Nevertheless, many of the precautions observed during the administration of blood should be used with these products also. Circulatory overload can be a problem, as can allergic and hypersensitivity reactions.
- Dextran, especially the higher molecular weight products, may increase bleeding time; this may not be apparent for 6 to 9 hours after administration.

Total Parenteral Nutrition

- Hyperalimentation or Total Parenteral Nutrition (TPN) must be administered via a central line, which has been placed via the subclavian vein, or other vessel near the superior vena cava. This line is placed by the physician, using the strictest of aseptic techniques.
- Because the fluids administered for TPN are such good growth media for bacteria, the need to maintain asepsis at the insertion site, and prevent contamination of the system cannot be overemphasized.
- While hypertonic dextrose, amino acids, and fat emulsions constitute the backbone of TPN therapy, the rate of flow, additives (vitamins, minerals, electrolytes), and concentrations must be ordered specifically by the physician. The pharmacy and dietary department will also be of assistance.

250 Pocket Nurse Guide to Drugs

- No medications should ever be added to TPN once it has been prepared by the pharmacy, or administered via the TPN line. If IV medications must be given, a separate peripheral IV should be started and maintained.
- Monitor the patient's weight, intake and output, serum electrolytes, BUN and other renal parameters, blood and urine glucose, blood counts, and vital signs. Observe for signs of fluid overload: edema, dyspnea, cough, distended neck veins, moist breath sounds, changes in level of consciousness. Once a week, liver function studies, and serum albumin, calcium and magnesium should be monitored.
- The infusion rate should be maintained at a steady rate; an infusion monitoring device should be used. Erratic infusion rates may cause the patient to experience problems with hyper-and hypoglycemia, as the patient's pancreas attempts to produce insulin in response to the hypertonic dextrose. In some cases, patients may require insulin while on TPN (which may be added to TPN) to treat hyperglycemia. It should be added by the pharmacy, and administered as a continuous infusion with the TPN.
- If the central line should become occluded, dislodged, or otherwise stop functioning, many institutions have standing orders that a peripheral infusion of Dextrose 10% may be started immediately (to prevent sudden hypoglycemia in the patient).
- TPN fluids should be prepared in low contamination conditions, with a laminar flow hood being used.
- Some patients requiring parenteral nutrition are suitable candidates for home, self-administered TPN. The nurse must work carefully to instruct the patient and family.

Amino Acids

- Monitor the serum electrolytes, BUN, intake and output, liver function studies, and urine glucose. Observe for signs of fatty acid deficiency (hair loss, flaking skin).
- Vitamins, electrolytes, trace elements, heparin, and insulin may be administered via the same line, but other medica-

Fluids and Electrolytes **251**

tions should not. Do not premix with amino acid infusions, but administer via a Y-connector.

Fat Emulsions

- Fat emulsions may be administered via central peripheral IV lines.
- Fat emulsions should comprise no more than 60% of the total daily caloric intake for the patient.
- Careful review of package inserts is recommended prior to administering fat emulsions.
- Also review carefully the instructions accompanying the administration sets.
- Visually inspect all fat emulsions prior to using. If the emulsion has "cracked" (the oil and other products have separated), then it should not be used. Do not shake fat emulsions.
- There may be hyperlipidemia during therapy with fat emulsions. The lipidemia should clear between daily infusions, or the next dose should be withheld.
- If a fat emulsion is being infused via piggyback line to an infusion containing a standard in-line filter, the fat emulsion must be inserted below the level of the filter (i.e., closer to the patient). Fat emulsions should not be passed through standard in-line filters.
- Do not mix anything with fat emulsions.
- Begin the infusion slowly (e.g., 1 ml/min initially) and increase to the desired rate if no untoward effect has occurred after 15 to 30 minutes. Consult the manufacturer's literature.

Antiarrhythmic Drugs

17

Digitoxin (see also Ch. 15)
Digoxin (see also Ch. 15)
Deslanoside (see also Ch. 15)
Ouabain (see also Ch. 15)
Bretylium tosylate
Atropine
Phenytoin (see also Ch. 7)
Lidocaine (see also Ch. 11)

Quinidine sulfate
Quinidine gluconate
Quinidine polygalacturonate
Procainamide
Disopyramide phosphate
Propranolol (see also Ch. 13)
Verapamil (see also Ch. 13)

Actions of Antiarrhythmic Drugs

Cardiac arrthymias occur because of pacing disorders in automaticity or the appearance of ectopic foci, from impulse conduction disorders across the AV node or through contracting tissues, or from a combination of these mechanisms. Different antiarrhythmic drugs have various mechanisms of action for the treatment of these conditions.

Drugs that block beta-adrenergic receptors in the heart slow the rate at the SA node and slow conduction through the AV node. Anticholinergic drugs may have just the opposite effects by blocking the muscarinic receptors that allow the heart to respond to vagal nerve stimulation. Local anesthetics and other drugs may alter cardiac cell membranes to change the sodium ion influx that causes phase 0 of the action potential. Calcium channel blocking drugs primarily change the responses of cells highly dependent upon the so-called slow calcium current, e.g. AV nodal cells or cells in ischemic regions of the muscle. Many of the antiarrhythmic drugs in use have more than one action on the heart. Table 17-1 summarizes the mechanism of action for the antiarrhythmic drugs.

Indications for Antiarrhythmic Drugs

Many of the drugs used to treat cardiac arrhythmias also have other clinical uses, in addition to their specific indications for different types of arrhythmias. These other indications are discussed as appropriate in other chapters.

Digitoxin and *digoxin* are used to slow conduction through the AV node, administered intravenously in emergencies and continued orally in maintenance doses. *Deslanoside* and *ouabain* are occasionally used as emergency medications. *Bretylium* is used primarily for ventricular tachycardia. *Atropine* is used to treat sinus bradycardia with reduced cardiac output, to increase heart rate, and to lessen heart block in some cases. *Phenytoin* is used primarily for digitalis-induced arrhythmias. *Lidocaine* is used for ventricular arrhythmias in a continuous infusion. *Quinidine, lidocaine,* and *procainamide* are used for ventricular premature contractions; *disopyramide* is used similarly. *Lidocaine* is the treatment of choice for ventricular arrhythmias, especially after myocardial infarction. *Propranolol* is used to increase the refractory period of the AV node; it may be added to digitalis to slow ventricular rates with atrial flutter. *Verapamil* is used to delay conduction through the AV node.

Nurse Alert for Antiarrhythmic Drugs

- At high doses, any antiarrhythmic drug may cause different kinds of arrhythmias; the safety margin for all antiarrhythmics is very narrow.
- *Phenytoin* may cause dangerous myocardial depression if administered intravenously too rapidly.
- Toxic reactions to *lidocaine* are particularly common in patients with reduced hepatic function and may include respiratory depression, convulsions, and coma.
- Be careful not to use *lidocaine* packaged with epinephrine as a local anesthetic; lidocaine is packaged separately for antiarrhythmic treatment.
- *Propranolol, quinidine, procainamide,* and *disopyramide* are depressant antiarrhythmics and may dangerously sup-

Text continued on p. 262

Table 17-1   Actions of antiarrhythmic drugs

Drug	Mechanism of Antiarrhythmic Action	Summary of Cardiac Actions		
		Conduction Velocity	Automaticity	Contractility
Digitalis	Slows conduction through the AV node	Slowed	Increased at high doses	Increased
Bretylium	Prolongs the effective refractory period	No change	No change or slight increase	No change or slight increase
Atropine	Blocks the effects of vagus nerve stimulation	Hastened	Increased	No change
Phenytoin	Depresses spontaneous depolarization in ventricular and atrial but not nodal tissue	No change or slightly hastened	Decreased	No change
Lidocaine	Increases the electrical threshold for ventricular stimulation	No change	Decreased	No change
Quinidine	Suppresses automaticity, especially in ectopic foci, by membrane-stabilizing and anticholinergic effects	Slowed	Decreased	Decreased

Procainamide	As for quinidine	Slowed	Decreased	Decreased
Disopyramide	As for quinidine	No change or slightly slowed	Decreased	Decreased
Propranolol	Beta-adrenergic blockade and membrane-stabilizing effects that increase AV nodal refractory period	Slowed	Decreased	Decreased
Verapamil	Blocks calcium channels and slows conduction through AV node	Slowed	No change or slightly decreased	Decreased

Table 17-2 Administration of antiarrhythmic drugs

Generic Name	Trade Name	Dosage and Administration	Comments
Digitoxin	Crystodigin De-Tone Purodigin*	ORAL, INTRAVENOUS: *Adults*—load with 0.6 mg, followed by 0.4 mg, then 0.2 mg every 4 to 6 hr until total dose of 1.2 to 1.8 mg; maintain with 0.05 to 0.2 mg daily. *Children*—individualize dose for age and weight.	Effective serum levels 14 to 26 ng/ml; degraded by the liver; half-time for elimination about 7 days.
Digoxin	Lanoxin	ORAL: *Adults*—load with 0.5 to 0.75 mg, followed by 0.25 to 0.5 mg every 6 to 8 hr up to a total dose of 1 to 1.5 mg; maintain with 0.125 to 0.5 mg daily. *Children*—individualize dose for age and weight. INTRAVENOUS: *Adults*—load with total dose of 1 mg delivered in divided doses over 8 to 12 hr; maintain with 0.125 to 0.5 mg daily. *Children*—individualize dose for age and weight.	Effective serum level 1 to 2 ng/ml, toxic at 3 ng/ml; excreted by the kidney; elimination half-time about 36 hr.

Antiarrhythmic Drugs 257

Deslanoside	Cedilanid-D	INTRAMUSCULAR, INTRAVENOUS: *Adults*—load with 0.8 mg followed by 0.4 mg every 2 to 4 hrs up to a total dose of 2 mg. *Children*—individualize dose for age and weight.	Onset of action within 30 min; maximal effect within 3 hr of dose.
Ouabain		INTRAVENOUS: *Adults*—250 μg for loading, 100 μg hourly to maintain, with total dose no more than 1 mg daily.	Onset of action within 10 min; maximal effect within 2 hr of dose.
Bretylium tosylate	Bretylol	INTRAMUSCULAR: *Adults*—5 to 10 mg/kg repeated in 1 to 2 hr, then every 6 to 8 hr. One site should receive no more than 5 ml of undiluted drug. INTRAVENOUS: *Adults*—5 to 10 mg/kg every 15 to 30 min to a maximal dose of 30 mg/kg.	Bretylium is excreted unchanged by the kidneys.

cont'd. next page

*Available in U.S. and Canada
†Available in Canada only

258 Pocket Nurse Guide to Drugs

Table 17-2 Administration of antiarrhythmic drugs—cont'd.

Generic Name	Trade Name	Dosage and Administration	Comments
Atropine		INTRAVENOUS: *Adults*—0.4 to 1 mg every 1 to 2 hr as needed. *Children*—0.01 to 0.03 mg/kg of body weight.	Rapidly effective; excreted by the kidney within 12 hr of administration.
Phenytoin	Dilantin*	ORAL: *Adults*—1 Gm every 12 hr to load, then 100 mg every 6 hr. *Children*—initially 10 to 15 mg/kg daily in 2 or 3 doses; maintain with 5 to 10 mg/kg daily in 2 or 3 doses. INTRAVENOUS: *Adults*—100 mg given over 10 min. Repeat if necessary at 5 to 15 min intervals. Dose held under 1 Gm.	Effective serum level 10 to 18 μg/ml; serum half-life 2 days; phenobarbital increases liver metabolism of phenytoin; coumarin anticoagulants, isoniazid, and paraaminosalicylic acid (PAS) may increase serum levels of phenytoin
Lidocaine	Xylocaine HCl for cardiac arrhythmias*;	INTRAMUSCULAR: *Adults*—emergency use, 4 to 5 mg/kg, or 3 ml of 10% solution (300 mg).	Effective serum level 1 to 5 μg/ml; serum half-life 15 to 20 min; metabolized in liver;

Generic	Brand	Dosage	Remarks
	Lidocaine without preservatives*	INTRAVENOUS: *Adults*—50 to 100 mg bolus, then drip at 1 to 5 mg per min. *Children*—5 mg/ml infused to give a dose of 0.03 mg/kg each min.	toxicity increased by reduced liver blood flow or function.
Quinidine sulfate	Cin-Quin Quinidex Extentabs* Quinora	ORAL: *Adults*—200 to 400 mg 4 times daily. *Children*—6 mg/kg every 4 to 6 hr. ORAL: *Adults*—extended release form—300 to 600 mg every 8-12 hours.	Test dose of 200 mg should be given to test for idiosyncratic reactions; effective serum level 3 to 6 μg/ml; serum half-life about 6 hr.
Quinidine gluconate	Duraquin Quinaglute Duro-Tabs* Quinate†	ORAL: *Adults*—324 to 972 mg (1 to 3 tablets) 2 or 3 times daily. INTRAMUSCULAR: *Adults*—200 to 400 mg every 4 to 6 hr. INTRAVENOUS: *Adults*—10 mg each minute up to 400 mg with ECG and blood pressure monitoring.	More slowly absorbed than quinidine sulfate.

cont'd. next page

*Available in U.S. and Canada
†Available in Canada only

Table 17-2   Administration of antiarrhythmic drugs—cont'd.

Generic Name	Trade Name	Dosage and Administration	Comments
Quinidine polygalacturonate	Cardioquin*	ORAL: *Adults*—as for quinidine sulfate (1 tablet of 275 mg is equivalent to 200 mg of quinidine sulfate).	Less irritating to gastrointestinal tract than other forms of quinidine.
Procainamide	Procan Pronestyl* Sub-Quin	ORAL: *Adults*—250 to 500 mg every 3 to 6 hr. *Children*—50 mg/kg daily in 4 to 6 doses. INTRAMUSCULAR: *Adults*—250 to 1000 mg every 6 hr. INTRAVENOUS: *Adults*—100 mg over 5 min as needed.	Effective serum level 4 to 8 μg/ml; serum half-life about 3 hr.
Procainamide sustained release	Procan-SR Pronestyl-SR	ORAL: *Adults*—50 mg/kg/day divided into 4 doses	Absorption is variable and may be extremely low in a few patients
Disopyramide	Norpace*	ORAL: *Adults*—100 to 150 mg every 6 hr.	Effective serum level 2 to 4 μg/ml; serum half-life less than 4 hr; kidneys eliminate 80% of the active drug and metabolites.
Propranolol	Inderal*	ORAL: *Adults*—10 to 80 mg 4 times daily. *Children*—0.5 to 4 mg/kg daily in 4 doses.	Effective serum level is highly variable; serum half-life 2½ to 4 hr; metabolized in the liver.

Antiarrhythmic Drugs

Verapamil	Calan Isoptin	INTRAVENOUS: *Adults*—1 mg each minute up to 10 mg or 0.1 to 0.15 mg/kg administered in increments of 0.5 to 0.75 mg every 1 to 2 minutes with ECG and blood pressure monitoring. *Children*—0.01 to 0.15 mg/kg over 3 to 5 min with ECG and blood pressure monitoring. ORAL: *Adults*—240 to 480 mg daily divided into 3 or 4 doses. INTRAVENOUS: *Adults*—Initially 5 to 10 mg over 2 to 5 min, repeated if necessary at 30 min. Maintenance with 0.005 mg/kg/min. *Infants to 1 yr*—0.1 to 0.2 mg/kg over 2 min, repeated if necessary at 30 min. *Children*—0.1 to 0.3 mg/kg over 2 min., repeated if necessary at 30 min.	Therapeutic serum levels are 0.08 to 0.3 μg/ml; verapamil is extensively metabolized by the liver.

*Available in U.S. and Canada
†Available in Canada only

262   **Pocket Nurse Guide to Drugs**

press cardiac function in patients already suffering a loss of function.

- *Propranolol* may precipitate severe bronchospasm, particularly in patients with asthma or allergies.
- *Disopyramide* should be used cautiously in patients with glaucoma, myasthenia gravis, or urinary retention problems.

Parenteral Administration

Bretylium

- Bretylium may be given undiluted for life-threatening emergencies. For other arrhythmias, dilute the contents of 1 ampule (500 mg) with at least 50 ml of dextrose 5% in water or sodium chloride, and infuse the prescribed dose over at least 8 minutes.

Atropine

- Atropine may be given undiluted but can be diluted in at least 10 ml of sterile water. Do not add to intravenous infusions. It is incompatible with many medications, so do not mix with other medications in a syringe; consult the pharmacy.
- Administer at a rate that does not exceed 0.6 mg per minute.
- If possible, the patient should be attached to a cardiac monitor during intravenous infusion.

Phenytoin

- Use only the diluent supplied by the manufacturer to dilute the powder. Do not add to intravenous infusions or mix with other drugs.
- Do not exceed an intravenous administration rate of 50 mg per minute.
- Flush IV tubing prior to and after administration of the drug with normal saline to avoid mixing the drug with the infusing fluids.
- The patient should be on a cardiac monitor; intravenous administration can cause cardiac arrest.

Antiarrhythmic Drugs 263

Lidocaine

- A 100 mg bolus can be given at a rate of 15 to 50 mg per minute.
- For infusions, add 1 Gm of lidocaine to 1000 ml of 5% dextrose in water (results in a concentration of 1 mg/ml) or add 1 Gm of lidocaine to 500 ml of 5% dextrose in water, giving a concentration of 2 mg/ml.
- A microdrip infusion set and an electronic infusion monitor should be used for constant infusion.
- The patient should be attached to a cardiac monitor.
- The rate of infusion is determined in part by the cardiac response seen on the monitor.
- The blood pressure and pulse should be monitored.
- Emergency drugs and resuscitation equipment should be readily available.

Quinidine

- The oral and intramuscular routes are preferred over the intravenous.
- Dilute 10 ml (800 mg) in 40 to 50 ml of 5% dextrose in water.
- Do not add to intravenous solutions or mix with other drugs in a syringe.
- Administer at a rate not to exceed 1 ml per minute (10 mg).

Procainamide

- Dilute before intravenous administration. For direct infusion, dilute 100 mg with 10 ml of 5% dextrose in water or sterile water for injection. For constant infusion, add 1 Gm to 500 ml 5% dextrose in water.
- Do not mix with other drugs or infusions.
- The rate of infusion should not exceed 25 to 50 mg per minute.
- If being given via infusion, use a microdrip infusion administrations set and an electronic infusion monitor.
- Monitor the blood pressure; if a drop of greater than 15mm Hg occurs, stop the infusion and notify the physician.
- Keep the patient supine.

264   Pocket Nurse Guide to Drugs

Table 17-3   Side effects of antiarrhythmic drugs

Digitalis	Bradycardia, premature ventricular beats, AV nodal tachycardia, anorexia, nausea
Bretylium	Bradycardia, hypotension, precipitation of anginal attacks, anginal pain, diarrhea, rash, flushing, fever, sweating; nausea and vomiting when administered intravenously too rapidly
Atropine	Dry mouth, cycloplegia, mydriasis, fever, urinary retention, confusion, blurred vision, tachycardia; constipation with long-term administration
Phenytoin	Rapid intravenous injection causes severe myocardial toxicity; chronic use produces cerebellar side effects and gingival hyperplasia; high blood levels may cause nausea, dizziness, or drowsiness; hyperglycemia
Lidocaine	Central nervous system effects such as confusion, drowsiness, convulsions, tinnitus, slurred speech, paresthesias, muscle twitching, respiratory depression, hypotension
Quinidine	Peripheral vasodilation, hypotension, paradoxical ventricular tachycardia, decreased cardiac output, cinchonism, allergy, fever, nausea, vomiting, diarrhea, abdominal cramps, hepatitis, hemolytic anemia, thrombocytopenia, agranulocytosis; lupus-like syndrome with long-term use, including arthritis and arthralgias, myalgias, and pericarditis
Procainamide	Hypotension, decreased cardiac output, ventricular tachycardia, lowered resistance to infection, allergy, anorexia, nausea, vomiting, skin rash, fever; gastrointestinal distress; chronic use causes collagen disorders resembling systemic lupus erythematosus, including polyarthralgia, pleuritic pain, and arthritis

Antiarrhythmic Drugs 265

Table 17-3 Side effects of antiarrhythmic drugs—cont'd.

Disopyramide	Anticholinergic effects: dry mouth, constipation, urinary hesitancy or retention, blurred vision; hypoglycemia
Propranolol	Bradycardia, lowered cardiac output; congestive heart failure; bronchospasm in persons with asthma
Verapamil	Hypotension, bradycardia, asystole with intravenous route; gastrointestinal disturbances, lightheadedness, headache, nervousness with oral drug

- The antidote for hypotension is phenylephrine or levarterenol.

Nursing Implications for Antiarrhythmic Drugs

Digitalis

- Digitalis preparations are discussed at length in Chapter 15.

Bretylium

- This drug is usually reserved for patients who do not respond to conventional antiarrhythmia therapy, but may be the first drug used to treat ventricular fibrillation.
- Monitor the vital signs, blood pressure and ECG during therapy. Initially there may be an increase in blood pressure, especially if the patient is also receiving vasopressors, then the blood pressure drops, especially the supine pressure. This is the most common side effect of the drug. If the systolic blood pressure falls below 75, it may be necessary to treat with dopamine or norepinephrine, but monitor the blood pressure closely. Bretylium enhances the vasopressor effects of catcholamines. Keep the patient supine.
- This drug should not be used to treat digitalis-induced arrhythmias because the initial release of norepinephrine caused by the bretylium may aggravate the digitalis toxicity.
- When administered intravenously too rapidly, the drug may

Pocket Nurse Guide to Drugs

cause nausea and vomiting. For this reason, in conscious patients it is preferable to dilute the drug and administer it over at least 8 minutes.

- This drug may be given intramuscularly. No more than 5 ml should be administered in one injection; rotate injection sites.
- There may be a delay in antiarrhythmic action, from several minutes up to hours, although ventricular fibrillation seems to respond very quickly.

Atropine

- Assess pulse and blood pressure after administering.
- With long term administration, constipation may be a problem, but it can often be relieved with dietary modifications.

Phenytoin

- Phenytoin is also discussed in Chapter 7.
- Early signs of toxicity include nystagmus, vertigo, ataxia, nausea, and vomiting. Overdose should be treated symptomatically. Monitor serum levels if available; effective therapeutic blood levels range from 10 to 20 μg/ml.
- Hyperglycemia has been reported. Monitor the blood glucose and urine glucose levels. Adjustment of insulin dosages in diabetics may be necessary.
- The safety of this drug in pregnancy is not known.
- Concomitant use of coumarin anticoagulants, disulfuram, phenylbutazone, sulfaphenazole, antihistamines, chloramphenicol, diazepam, diazoxide, valproate, or isoniazid may increase the risk of phenytoin toxicity. Barbiturates, alcohol, folic acid, and loxapine may enhance the rate of metabolism of phenytoin, resulting in decreased phenytoin activity per dose.
- The intramuscular route should be avoided because of erratic absorption.
- There is an oral suspension available. Shake the suspension thoroughly before pouring the desired dose; instruct patients and families to do the same.

Lidocaine

- Monitor the vital signs and blood pressure. Side effects are much more common in the elderly, and may be prevented by using lower doses.
- Depression of cardiac activity as manifested by prolonged P-R intervals and widened QRS complexes are indications for discontinuing therapy.
- If possible, monitor serum drug levels. Therapeutic plasma levels vary from 1.2 to 5 μg/ml.
- Lidocaine clearance is reduced with concomitant administration of cimetidine or propranolol; this may necessitate decreasing the dose of lidocaine.
- The intravenous route is preferred over the intramuscular route.
- For intramuscular injection: The deltoid is the preferred site.
- Intravascular injection must be avoided; aspirate before injecting any medication and pause during injection to aspirate again several times.
- The patients should be attached to a cardiac monitor.
- Monitor the pulse and blood pressure frequently.
- Emergency drugs and resuscitation equipment should be available. The intramuscular route can result in elevation of the serum creatinine phosphokinase (CPK) levels, thus reducing the value of this diagnostic test in patients who may have myocardial damage.

Quinidine

- A test dose of 1 tablet or 200 mg intramuscularly should always precede full-dose administration to test for idiosyncratic response.
- Instruct the patient to report any fever, sore throat, infection, bleeding, or bruising. Encourage the patient to return for regular follow-up visits with the health care provider.
- When initiating therapy, it is preferable to have the patient on a cardiac monitor. The drug should be discontinued, at least temporarily, if any of the following occur: disappear-

268 Pocket Nurse Guide to Drugs

ance of P waves; widening of the QRS complex by more than 25%; resumption of sinus rhythm; severe side effects.

- Quinidine effectiveness is enhanced by normal potassium levels; the effectiveness is reduced in the presence of hypokalemia. Monitor the serum electrolyte levels.
- Hypotension can be a problem; monitor the blood pressure at regular intervals until the patient's condition is stabilized.
- Taking the drug with meals or food may reduce side effects.
- Elevated serum digoxin levels have been reported in patients taking both quinidine and digoxin. The effect of quinidine on digitoxin levels is not clear.
- Patients taking quinidine as well as phenobarbital, phenytoin, or rifampin may need an increase in quinidine dosage. The action of the coumarin anticoagulants or neuromuscular blocking agents may be enhanced by quinidine.
- Intramuscular injections are painful, increase serum creatinine phosphokinase (CPK) levels, and are erratically and incompletely absorbed.
- Monitor serum drug levels if possible. Therapeutic plasma levels vary with the method used.

Procainamide

- Major side effects include precipitous drop in blood pressure, prolongations of the P-R interval, widening of the QRS, prolongation of the Q-T interval, ventricular tachycardia or fibrillation, and agranulocytosis. Monitor the ECG when initiating therapy and at regular intervals while the patient is on long-term therapy. Teach the patient to report any unexplained fever, sore throat, rash or fatigue.
- Antinuclear antibody titers (ANA titers) should be measured before beginning therapy and at regular intervals.
- Administration of oral doses with meals or food may reduce gastric irritation.
- Concomitant administration of procainamide with cimetidine may result in an altered patient response to the antiarrhythmic. Observe the patient carefully when both drugs are being used.
- Monitor serum drug levels if available. Therapeutic blood

Antiarrhythmic Drugs 269

levels range between 4 and 10 μg/ml, but may occasionally require higher levels.

Disopyramide

- This drug can cause hypotension. Monitor the blood pressure frequently until the dose is established. In the individual with a poorly compensating heart, hypotension may be severe; vasopressors should be readily available.
- If widening of the QRS complex is greater than 25% of the original value or if prolongation of the Q-T interval or first-degree heart block develop, the drug should be discontinued and the patient reevaluated.
- Disopyramide does not increase serum digoxin levels as does quinidine.
- The safe use of this drug in pregnancy has not been established; the drug is excreted in breast milk.
- Concomitant administration with phenytoin may decrease serum levels of disopyramide; observe the patient carefully for an increase in arrythmias.
- An oral suspension can be made (see manufacturer's literature). Store the suspension in the refrigerator; shake thoroughly before preparing the prescribed dose. Instruct patients and families to do the same.
- There are regular and sustained release preparations of this drug. The two are not interchangeable without some adjustment of the dosing frequency. Instruct patients to be alert to the dosage form prescribed, and to take it as ordered.
- Monitor serum drug levels if available. Therapeutic levels are from 2 to 5 μg/ml, or higher for severe arrhythmias.

Propranolol

This drug is discussed in Chapter 13.

Verapamil

This drug is discussed in Chapter 13.

Anticoagulant, Thrombolytic, and Hemostatic Drugs

18

Anticoagulants
  Heparin
  Dicumarol
  (bishydroxycoumarin)
  Phenprocoumon
  Warfarin
  Anisindione
  Phenindione
Thrombolytics
  Streptokinase
  Urokinase

Hemostatic agents
  Systemic agents
    Aminocaproic acid
    Phytonadione (vitamin K_1)
    Menadione (vitamin K_3)
    Menadiol sodium
    diphosphate
    Menadione sodium
    bisulfite
  Local agents
    Absorbable gelatin sponge
    Absorbable gelatin film
    Oxidized cellulose
    Oxidized regenerated
    cellulose
    Microfibrillar collagen
    hemostat
    Thrombin

Anticoagulants

Actions of Anticoagulants

Anticoagulants interfere with any of the stages leading to the formation of fibrin. Heparin activates antithrombin III to neutralize factor Xa and stop coagulation at stage I and prevent thrombin activity at stage III. Oral anticoagulants prevent the synthesis of factors II, VII, IX, and X, which are necessary for stage I, and prevent the synthesis of prothrombin at stage II.

Indications for Anticoagulants

Anticoagulants are used in patients with recent thrombus, immobilized after certain types of surgery, with certain cardiac valve diseases, or on hemodialysis. Heparin is generally used only with inpatients to achieve anticoagulation, to prevent postoperative thromboembolism, and to prevent coagulation of laboratory samples and stored blood. Oral anticoagulants are the choice for outpatient therapy.

Nurse Alert for Anticoagulants

- Blood coagulation studies must be monitored carefully and the dosage titrated; monitor the patient for bleeding and check the stool for occult blood.
- Drug interactions are particularly common with coumarins.
- Caution patients to avoid activities with a high risk of injury.
- Pregnant women and women of childbearing age should be counseled regarding the risks associated with anticoagulants, including birth defects.
- Caution patients against the use of alcohol while taking oral anticoagulants.

Parenteral Administration of Anticoagulants

Intravenous Administration of Heparin

- Check the intravenous catheter frequently to ascertain that it is still in the vein.
- If the heparin is being given via constant infusion, an electronic infusion monitor should be used to regulate the flow. The infusion rate should be checked frequently (at ½- to 1 hour intervals).
- Heparin is incompatible with many other medications. It should be administered via fresh tubing, or the tubing should be flushed before and after administration. Consult with the pharmacy if in doubt.

272 Pocket Nurse Guide to Drugs

Table 18-1 Administration of anticoagulants

Generic Name	Trade Name	Dosage and Administration	Duration
Heparin	Hepathrom, Heprinar, Lipo-Hepin, Liquaemin, Panheprin, Calcilean†	SUBCUTANEOUS: 10,000 to 20,000 units, then 8000 to 10,000 units every 8 hr or 15,000 to 20,000 units every 12 hr. INTRAVENOUS: *Intermittent*—10,000 units, then 5000 to 10,000 units every 4 to 6 hr. *Continuous*—20,000 to 40,000 units daily in 1000 ml. SUBCUTANEOUS: 5000 units 2 hr before surgery, then every 8 to 12 hr until ambulatory.	Duration depends on dose and route of administration, but is on the order of hours.
Heparin and Dihydroergotamine (DHE)	Embolex	Heparin 5000 units and DHE 0.5 mg every 12 hours.	To prevent embolus formation post-surgery, DHE increases venous tone; heparin retards coagulation.
Oral Anticoagulants: Coumarins			
Dicumarol (bishydroxycoumarin)		ORAL: 200 to 300 mg day 1; 25 to 200 mg daily for maintenance.	Half-life is 1 to 2 days. Peak effect in 1 to 4 days.

Anticoagulant, Thrombolytic, and Hemostatic Drugs

(continued) Anticoagulant effect persists 2 to 10 days after discontinuance.

Drug	Brand	Dosage	
Phenprocoumon	Liquamar	ORAL: 24 mg day 1; 0.75 to 6 mg daily for maintenance.	Half-life is 6½ days. Peak effect in 2 to 3 days. Anticoagulant effect persists 4 to 7 days after discontinuance.
Warfarin	Athrombin* Coumadin Panwarfin	ORAL, INTRAMUSCULAR, INTRAVENOUS: 10 to 15 mg daily until prothrombin time is in therapeutic range. 2 to 10 mg daily for maintenance. A loading dose of 40 to 60 mg (20 to 30 mg in the elderly) may be given initially.	Half-life is 2 days. Peak effect in 1 to 3 days. Anticoagulant effect persists 4 to 5 days after discontinuance.
Oral Anticoagulants: Indandiones			
Anisindione	Miradon	ORAL: 300 mg day 1, 200 mg day 2; 100 mg day 3; 25 to 250 mg daily for maintenance.	Half-life is 3 to 5 days. Peak effect in 2 to 3 days. Anticoagulant effect persists 1 to 3 days after discontinuance.
Phenindione	Hedulin Danilone†	ORAL: 300 mg day 1, 200 mg day daily for maintenance.	Half-life is 5 hr. Peak effect in 1 to 2 days. Anticoagulant effect persists 2 to 4 days after discontinuance.

*Available in U.S. and Canada

274   **Pocket Nurse Guide to Drugs**

Parenteral Administration of Warfarin

- Warfarin is available for intravenous or intramuscular use, although this use is much less common than oral administration.
- Diluent is supplied by the manufacturer and makes a solution of 25 mg/ml.
- For intravenous use, give via intravenous injection and do not mix with intravenous fluids. Flush tubing before and after administration.
- Warfarin is compatible with heparin in a syringe but incompatible with many other medications; consult the pharmacy.
- Rate of administration should not exceed 25 mg (1 ml) per minute.

Side Effects of Anticoagulants

The major side effect of *heparin* is hemorrhage; hypersensitivity reactions may include chills, fever, urticaria, asthma, rhinitis, lacrimation, anaphylaxis, alopecia, burning sensation in the feet, myalgias, bone pain, and thrombocytopenia. The *coumarins* may cause hemorrhage, diarrhea, dermatitis, alopecia, and rarely agranulocytosis and elevated serum transaminase. Frequent side effects of the *indandiones* include rashes, depression of bone marrow, hepatitis, and renal damage; less frequent side effects are jaundice, agranulocytosis, dermatitis, and red cell aplasia; alkaline urine has an orange color.

Nursing Implications for Anticoagulants

General

- Teach patients receiving anticoagulants why they are taking the medication, the importance of taking the correct dose as directed, and precautions to observe to avoid bleeding.
- Patients should use electric razors while taking anticoagulants because there is less risk of cutting themselves.
- Teach patients to report any signs of bleeding from any site: nosebleeds, hematuria, bloody or tarry stools, bleeding

Anticoagulant, Thrombolytic, and Hemostatic Drugs 275

gums, change in menstrual flow, excessive bruising, or excessive bleeding from any cut or scratch.

- Patients should not go barefoot.
- Patients should brush their teeth gently, with a soft-bristle brush, and floss gently. Patients may find it necessary to forego flossing while on anticoagulant therapy, and some may even have to give up tooth-brushing because of excessive bleeding from gums. Note that excessive bleeding may indicate over-medication and should be reported.
- Remind patients to keep all health care providers, especially dentists, informed of any medications they are taking.
- Patients should obtain and wear a medical alert bracelet or tag stating their anticoagulant medication.
- Keep in mind the possibility of drug interactions between the anticoagulants and many other drugs, therefore patients should not take any medications without clearance from their physicians. Point out to the patient that this includes even over-the-counter preparations such as aspirin, cold remedies, and cough remedies. Aspirin is of particular danger because of its potent antiplatelet effects.

Heparin

- Many hospitals require that heparin doses be checked by two professionals before administration.
- Blood tests used to monitor heparin therapy include the Lee-White clotting time (desired goal of therapy is 20 minutes or the physician's preference) and the partial thromboplastin time (PTT) or activated PTT (aPTT), the desired goal of therapy being 1½ to 2 times normal.
- It is often customary to obtain the necessary coagulation studies daily or more often when therapy is being initiated. The blood is drawn before a scheduled time of heparin administration, and based on the laboratory results, the heparin dose for that day is determined. Patients on continuous intravenous heparin therapy are usually monitored with at least daily laboratory work. Check for new laboratory results and new heparin orders before each dose of heparin is administered. The physician should always be

Pocket Nurse Guide to Drugs

notified if the level of anticoagulation is not within the therapeutic range.

- Patients on low-dose heparin therapy will have slight, if any, alteration in the clotting time or PTT. Platelet counts need to be monitored to detect thrombocytopenia secondary to heparin therapy. Thrombocytopenia increases the risk of hemorrhage.

- When a patient is on heparin therapy while an oral anticoagulant is begun, it is necessary to monitor the anticoagulant activity resulting from both drugs. In addition to the clotting time and PTT, the prothrombin time (PT or pro time) will be added to the necessary lab work. The PT should be within the therapeutic range before heparin is discontinued.

- Read the label on the heparin carefully because there are many strengths available.

- The antidote for heparin overdose is protamine sulfate, which should be kept available. If anticoagulation is still needed, heparin therapy can be resumed after 24 to 36 hours.

- If possible, intravenous heparin therapy should be discontinued a couple of days before surgery.

- If possible, the intramuscular route of administration for any medications should be avoided during heparin therapy because of the danger of intramuscular bleeding. If absolutely unavoidable, intramuscular injections should be scheduled for times when the coagulation time is the shortest, such as ½ to 1 hour before the next dose of heparin. This is of little concern for patients on low-dose heparin therapy.

- Routine analyses of stool and urine for occult blood may be done on patients receiving heparin.

- In some patients, heparin therapy may cause thrombocytopenia. Monitor the platelet count, in addition to the usual blood studies for monitoring heparin activity. Symptoms of severe thrombocytopenia would be bleeding from the gums, urinary tract, or gastrointestinal tract and bruising; these are the same symptoms seen with heparin overdose.

Oral Anticoagulants

- The anticoagulant activity of the coumarins and indandiones is monitored by using the prothrombin time (PT or pro time), the desired goal being 1½ to 2½ times normal, or when expressed as a percent, 20% to 30% of the normal prothrombin activity.
- Overdose of the coumarins and indandiones is treated with vitamin K_1 phytonadione (Aquamephyton), if further therapy with the anticoagulant is necessary. If immediate and/or partial reversal of hemorrhage is necessary, fresh frozen plasma is transfused.
- Patients taking oral anticoagulants should be instructed not to "double up" if a dose is missed.
- The patient and family should be helped to understand the importance of returning for regular follow-up visits to monitor the anticoagulant activity. Blood work should be done routinely to evaluate the prothrombin time, liver function tests, hemoglobin, white cell count, and platelet count.
- The patient on long-term anticoagulant therapy should wear a necklace or bracelet and have a card available indicating that anticoagulants are being used.

Thrombolytics

    Streptokinase
    Urokinase

Actions of Thrombolytics

Thrombolytic drugs speed the degradation of fibrin in clots by activating profibrinolysin.

Indications for Thrombolytics

Thrombolytic therapy is used in acute care settings to dissolve clots in patients with acute pulmonary embolism, deep vein thrombosis, peripheral arterial occlusion, occluded renal dialysis shunts or catheters, and for lysis of coronary artery thrombi.

Table 18-2 Administration of thrombolytics

Generic Name	Trade Name	Dosage and Administration
Streptokinase	Streptase	Loading dose of 250,000 IU in 30 min, then intravenous infusion of 100,000 IU hr. Dosage is continued for 24 to 72 hr for pulmonary embolism and for 72 hr for deep vein embolism.
Urokinase	Abbokinase	Loading dose of 2000 IU/lb in 10 min by intravenous infusion, then 2000 IU/lb/hr for 12 hr.

Nurse Alert for Thrombolytics

- The patient must be monitored for signs of clot dissolution and switched as soon as possible to heparin therapy.
- The hematocrit should be checked daily.
- Check the patient frequently for signs of bleeding.
- Thrombolytics are contraindicated within 10 days of surgery, following delivery, liver or kidney biopsy, or spinal puncture, and when dissecting aneurysm or active tuberculosis with cavitation is suspected.
- Thrombolytics are contraindicated in pregnancy unless absolutely necessary.

Side Effects of Thrombolytics

Streptokinase frequently causes mild allergic reactions with itching, flushing, nausea, headache, and fever. *Streptokinase* and *urokinase* may both cause bleeding, a more common side effect than with heparin therapy.

Nursing Implications for Thrombolytics

- If bleeding occurs, the drug should be stopped. Red blood cells and plasma volume expanders other than dextran may be given. Aminocaproic acid can be used.

Anticoagulant, Thrombolytic, and Hemostatic Drugs **279**

- A drop in hematocrit will be experienced by 20% to 30% of patients even if clinical bleeding has not occurred.
- Antibodies from a prior streptococcal infection may inactivate the streptokinase. Thus the efficacy of therapy should be checked by a prolonged thrombin time demonstrating fibrin breakdown products. Rarely, in persons having recently recovered from streptococcal infections, the drug may be completely inactivated and urokinase should be used.
- Instructions are supplied by the manufacturer for the correct dose of medication based on the desired dose and the patient's weight. Collaborate with the pharmacy in the use of these drugs.
- The same precautions that would be observed in administering heparin via constant infusion should be observed with either of these drugs.
- After initial treatment with either of these drugs, the patient is then switched to heparin therapy.
- Intramuscular injections of any medication are absolutely contraindicated because of the possibility of intramuscular bleeding. Venipunctures should be minimized, and pressure must be applied to the site for a minimum of 15 minutes.

Hemostatic Agents

Systemic agents
Aminocaproic acid
Phytonadione (vitamin K_1)
Menadione (vitamin K_3)
Menadiol sodium diphosphate
Menadione sodium bisulfite
Local agents
Absorbable gelatin sponge
Absorbable gelatin film
Oxidized cellulose
Oxidized regenerated cellulose
Microfibrillar collagen hemostat
Thrombin

280   Pocket Nurse Guide to Drugs

Table 18-3   Administration of hemostatic agents

Generic Name	Trade Name	Dosage and Administration
Systemic Hemostatic Agents		
Aminocaproic acid	Amicar*	ORAL, INTRAVENOUS: *Adults*—5 to 6 Gm initially orally or by slow intravenous infusion, then 1 Gm hourly or 6 Gm every 6 hr. Maximum in 24 hr is 30 Gm. Reduced dosage is used with low renal output or renal disease. *Children*—100 mg/kg every 6 hr for 6 days.
Phytonadione (vitamin K_1)	Aquamephyton* Konakion* Mephyton	ORAL, INTRAMUSCULAR, SUBCUTANEOUS: *Adults* and *children*—2.5 to 25 mg. INTRAMUSCULAR, SUBCUTANEOUS, INTRAVENOUS: *Newborns*—0.5 to 1 mg immediately after birth. Alternatively the mother is given 1 to 5 mg 12 to 24 hr before delivery.
Menadione (Vitamin K_3)		ORAL, INTRAMUSCULAR: *Adults* and *children*—2 to 10 mg daily.
Menadiol sodium diphosphate	Synkayvite*	ORAL, INTRAMUSCULAR, SUBCUTANEOUS, INTRAVENOUS: *Adults*—5 to 15 mg once or twice daily. *Children*—5 to 10 mg once or twice daily.
Menadione sodium bisulfite		INTRAMUSCULAR, SUBCUTANEOUS, INTRAVENOUS: 2.5 to 10 mg daily.

*Available in U.S. and Canada

Anticoagulant, Thrombolytic, and Hemostatic Drugs **281**

Table 18-3 Administration of hemostatic agents—cont'd.

Generic Name	Trade Name	Dosage and Administration
Local Hemostatic Agents		
Absorbable gelatin sponge	Gelfoam	Blocks and cones of various sizes. Also a sterile (surgical) and nonsterile (dental) powder.
Absorbable gelatin film	Gelfilm	Thin film strips.
Oxidized cellulose	Oxycel	Gauze-type pads or strips. Also as sponges 2 × 1 × 1 inch.
Oxidized regenerated cellulose	Surgicel	Knitted fabric strips.
Microfibrillar collagen hemostat	Avitene	Sterile powder. 1 Gm should cover 50 × 50 cm (20 × 20 inches) to control light bleeding.
Thrombin	Thrombin, Topical	Sterile powder. Packaged by units. May be dissolved in sterile saline solution and applied in absorbable gelatin sponge.

Actions of Hemostatic Agents

Epsilon aminocaproic acid inhibits the activation of profibrinolysin and inhibits the dissolution of blood clots. Vitamin K is used in replacement therapy required for the synthesis of clotting factors, II, VII, IX, and X in the liver. The local absorbable hemostatics provide a surface to promote platelet adhesion and thereby promote blood clotting locally.

Indications for Hemostatic Agents

Hemostatic therapy is used in general for patients in whom the retention or formation of a blood clot is desirable, or who have been overmedicated with an anticoagulant. Aminocaproic acid may be used as an antidote for streptokinase or urokinase overdose or in special surgical situations. Phytonadione is used in emergencies for oral anticoagulant overdose. Menadiol sodium diphosphate is used to correct secondary hypoprothrombinemia. Menadione sodium bisulfite is used to correct severe vitamin K deficiency. Absorbable gelatin sponge, microfibrillar collagen hemostat, and thrombin are used to control bleeding in a wound or at an operative site. Absorbable gelatin film is used to repair membranes in neural, thoracic, and ocular surgery. Oxidized cellulose and oxidized regenerated cellulose are used to control hemorrhage and absorb blood.

Nurse Alert for Hemostatic Agents

- Coagulation studies and hematocrit should be monitored.
- Observe the patient for signs that bleeding is stopping.
- Aminocaproic acid may present risks in pregnancy and should be used cautiously.
- Menadione is contraindicated in newborns, women in advanced pregnancy, and patients with glucose-6-phosphate dehydrogenase deficiency.

Parenteral Administration of Hemostatic Agents

Parenteral Administration of Aminocaproic Acid

- The drug is supplied at a concentration of 1 Gm/4 ml, but should be diluted before administration with normal saline, sterile water, 5% dextrose in water or saline, or lactated Ringer's solution. Dilute until the ordered dose is in a volume of 50 to 100 ml.
- The dose is usually 5 to 6 Gm during the first hour and then 1 Gm per hour afterwards. The patient should be reevaluated after 8 hours of therapy if not before.
- Rapid infusion of the undiluted drug can cause hypotension, bradycardia, or arrhythmias. Monitor the pulse and pressure frequently during administration, and, if possible, have the patient attached to a cardiac monitor.

Intravenous Administration of Vitamin K_1, Phytonadione

- Read the labels carefully; vitamin K_3, menadione (Konakion), is for intramuscular use only.

Anticoagulant, Thrombolytic, and Hemostatic Drugs **283**

- Vitamin K_1, phytonadione (Aquamephyton), should be diluted for intravenous administration with normal saline solution, 5% dextrose in water, or 5% dextrose in normal saline solution only; other diluents should not be used.
- The rate of administration should not exceed 1 mg per minute.
- The intravenous route should be used only in emergencies because severe reactions and fatalities have occurred with this route of administration. Reactions have included anaphylaxis, shock, cardiac arrest, respiratory arrest, and, less seriously, flushing, excessive sweating (hyperhidrosis), and a feeling of chest constriction. Patients should be monitored carefully during and after intravenous administration, including evaluation of vital signs, blood pressure, and electrocardiogram.
- The drug is incompatible with many drugs; check with the pharmacy if in doubt.

Both menadiol diphosphate sodium and menadione bisulfate sodium can be administered intravenously and produce a rapid response via this route, but phytonadione is the preparation of choice. Menadiol phosphate sodium may be given undiluted or added to most intravenous infusions; the rate of administration should not exceed 75 mg per minute. Menadione bisulfate sodium may be given undiluted but should *not* be added to intravenous solutions; the rate of administration should not exceed 2 mg per minute. Both drugs are incompatible with several other drugs; consult the pharmacy. Although severe side effects are less frequent with these preparations than with phytonadione, side effects are still possible, and patients should be monitored carefully.

Side Effects of Hemostatic Agents

Aminocaproic acid may cause minor side effects including nausea, cramps, dizziness, headache, ringing in the ears, or stuffy nose. *Vitamin K* administered intravenously may cause a reaction including flushing, a heavy feeling in the chest, sweating, vascular collapse, and anaphylaxis; intramuscular and subcutaneous administration may cause pain and bleeding at the injection site.

Nursing Implications for Hemostatic Agents

- The daily requirement for vitamin K has not been established but has been estimated at 0.03 μg/kg for adults and 5 μg/kg for children. Although it is not stored in the body for long periods, vitamin K deficiency is rare in adults on the basis of dietary deficiency alone. Dietary sources include tomatoes, green leafy vegetables, meats, dairy products, cereals, and fruits.
- Patients with bile deficiency who are receiving oral phytonadione or menadione need concomitant administration of bile salts for drug absorption.
- Regular determinations of the plasma prothrombin time (PT or pro time) will be made to evaluate the effectiveness of therapy.
- Menadione (K_3) and phytonadione (K_1) are preferred for treatment of hypoprothrombinemia secondary to oral anticoagulant overdose.
- For treatment and prevention of hemorrhagic disease in the newborn, phytonadione is preferred.
- Intramuscular injection of vitamin K_1 or K_3 can cause pain at the injection site, nodule formation, and bleeding from the injection site. In older children and adults, the gluteus maximus is the preferred intramuscular injection site. In infants and small children, the anterolateral aspect of the thigh is preferred.
- Vitamins K_1 and K_3 are light sensitive and should be stored in a dark place. Doses should be administered as soon as prepared and unused portions discarded. If K_1 is being administered via the intravenous route, the tubing and container should be covered with foil or light-resistant paper.
- The concomitant use of red blood cells and fresh frozen plasma may be necessary in cases of frank or severe hemorrhage resulting from excessively prolonged prothrombin times.

Antilipemics

19

Cholestyramine resin
Colestipol hydrochloride
Clofibrate
Gemfibrozil

Niacin (nicotinic acid)
Dextrothyroxine
Probucol

Actions of Antilipemics

Cholestyramine resin and *colestipol* bind bile acids, increasing the amount of fecal bile acid and increasing the excretion of cholesterol. *Clofibrate* and *gemfibrozil* inhibit triglyceride synthesis in the liver; clofibrate also inhibits the breakdown of triglycerides in fat tissue. *Niacin* inhibits the synthesis of very low density lipoproteins in the liver. *Dextrothyroxine* increases the degradation of low density lipoproteins and thereby lowers plasma cholesterol levels. *Probucol* lowers cholesterol probably by inhibiting cholesterol biosynthesis in the liver.

Indications for Antilipemics

The antilipemics may be used to treat the different types of hyperlipidemia by reducing blood lipid concentrations, although this decrease has not been shown to reverse or halt atherosclerosis already present. *Cholestyramine* and *colestipol* are used for type II hyperlipidemia. *Clofibrate* is used to treat types III, IV, and V hyperlipidemia, and type II if the level of very low density lipoproteins is elevated. *Niacin* is used for types II, III, IV, and V hyperlipidemia. *Dextrothyroxine* and *probucol* are used for type II hyperlipidemia.

285

Pocket Nurse Guide to Drugs

Table 19-1   Administration of antilipemics

Generic Name	Trade Name	Dosage and Administration
Cholestyramine resin	Questran†	ORAL: *Adults*—4 Gm 4 times daily (at meals and bedtime). May be increased to 6 Gm 4 times daily. Alternatively, the dosage may be divided into 2 or 3 doses. Material must be mixed with a liquid (1 oz for each gram). *Children*—over 6 yr, 8 Gm twice daily with meals. Total maximum dosage, 24 Gm daily.
Colestipol hydrochloride	Colestid	ORAL: *Adults*—15 to 30 Gm daily in 2 to 4 doses with meals. Mix 1 oz liquid with each 4 to 6 Gm. *Children*—not established.
Clofibrate	Atromid-S†	ORAL: *Adults*—500 mg 3 to 4 times daily.
Gemfibrozil	Lopid†	ORAL: *Adults*—600 mg twice daily, 30 minutes before meals.
Niacin (nicotinic acid)	Nicobid* Niac* Nicolar Wampocap	ORAL: *Adults*—initially 100 mg 3 times daily, increasing to a total of 2 to 6 Gm daily in divided doses with or after meals.
Dextrothyroxine	Choloxin†	ORAL: *Adults*—with normal thyroid function, initially, 1 to 2 mg daily. May be increased monthly by 1 to 2 mg to a maximum of 8 mg daily (4 mg daily maximum in patients taking digitalis). *Children*—initially, 0.05 mg/kg body weight. May be increased monthly by 0.05 mg/kg to a maximum daily dose of 4 mg.

†Available in U.S. and Canada
*Time-released forms.

Table 19-1 Administration of antilipemics—cont'd.

Generic Name	Trade Name	Dosage and Administration
Probucol	Lorelco†	ORAL: *Adults*—500 mg twice daily (with breakfast and dinner). *Children*—not established.

†Available in U.S. and Canada
*Time-released forms.

Nurse Alert for Antilipemics

- Clofibrate is contraindicated in pregnancy or lactation; the other antilipemics should be used with caution in pregnancy to prevent birth defects, and in lactation.
- Clofibrate and gemfibrozil should be used with caution in patients with liver or kidney disease.
- Dextrothyroxine is contraindicated in pregnancy and in patients with hypertension, heart, renal, or liver disease.
- Gemfibrozil is contraindicated in patients with pre-existing gall bladder disease.

Side Effects of Antilipemics

Cholestyramine resin and *colestipol* may cause bloating, nausea, and constipation at the start of therapy and interference with the absorption of fat-soluble vitamins, digitalis, thyroxine, and coumarin anticoagulants. *Clofibrate* and *gemfibrozil* commonly cause abdominal distress, flatulence, loose stools, muscle cramps, headache, fatigue, and urticaria; less common side effects include alopecia, increased or decreased incidence of angina, cardiac arrhythmias, impotence and decreased libido, proteinuria, and alterations in blood values. *Niacin* commonly causes flushing, itching, and gastrointestinal upset and may cause or aggrevate peptic ulcer, glucose intolerance, and gout. *Dextrothyroxine* may cause dizziness, diarrhea, altered taste sense, weight loss, nervousness, insomnia, sweating, menstrual irregularities, hypersensitivity marked by itching or rash, and may aggravate angina. *Probucol* may cause diarrhea, gas, abdominal pain, nausea, and vomiting.

288 **Pocket Nurse Guide to Drugs**

Nursing Implications for Antilipemics

- Patients requiring diet modification will probably benefit from referral to a dietitian.
- If patient noncompliance with dietary restriction occurs, be nonjudgmental and continue to individualize the health care teaching and patient approaches.
- In hereditary hyperlipidemia, it will be necessary to screen children for the presence of the hyperlipidemia and to place them on special diets also.
- Many of the drugs used to lower blood lipid levels need to be taken for 3 months or more before effects can be seen. Drugs should not be continued indefinitely if there is no positive response to them.
- If a drug does produce a desired effect in lowering blood lipid levels, it is important that the patient understand that it may be necessary to continue treatment for years.

Cholestyramine and Colestipol

- These two drugs should be taken before meals. Oral administration of cholestyramine or colestipol:
  a. Neither drug should be taken in its dry form. Always mix with fluid or with food or fruit having a high fluid content.
  b. Fill a glass with 4 to 6 ounces of water, milk, or juice. Put the correct dose of medication on top of the fluid and let it stand, without stirring, for 1 to 2 minutes. This allows the medicine to absorb moisture and will help prevent lumps. Stir and drink the mixture while the drug is still suspended. Add a little more of the selected beverage to rinse the glass, and drink this also.
  c. Applesauce, crushed pineapple, and soups with high fluid content may also be used.
  d. Carbonated beverages may be used, but the addition of the medication will cause excessive foaming initially, so a large glass should be used.
- Because these two drugs interfere with absorption of the fat-soluble vitamins, supplemental vitamins may be necessary. Vitamin K deficiency would be manifested by a tendency to bleed.

Because cholestyramine or colestipol may absorb other drugs given with them, other medications that the patient receives should be given 1 hour before or 4 to 6 hours after but not at the same time as cholestyramine or cholestipol. If therapeutic dosage levels for a drug have been determined while a patient was receiving cholestyramine or colestipol and the antilipemic drug is then discontinued, the dose of the other medication may then be too high. This has occurred with digitalis preparations and oral anticoagulants.

If constipation is a chronic problem, dietary manipulation may help, or a stool softener can be prescribed. It may be necessary to reduce the dose of the antilipemic drug.

These two drugs may be prescribed to treat the pruritus of biliary stasis. When the drug is discontinued, the pruritus may reappear.

Clofibrate and Gemfibrozil

Long-term follow-up of the effects of these drugs includes careful questioning about side effects and blood analysis, urinalysis, and cardiac assessment.

The patient with chest pain may have elevated serum transaminase levels because of chronic clofibrate use, myocardial damage, or both.

Caution must be used in titrating the dose of other drugs, which may be displaced from albumin binding sites by clofibrate or gemfibrozil. A specific example is coumarin.

Displacement of tolbutamide may result in more frequent episodes of hypoglycemia.

Niacin Preparations

Some patients will find that taking niacin preparations with meals or in a sustained-release form will decrease the severity of side effects.

Patients taking beta adrenergic antagonists such as propranolol (Inderal) for hypertension may have an increased incidence of hypotensive episodes when niacin is added to their medications.

Many patients with type III, IV, and V hyperlipidemias already suffer from gout or diabetes and will be unable to

290   **Pocket Nurse Guide to Drugs**

tolerate aggravation of these diseases by the niacin preparations.

- Nicotinamide (niacinamide), the niacin component of many multivitamin preparations, does not produce the characteristic blushing (vasodilation) seen with other niacin formulations. Nicotinamide does not lower plasma cholesterol levels, so this preparation is useful only in vitamin replacement or in treatment of pellagra, a disease caused specifically by niacin deficiency.
- Preparations are available for intramuscular and intravenous administration, although oral administration is the usual route. Intravenous nicotinic acid may be given undiluted or diluted in sodium chloride. The rate of administration should not exceed 2 mg per minute.

Dextrothyroxine

- Treatment with dextrothyroxine mimics treatment with any thyroid medication. Overdose would result in symptoms of hyperthyroidism. The necessary dose of anticoagulant is usually less in patients receiving this drug, and diabetics will often find it necessary to readjust their insulin dosage.
- Note that patients taking digitalis preparations concomitantly with dextrothyroxine are particularly susceptible to cardiac side effects. The patient receiving digitalis should not exceed a total dose of 4 mg of dextrothyroxine. The effects of both drugs should be monitored carefully (Chapters 15 and 19).

Probucol

- Absorption of probucol is increased if the drug is taken with meals.
- So far there have been no reported drug interactions with anticoagulants or hypoglycemic agents in patients also receiving probucol.

Drugs to Treat Nutritional Anemias

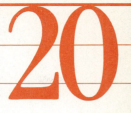

Iron deficiency anemia
   Ferrous sulfate
   Ferrous gluconate
   Ferrocholinate
   Ferrous fumarate
   Ferroglycine sulfate
   Iron-dextran

Antidote for iron toxicity
   Deferoxamine mesylate
Megaloblastic macrocytic anemias
   Vitamin B_{12} (cyanocobalamin)
   Hydroxocobalamin
   Folic acid
   Leucovorin calcium

Iron Deficiency Anemia

Actions of Drugs for Iron Deficiency Anemias

Iron in dietary or replacement sources is an essential component of hemoglobin, necessary to carry oxygen, and of myoglobin, the oxygen-carrying protein of muscle. Deferoxamine combines with iron in the plasma to form a complex that is excreted.

Indications for Drugs for Iron Deficiency Anemias

Iron preparations are generally used for replacement therapy in iron deficiency anemias, which may result from blood loss or rapid growth as in pregnancy and childhood and adolescence. Iron-dextran injections are reserved for use in severe iron deficiency anemias when oral iron is contraindicated or unsuccessful. Deferoxamine is used to manage acute iron intoxication or administered long term to manage secondary hemochromatosis.

Table 20-1 Administration of drugs for iron deficiency anemias

Generic Name	Trade Name	Dosage and Administration
Iron Salts for Iron Deficiency Anemia		
Ferrous sulfate (20% elemental iron)	Feosol Fer-In-Sol* Fero-Gradumet Mol-Iron	Replacement therapy requires 90 to 300 mg of elemental iron daily in divided doses before meals if tolerated or with meals.
Ferrous gluconate (11.6% elemental iron)	Fergon* Ferralet Plus Entron	See above.
Ferrocholinate (12% elemental iron)	Chel-Iron Ferrolip Plus Kelex	See above.
Ferrous fumarate (33% elemental iron)	Ferranol Fumerin Feostat Various others	See above.
Ferroglycine sulfate (16% elemental iron)	Ferronord	See above.

Iron-dextran injection	Imferon	INTRAVENOUS: *Adults and children*—no more than 100 mg daily, no faster than 50 mg (1 ml) per minute of the undiluted solution, or dilute in 500 to 1000 ml normal saline solution and administer by drip over 10 hr.

Antidote for Iron Toxicity

Deferoxamine mesylate	Desferal* Mesylate	INTRAMUSCULAR: preferred route; 1 Gm followed by 0.5 Gm at 4 hr and 8 hr. INTRAVENOUS: in face of cardiovascular collapse; as for intramuscular but infused at 15 mg kg/hr. Not to exceed 6 Gm in 24 hr.

*Available in U.S. and Canada

Nurse Alert for Drugs for Iron Deficiency Anemias

- Iron toxicity causes acute nausea and vomiting, metabolic acidosis and cardiovascular collapse, and eventually tissue injury and death if untreated.
- Chronic iron toxicity from overload may occur with parenteral iron or frequent blood transfusions, resulting in a bronze skin color, diabetes mellitus, liver damage, and heart failure and death if untreated.
- To decrease the risk of anaphylaxis, give a small test dose the first day with full strength doses to begin the next day; appropriate medications and resuscitation equipment should be available when iron is administered parenterally.
- Oral iron is contraindicated with gastrointestinal disease.

Side Effects of Drugs for Iron Deficiency Anemias

Oral iron preparations may cause gastrointestinal irritation if taken on an empty stomach. The regular use of iron preparations may cause either diarrhea or constipation. Parenteral iron may cause allergic or anaphylactic reactions, arthralgias, myalgia, headache, transitory paresthesia, nausea, shivering, rash, and pain at the injection site. Intravenous iron may cause flushing, hypotension, and phlebitis. Deferoxamine will turn the urine pink or red.

Nursing Implications for Drugs for Iron Deficiency Anemias

- Iron preparations should be taken on an empty stomach. If the drug cannot be taken on an empty stomach due to gastrointestinal irritation, then the patient may be advised to take the drug with meals. Absorption is significantly reduced in the presence of milk, antacids, tetracycline, many cereals, and eggs. Since the absorption is increased with the ingestion of ascorbic acid (vitamin C), some patients may wish to take the iron with orange or another citrus juice.
- Inform the patient that the color and consistency of feces may change during iron therapy. Feces will be dark green or black in color and more tarry in consistency than usual. If

Drugs to Treat Nutritional Anemias   295

there is doubt about whether the cause of a change in color or consistency in stools is due to blood or to ingestion of iron, the stool should be tested for blood.

- Decreasing the dose of iron while increasing the frequency of taking the iron may decrease the incidence or severity of side effects.

- Liquid iron preparations may stain the teeth so should be taken through a straw. Dilute the preparation well with water or fruit juice (see the individual manufacturer's suggestions), and rinse the mouth out well after taking the dose.

- Intramuscular iron dextran: These preparations should only be administered in the large muscle mass of the buttocks to avoid possible staining of the skin in more frequently visible areas. The following method of administration is suggested to help reduce the possibility of staining. After drawing up the ordered dose, add 0.1 ml of air to the syringe. Discard the needle used to draw up the medication and obtain a new one. Use the Z-tract method of intramuscular administration, and inject all of the medication and the 0.1 ml of air, the desired effect of the air being to flush any remaining medication out of the needle; then withdraw the needle.

- After an initial test dose, intravenous iron should be injected slowly via direct intravenous push at a rate not to exceed 1 ml (50 mg) per minute.

- Parenteral iron preparations should not be used concurrently with oral preparations, as the incidence of toxic reactions to the parenteral forms is increased in this situation.

- Review with the patient the dietary history and instruct as appropriate about modifications that could be made to increase the intake of iron-rich foods.

- Remind patients to keep iron preparations and all drugs out of the reach of children. Instruct patients about the signs and symptoms of acute iron overdose and emphasize the importance of seeking prompt medical attention if overdose is suspected.

- The intramuscular route is preferred for deferoxamine, although it may cause pain at the injection site. If administered intravenously, the rate of administration

should not exceed 15 mg/kg/per hour. Monitor the vital signs.
- Treatment of iron overdose should be done in the acute care setting where equipment and personnel are available for appropriate monitoring of cardiovascular functioning and treatment of possible circulatory collapse.

Megaloblastic Macrocytic Anemias

Vitamin B_{12} (cyanocobalamin)
Hydroxocobalamin
Folic acid
Leucovorin calcium

Actions of Drugs for Megaloblastic Macrocytic Anemias

Vitamin B_{12} and folic acid in dietary or replacement sources are needed in the synthesis of thymidylate, a component of DNA; deficiency results in release of red blood cells which are large and immature (macrocytic, megaloblastic).

Indications for Drugs for Megaloblastic Macrocytic Anemias

Vitamin B_{12} in intramuscular injections is used for pernicious anemia, not as a general tonic for the elderly, for neurological disorders, general malnutrition, or loss of appetite. Folic acid preparations are used in replacement therapy for folic acid deficiency for individuals with poor diets, chronic alcoholics, pregnant women, and nursing mothers. Leucovorin is used to protect normal tissue when given with methotrexate or pyramethamine.

Nurse Alert for Drugs for Megaloblastic Macrocytic Anemias

- With vitamin B_{12} observe the patient carefully after first doses, monitoring vital signs after parenteral administration.

Drugs to Treat Nutritional Anemias **297**

Table 20-2 Administration of drugs for megaloblastic macrocytic anemias

Generic Name	Trade Name	Dosage and Administration
Vitamin B$_{12}$ (Cyanocobalamin) for Pernicious Anemia		
Vitamin B$_{12}$ (cyanocobalamin)	Betalin 12 Crystalline Redisol Rubramin PC Sytobex	INTRAMUSCULAR: 30 to 50 μg daily for 5 to 10 days, then 100 to 200 μg monthly.
Hydroxocobalamin	AlphaRedisol	As for cyanocobalamin.
Folic Acid for Anemia		
Folic acid	Folvite	ANY ROUTE: *Adults or children*—1 mg daily.
Leucovorin calcium	Leucovorin Calcium	For megaloblastic anemia: 1 mg daily. To counter folic acid antagonists: give in amounts equal to the weight of antagonist.

■ To test for reactions it may be appropriate to use a small test dose the day before the first full dose is administered.

Side Effects of Drugs for Megaloblastic Macrocytic Anemias

Vitamin B$_{12}$ injections are virtually free of side effects; rare side effects include diarrhea, itching, a feeling of swelling throughout the body, pulmonary edema, congestive heart failure, and anaphylactic shock. Folic acid is nontoxic and has no significant side effects.

Nursing Implications for Drugs for Megaloblastic Macrocytic Anemias

■ Patients with pernicious anemia need to be taught about the disease.
■ Cyanocobalamin should never be given intravenously.

Pocket Nurse Guide to Drugs

- In those rare cases in which vitamin B_{12} deficiency is due to dietary causes, review the diet with the patient and instruct the patient about possible sources of the vitamin from the diet.
- Review with patients their usual dietary intake, and instruct as needed about sources of folic acid.
- Leucovorin should be reconstituted as directed on the vial. Use the reconstituted solution as soon as possible; precipitation may occur if it is left standing.

PART IV

GASTRO-INTESTINAL SYSTEM DRUGS

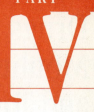

Drugs Affecting Motility and Tone

21

Drugs to increase tone and motility
    Bethanechol chloride
    Metoclopramide
    Neostigmine methylsulfate
Anticholinergic and
antispasmodic drugs
to decrease motility
    Atropine
    Belladonna extract, leaf,
    tincture
    Hyoscyamine hydrobromide
    Hyoscyamine sulfate
    Homatropine methylbromide
    Methscopolamine bromide
    Anisotropine methylbromide

Clidinium bromide
Diphemanil methylsulfate
Glycopyrrolate
Hexocyclium methylsulfate
Isopropamide iodide
Mepenzolate bromide
Methantheline bromide
Oxyphenonium bromide
Oxyphencyclimine
hydrochloride
Propantheline bromide
Tridihexethyl chloride
Dicyclomine hydrochloride
Methixene hydrochloride
Thiphenamil hydrochloride

Actions of Drugs Affecting Tone and Motility

Of the drugs to *increase* motility and tone, the cholinomimetic drugs bethanechol and neostigmine act on the parasympathetic nervous system by muscarinic stimulation. Metoclopramide is a dopamine antagonist that stimulates the motility of the upper gastrointestinal tract without stimulating gastric, biliary, or pancreatic secretions.

Of the drugs to *decrease* tone and motility, the anticholinergic drugs block muscarinic receptors and inhibit gastric acid secretion and depress motility, and the antispasmodic drugs relax the smooth muscle of the gastrointestinal tract without anticholinergic effects.

Indications for Drugs Affecting Motility and Tone

Drugs to *increase* tone and motility are generally indicated to stimulate an atonic intestine or bladder. Metoclopramide is used to treat diabetic gastroparesis to increase gastric emptying; also to facilitate intubation of the small intestine for biopsy, and to stimulate gastric emptying and intestinal transit of barium in radiologic examinations.

The anticholinergic drugs to *decrease* tone and motility are generally indicated for peptic ulcer and hyperactive bowel disorders, to reduce gastrointestinal motility and gastric acid secretion. Diphemanil methylsulfate also aids in controlling excessive sweating. Oxyphencyclimine hydrochloride and propantheline bromide also reduce motility in the genitourinary and biliary tracts. The antispasmodic drugs control hypermotility but not gastric secretion.

Nurse Alert for Drugs Affecting Motility and Tone

- *Bethanechol* is contraindicated in cases of mechanical obstruction of the gastrointestinal or urinary tracts because of the danger of rupture following induced hypermotility.
- *Bethanechol* and *neostigmine* should be used with caution in patients with epilepsy, Parkinson's disease, bradycardia, ulcer, heart disease, or pregnancy.
- *Metoclopramide* is contraindicated for patients receiving thioxanthene, phenothiazene, or butyrophenone compounds, or within two weeks of tricyclic antidepressants, adrenergic agents, or MAO inhibitors; for patients with mechanical obstruction, perforation, or possible hemorrhage; and for patients with pheochromocytoma, epilepsy, or extrapyramidal symptoms. Caution patients on metoclopramide to avoid use of alcohol, tranquilizers, sleeping medications and narcotic analgesis and to avoid activities requiring mental alertness until individual effects are established.
- *Anticholinergic* and *antispasmodic* drugs are contraindicated in patients with myasthenia gravis, tachycardia, or a history of heart disease with tachycardia. Use with caution

Text continued on p. 307

Table 21-1 Administration of drugs affecting motility and tone

Generic Name	Trade Name	Dosage and Administration
Drugs to Increase Tone and Motility		
Bethanechol chloride	Urecholine* Duvoid Myotonachol	ORAL: *Adults*—10 to 30 mg every 6 to 8 hr. SUBCUTANEOUS: *Adults*—2.5 to 5 mg every 6 to 8 hr; maximum, 10 mg/day. Never give IV or IM Onset: 30 min.
Metoclopramide	Reglan	INTRAVENOUS: *Adults*—10 mg injected over one to two min. *Children* under 6 yr: 0.1 mg/kg. *Children* 6-14 yrs: 2.5 to 5 mg. ORAL: *Adults*—10 mg 4 times daily, 30 min before bedtime. *Children* under 6 yr: 0.1 mg/kg as a single dose. *Children* 6-16: 0.5 mg/kg daily in 3 divided doses.
Neostigmine methylsulfate	Prostigmin Methylsulfate*	SUBCUTANEOUS, INTRAMUSCULAR: *Adults*—0.25 to 0.5 mg every 3 to 4 hr to stimulate bladder or gastrointestinal tract. Onset: 10 to 20 min.
Anticholinergic Drugs—Antispasmodic Drugs: to Decrease Tone and Motility		
Belladonna Alkaloids (Uncharged)		
Atropine sulfate		ORAL, SUBCUTANEOUS: *Adults*—0.3 to 1.2 mg every 4 to 6 hr. SUBCUTANEOUS: *Children*—0.01 mg/kg every 4 to 6 hr.

Belladonna extract		ORAL: *Adults*—15 mg every 8 hr.
Belladonna fluid extract		ORAL: *Adults*—0.06 ml every 8 hr.
Belladonna leaf		ORAL: *Adults*—30 to 200 mg.
Belladonna tincture		ORAL: *Adults*—0.6 to 1 ml every 6 to 8 hr. *Children*—0.03 ml/kg in 3 or 4 divided doses.
Hyoscyamine hydrobromide (L-isomer of atropine)		ORAL, INTRAMUSCULAR, SUBCUTANEOUS, INTRAVENOUS: *Adults*—0.25 mg every 6 to 8 hr.
Hyoscyamine sulfate	Anaspaz Levsin	ORAL: *Adults*—0.125 to 0.25 mg every 4 to 6 hr. *Children*—2 to 10 yr, ½ adult dosage; under 2 yr, ¼ adult dosage. INTRAMUSCULAR, SUBCUTANEOUS, INTRAVENOUS: *Adults*—0.25 to 0.5 mg every 4 to 6 hr.

Charged Derivatives of Atropine

Homatropine methylbromide	Sed-Tensse	ORAL: *Adults*—2.5 to 10 mg every 6 hr. *Children*—3 to 6 mg every 6 hr. *Infants*—0.3 mg dissolved in water every 4 hr.
Methscopolamine bromide	Pamine	ORAL: *Adults*—2.5 to 5 mg every 6 hr. *Children*—0.2 mg/kg every 6 hr. INTRAMUSCULAR, SUBCUTANEOUS: *Adults*—0.25 to 1 mg every 6 to 8 hr. Onset: 1 hr.

cont'd. next page

*Available in U.S. and Canada
†Available in Canada only

Table 21-1 Administration of drugs affecting motility and tone—cont'd.

Generic Name	Trade Name	Dosage and Administration
Synthetic Substitutes for Atropine		
Anisotropine methylbromide	Valpin	ORAL: *Adults*—50 mg 3 times daily. Onset: 1 hr.
Clidinium bromide	Quarzan	ORAL: *Adults*—2.5 to 5 mg 3 or 4 times daily before meals and at bedtime. Reduce dosage to 2.5 mg 3 times daily before meals for *elderly* patients.
Diphemanil methylsulfate	Prantal	ORAL: 100 to 200 mg every 4 to 6 hr initially, then 50 to 100 mg every 4 to 6 hr for maintenance. Onset: 1 to 2 hr. Timed-release, 100 to 200 mg every 8 hr.
Glycopyrrolate	Robinul*	ORAL: 1 to 2 mg 3 times daily initially, then 1 to 2 mg 2 times daily for maintenance. Onset: 1 hr. INTRAMUSCULAR, SUBCUTANEOUS, INTRAVENOUS: 0.1 to 0.2 mg every 4 hr. Onset: 10 min.
Hexocyclium methylsulfate	TRAL	ORAL: *Adults*—25 mg 4 times daily before meals and at bedtime. May be taken twice daily in combined release capsules.
Isopropamide iodide	Darbid*	ORAL: *Adults* and *children* over 12 yrs—5 mg every 12 hr, may increase to 10 mg every 12 hrs for severe symptoms.

Generic name	Trade name	Dosage
Mepenzolate bromide	Cantil*	ORAL: *Adults*—25 mg 4 times daily. Increase to 50 mg if necessary.
Methantheline bromide	Banthine	ORAL: *Adults*—50 to 100 mg every 6 hr initially; reduce by ½ for maintenance. *Children*—6 mg/kg daily in 4 doses. Onset: 30 min. INTRAMUSCULAR: *Adults*—50 mg every 6 hr. *Children*—6 mg/kg daily in 4 doses. Onset: 30 min.
Oxyphenonium bromide	Antrenyl	ORAL: *Adults*—10 mg 4 times daily. Use 5 mg for *elderly* patients.
Oxyphencyclimine hydrochloride	Daricon*	ORAL: 10 mg 2 times daily; can be increased to 50 mg if tolerated.
Propantheline bromide	Banlin† Pro-Banthine* Propanthel*	ORAL: *Adults*—15 mg 3 times daily plus 30 mg at bedtime or 30 mg timed-release every 8 to 12 hr. *Children*—1.5 mg/kg daily every 6 hr. INTRAMUSCULAR OR INTRAVENOUS: *Adults*—30 mg every 6 hr.
Tridihexethylchloride	Pathilon	ORAL: 25 mg 3 times daily before meals and 50 mg at bedtime. Timed-release, 75 mg every 6 to 12 hr. INTRAMUSCULAR, SUBCUTANEOUS, INTRAVENOUS: *Adults*—10 to 20 mg every 6 hr.

cont'd. next page

*Available in U.S. and Canada
†Available in Canada only

Table 21-1 Administration of drugs affecting motility and tone—cont'd.

Generic Name	Trade Name	Dosage and Administration
Antispasmodic Drugs		
Dicyclomine hydrochloride	Antispas Bentyl Bentylol†	ORAL OR INTRAMUSCULAR: *Adults*—10 to 20 mg 3 or 4 times daily. *Children*—10 mg 3 or 4 times daily. *Infants*—5 mg 3 or 4 times daily.
Methixene hydrocloride	Trest*	ORAL: 1 mg 2 to 3 times daily.
Thiphenamil hydrochloride	Trocinate	ORAL: *Adults*—400 mg every 4 hr. *Children*—over 6 yr, 200 mg every 4 hr.

*Available in U.S. and Canada
†Available in Canada only

Drugs Affecting Motility and Tone **307**

in pregnancy, prostatic hypertrophy, pyloric obstruction, obstruction of the bladder neck, or severe cardiac disease.
- Caution patients to avoid activities requiring mental alertness until effects are established. Caution patients that perspiration is inhibited and heatstroke or heat exhaustion is more likely with strenuous activity at high temperatures.

Side Effects of Drugs Affecting Motility and Tone

Bethanechol may cause salivation, flushing, sweating, diarrhea, nausea, belching, and abdominal cramps. *Metoclopramide* may produce restlessness, drowsiness, fatigue, lassitude, constipation, diarrhea, rashes, anxiety, dry mouth, swelling around mouth or eyes, and hirsutism.

Anticholinergic drugs may cause dry mouth, photophobia and dilated pupils, blurred vision, tachycardia, constipation, and acute urinary retention; in toxic doses, atropine and oxyphencyclamine may cause CNS stimulation including restlessness, tremor, irritability, delirium, or hallucinations. Side effects of the *antispasmodics* include constipation or diarrhea, rash, euphoria, dizziness, drowsiness, headache, nausea, and weakness.

Nursing Implications for Bethanechol and Neostigmine

- Atropine sulfate (0.5 to 1.0 mg) should be on hand to counteract excessive cholinergic side effects in patients receiving bethanechol or neostigmine subcutaneously for an atonic bladder or gastrointestinal tract.
- Check dosages carefully. The oral dose of bethanechol may be as high as 50 mg, whereas the subcutaneous dose should not exceed 5 mg.
- Oral doses of bethanechol should be taken when the stomach is empty; if taken with meals or just after eating, nausea and vomiting may occur.
- Patients receiving subcutaneous bethanechol, especially the first dose, should not be left unattended for the first 10 minutes. The drug acts very rapidly, with results apparent in 5 to 15 minutes and if serious side effects are going to occur, they usually will do so within minutes.

308 **Pocket Nurse Guide to Drugs**

- In selected situations, the physician may order a test dose of one-half or less of the desired dose to monitor the patient's response. Monitor the blood pressure and pulse.
- Check the pulse before administering neostigmine. Notify the physician if the rate is below 80, and withhold the dose pending physician approval.

Nursing Implications for Metoclopramide

- Rarely, the drug will produce extrapyramidal reactions, especially in children and the elderly, and usually after long-term use. These reactions include Parkinsonism, dystonic movements, and tardive dyskinesia. While most side effects disappear when the medication is discontinued, tardive dyskinesia may not. Instruct the patient and family to report any unusual side effects, especially protrusion of the tongue, puffing of the cheeks, chewing movements, involuntary movements of the extremities or trunk. Diphenhydramine hydrochloride may be used to treat extrapyramidal reactions.

Nursing Implications for Anticholinergics and Antispasmodics

- Anticholinergic drugs may precipitate an attack of acute angle-closure glaucoma, although this is more common with parenteral forms. Patients with open-angle glaucoma who have their glaucoma under control with miotics can safely take anticholinergics.
- These drugs are usually taken before meals and at bedtime unless a timed-release form is being used.
- These medications should not be taken at the same time antacids are taken, because the antacid will slow absorption of the other drug.
- Urinary retention can occur occasionally, although this is more common in men with preexisting prostatic hypertrophy. Instruct the patient to report inability to void, increasing difficulty in initiating urination, or feelings of incomplete bladder emptying. It may help to instruct the patient to void at the time a dose is taken. In the hospital, monitor the fluid intake and output.

Drugs Affecting Motility and Tone   309

- Constipation often occurs, especially with long-term use. Instruct the patient to increase the daily fluid intake to at least 3000 ml and to add to the diet more roughage and fiber, if allowed. Increasing the level of activity may also help. If diarrhea occurs, it may indicate incomplete obstruction of the gastrointestinal tract and should be investigated. Instruct the patient to keep a record of bowel movements so that constipation, if it occurs, can be treated before becoming too severe. The patient should consult the physician if a bowel movement has not occurred in 3 days. Instruct the patient not to take cathartics or other aids to defecation without consulting the physician, since these drugs may be contraindicated in diseases that require anticholinergic therapy.
- Chewing gum, sucking on hard candies or commercially prepared saliva substitutes may help relieve a dry mouth. Consult the physician.
- Because side effects almost always occur at therapeutic doses, patient compliance may be poor and will need reinforcing.
- If a combination drug has been prescribed for the patient, review the side effects of each of the component parts of the combination with the patient.
- Neostigmine is used to treat overdose with any of these medications.
- Tincture of belladonna may be prescribed by the number of drops. Dilute the dose in 15 to 30 ml of water before administering to ensure that the patient receives the entire dose.

Drugs to Treat Ulcers

22

Antacids
   Aluminum carbonate
   Aluminum hydroxide gel
   Dihydroxyaluminum
   aminoacetate
   Dihydroxyaluminum sodium
   carbonate
   Calcium carbonate
   Magaldrate
   (hydroxymagnesium
   aluminate)
   Magnesium carbonate
   Magnesium hydroxide
   Magnesium oxide
   Magnesium phosphate
   Magnesium trisilicate

H_2 receptor antagonists
   Cimetidine
   Cimetidine hydrochloride
   Ranitidine
Agent to coat ulcer crater
   Sucralfate
See also anticholinergic drugs
(Ch. 23).

Actions of Drugs to Treat Ulcers

Antacids are weak bases that neutralize the hydrochloric acid secreted by the stomach. *Anticholinergic* drugs taken before eating depress the secretion of acid that occurs on eating. The *H_2 receptor antagonists* cimetidine and ranitidine act to block the secretion of hydrochloric acid by the parietal cells. *Sucralfate* binds to proteins in ulcerated tissue and thus protects the ulcer from the destructive action of the digestive enzyme pepsin.

Indications of Drugs to Treat Ulcers

Of the *antacids*, sodium bicarbonate is generally used only for short-term therapy; nonsystemic antacids are most effective when taken on an hourly or regular basis to neutralize gastric

310

acid. *Cimetidine* and *ranitidine* are used for stomach and duodenal ulcers and for various other conditions in which stomach acid impedes therapy, including the Zollinger-Ellison syndrome, benign gastric ulcers, esophageal ulcers, pancreatic insufficiency, and gastrointestinal hemorrhage. *Sucralfate* is used in the initial treatment of duodenal ulcers.

Nurse Alert for Drugs to Treat Ulcers

- *Antacids* can interfere with the absorption of tetracycline, warfarin, digoxin, quinine, and quinidine. Antacids should not be taken within 30 minutes before or after sucralfate. Because many antacids are high in sodium, they should be used cautiously in patients with cardiac disease, hypertension, or renal disease.
- *Cimetidine* may potentiate the effect of oral anticoagulants, theophylline, caffeine, phenobarbital, phenytoin, carbamazepine, propranolol, diazepam, and chlordiazepoxide. Cimetidine is not recommended in pregnancy unless the benefits outweigh the risks.
- *Sucralfate* should not be taken at the same time as digoxin or tetracycline, cimetidine, or phenytoin.

Side Effects of Drugs to Treat Ulcers

Of the *antacids*, the aluminum and calcium salts can be constipating and the magnesium salts laxative; most antacids combine the two but may still produce diarrhea or constipation. *Sodium bicarbonate* may lead to rebound hypersecretion of gastric acid and makes the blood and urine slightly alkaline. The side effects of *cimetidine* are mild and rare but include headache, dizziness, fatigue, muscle pain, and diarrhea or constipation; high doses may cause gynecomastia and impotence in men, and breast tenderness in women. In the elderly cimetidine may cause delusions, hallucinations, agitation, and other signs of confusion. *Ranitidine* may cause headache, malaise, dizziness, constipation, nausea, abdominal pain, rashes, and a decrease in white blood count. *Sucralfate* rarely causes side effects, the most common being constipation.

Table 22-1 Administration of drugs to treat ulcers

Generic Name	Trade Name	Dosage and Administration
Antacids		
Aluminum hydroxide gel	ALterna GEL Amphojel*	ORAL: *Adults*—5 to 30 ml up to 40 ml every 30 min if pain is severe.
Aluminum carbonate gel	Basaljel	ORAL: 5 to 10 ml or 2 caps every 2 hours up to 12 times daily.
Dihydroxyaluminum aminoacetate	Robalate*	ORAL: *Adults*—0.5 to 2 Gm 4 times daily.
Dihydroxyaluminum sodium carbonate	Rolaids	ORAL: *Adults*—1 to 2 tablets 4 times daily.
Calcium carbonate	Dicarbosil Titralac Tums	ORAL: *Adults*—1 to 4 Gm 1 and 3 hr after meals and at bedtime. Tablets should be chewed before swallowing.
Magaldrate	Riopan	ORAL: *Adults*—480 to 960 mg between meals and at bedtime.
Magnesium carbonate	Milk of Magnesia	
Magnesium hydroxide		
Magnesium oxide		
Magnesium phosphate		
Magnesium trisilicate		

H₂ Receptor Antagonists

Cimetidine	Tagamet*	ORAL: *Adults*—300 mg with meals and at bedtime until ulcer is healed (3 to 6 wk); then 300 mg at bedtime to inhibit nocturnal secretion.
Cimetidine hydrochloride	Tagamet Hydrochloride*	INTRAVENOUS: *Adults*—1 to 4 mg/kg/hr or 300 mg diluted and infused over 15 to 20 min. INTRAMUSCULAR: *Adults*—300 mg every 6 hr. ORAL, INTRAVENOUS: *Children*—20 to 40 mg/kg in divided doses.
Ranitidine	Zantac	ORAL: *Adults*—150 mg every 12 hrs.

Agent That Coats Ulcer Craters

Sucralfate	Carafate Sulcrate†	ORAL: *Adults*—1 Gm 4 times a day. Take 1 hr. before meals and 1 hr before bed.

*Available in U.S. and Canada.
†Available in Canada only.

314 Pocket Nurse Guide to Drugs

Nursing Implications for Drugs for Ulcers
Antacids

- Most patients will find it necessary to alternate aluminum and calcium salts with magnesium salts to regulate bowel movements. Even combinations tend to cause either constipation or diarrhea in many individuals.
- Read labels carefully and instruct patients to do the same. Many antacids are now available in several forms (e.g., double strength or with simethicone), and the names are almost identical. If in doubt, consult the pharmacist.
- Antacid tablets should be chewed, not swallowed whole.
- Liquid and tablet preparations should be followed by enough water to ensure that the dose reaches the stomach.
- Since antacids may interfere with the absorption of other drugs the patient may be taking, review the dosage schedules of all the prescribed medications, and rearrange the schedules as needed to prevent this problem. Remind patients to keep health care providers informed of all medications that are being taken, including antacids.

Cimetidine

- Cimetidine reduces liver metabolism and blood flow, leading to prolonged effects of the following drugs: oral anticoagulants, especially warfarin; theophylline and caffeine; phenobarbital, phenytoin, carbamazepine, propranolol, diazepam, chlordiazepoxide, and probably prazepam and clorazepate. The doses of all of these drugs may need to be reduced, and patients receiving them should be cautioned to observe for side effects of these drugs.
- Cimetidine may be given orally, in tablet or liquid forms. It may be given undiluted intramuscularly. For intravenous "push" infusion, dilute 300 mg with sodium chloride solution or other diluent (see manufacturer's instructions) to make a total volume of 20 ml; inject over 1 to 2 minutes. For intermittent infusion, dilute in an appropriate solution, and infuse over 15 to 20 minutes.
- Confusion, hallucinations, delusions, and agitation have been reported, especially in the seriously ill and/or elderly.

Drugs to Treat Ulcers 315

Because these two groups of patients are often expected to be disoriented, a drug source for the confusion is often overlooked. Caution patients and families to report any changes in behavior or level of functioning.
- Separate the administration of cimetidine and antacids or metoclopramide by at least one hour.
- Oral doses are best administered with or just before meals.

Ranitidine

- The safe use of this drug in pregnancy or lactation has not been established. Instruct patients to direct questions to their physicians.

Sucralfate

- Side effects are rare, the most frequent one being constipation. Instruct patients to keep a record of bowel movements and to include adequate amounts of fluid, bulk and roughage to prevent constipation. If patient is on antacids also, changing the brand of antacid may help prevent constipation.
- Antacids and sucralfate should not be taken within one-half hour of each other.
- Digoxin and tetracycline should be taken at a different time of day than sucralfate.
- The drug is most effective when taken on an empty stomach, 30 to 60 minutes before mealtime or at bedtime.

Antiemetic Drugs

23

Anticholinergic drugs
  Scopolamine
  Scopolamine hydrobromide
Antihistamine drugs
  Buclizine hydrochloride
  Cyclizine hydrochloride
  Cyclizine lactate
  Dimenhydrinate
  Diphenhydramine
  hydrochloride
  Hydroxyzine hydrochloride
  Hydroxyzine pamoate
  Meclizine hydrochloride
  Promethazine hydrochloride

Antidopaminergic drugs
  Chlorpromazine hydrochloride
  Droperidol
  Fluphenazine hydrochloride
  Haloperidol
  Perphenazine
  Prochlorperazine
  Prochlorperazine edisylate
  Prochlorperazine maleate
  Promazine hydrochloride
  Thiethylperazine maleate
  Triflupromazine hydrochloride
Miscellaneous drugs
  Benzquinamide hydrochloride
  Diphenidol hydrochloride
  Domperidone
  Metoclopramide
  Trimethobenzamide
  hydrochloride

Actions of Antiemetic Drugs

The action of antihistamines and anticholinergics in preventing motion sickness and vertigo is not clear but presumably reduces the stimulation of receptors in the labyrinth governing the sense of equilibrium. The antidopaminergic drugs act in the chemoreceptor trigger zone. Diphenidol acts on the aural vestibular apparatus. Benzquinamide and trimethobenzamide inhibit stimulation of the chemoreceptor trigger zone. Domperidone acts to prevent the loss of gastrointestinal tone in the early step of vomiting. Metoclopramide stimulates the gastrointestinal system to counteract the loss of tone in vomiting.

Antiemetic Drugs 317

Indications for Antiemetics

The antihistamines and the anticholinergic drug scopolamine are used prophylactically to prevent motion sickness and vertigo. Antidopaminergics are used to reduce the vomiting from chemotherapy and radiation therapy of cancer and toxins and to control postoperative vomiting. Dimenhydrinate and diphenhydramine are used to control the nausea and vomiting of pregnancy. Droperidol is used primarily as an anesthetic premedication because of its sedating effects. Diphenidol may also be used to prevent vertigo after surgery on the middle ear. Trimethobezamide and domperidone are also used with gastroenteritis. Metoclopramide is also used to reduce nausea and vomiting with cancer chemotherapy.

Nurse Alert for Antiemetic Drugs

- Antiemetics treat only symptoms; effort should always be made to find and treat the underlying cause of nausea and vomiting.
- Because all antiemetics may cause drowsiness, the patient should be cautioned against activities requiring mental alertness until individual effects are established; patients should also avoid drugs that cause CNS depression or drowsiness, such as alcohol, tranquilizers, sleeping medications, and narcotic analgesics.
- Antiemetics should be contraindicated in pregnancy except where clearly warranted. Diphenidol is contraindicated in patients with renal impairment, and in infants and children under 12 kg.
- Trimethobenzamide is contraindicated in patients with a history of seizures.

Side Effects of Antiemetics

The *anticholinergics* may cause drowsiness, dry mouth, blurred vision, and photophobia. *Dimenhydrinate* causes drowsiness, and *diphenhydramine* causes sedation. *Chlorpromazine* may cause hypotension on initial injection and drowsiness. *Droperidol* is highly sedating. *Promazine* and

Text continued on p. 324

Table 23-1 Administration of antiemetics

Generic Name	Trade Name	Dosage and Administration
Anticholinergic Drugs		
Scopolamine	Transderm-Scop	TOPICAL: *Adults*—one adhesive unit is placed behind the ear several hrs. before travel. Duration is 72 hrs.
Scopolamine hydrobromide		ORAL, SUBCUTANEOUS: *Adults*—0.6 to 1.0 mg. *Children*—0.006 mg/kg body weight.
Antihistaminic Drugs		
Buclizine hydrochloride	Bucladin-S	ORAL: *Adults*—50 mg 30 min before traveling and 4 to 6 hr later. For vertigo, 50 mg 2 times daily.
Cyclizine hydrochloride; cyclizine lactate	Marezine*	ORAL: *Adults*—50 mg 30 min before traveling and 4 to 6 hr later; maximum, 200 mg daily. *Children*—6 to 10 yr, 3 mg/kg body weight divided into 3 doses daily.
Dimenhydrinate	Dramamine*	INTRAMUSCULAR: *Adults*—50 mg as needed. *Children*—under 2 years, 1.25 mg/kg; older children, ⅓ to ½ adult dose. INTRAVENOUS: *Adults*—50 mg diluted in 10 ml saline solution, injected over 2 min. ORAL: *Adults*—50 to 100 mg every 4 hr. *Children*—5 mg/kg body weight divided into 4 doses; maximum, 150 mg daily. RECTAL: *Adults*—100 mg 1 to 2 times daily.
Diphenhydramine hydrochloride	Benadryl hydrochloride	DEEP INTRAMUSCULAR: *Adults*—10 mg, increased to 20 to 50 mg every 2 to 3 hr if needed; maximum, 400 mg daily. *Children*—

Antiemetic Drugs

Generic name	Trade names	Route and dosage
		5 mg/kg body weight divided into 4 doses; maximum, 300 mg daily. INTRAVENOUS: *Adults*—same as deep intramuscular. ORAL: *Adults*—50 mg 30 min before traveling, then 50 mg before each meal. *Children*—5 mg/kg body weight divided into 4 doses; maximum, 300 mg daily.
Hydroxyzine hydrochloride	Vistaject Atarax*	INTRAMUSCULAR: *Adults*—25 to 100 mg. *Children*—1 mg/kg body weight. ORAL: *Adults*—50 to 100 mg 4 times daily. *Children*—over 6 yr, 50 to 100 mg per day in divided doses; under 6 yr, 50 mg per day in divided doses.
Hydroxyzine pamoate	Vistaril	ORAL: *Adults*—25 to 100 mg 3 to 4 times daily. *Children*—over 6 yr, 50 to 100 mg daily divided into 4 doses; under 6 yr, 50 mg daily divided into 4 doses; or 1.1 mg/kg.
Meclizine hydrochloride	Antivert* Bonine	ORAL: *Adults*—25 to 50 mg once daily, taken 60 min or longer before traveling; 25 to 100 mg daily in divided doses for vertigo or radiation sickness.
Promethazine hydrochloride	Phenergan* Remsed Zipan	INTRAMUSCULAR, RECTAL: *Adults*—25 mg, then 12.5 to 25 mg as needed every 4 to 6 hr. *Children*—under 12 yr, no more than half the adult dose. ORAL: *Adults*—25 mg 2 times daily. *Children*—12.5 to 25 mg twice daily.

cont'd. next page

* Available in U.S. and Canada

† Available in Canada only

Table 23-1   Administration of antiemetics—cont'd.

Generic Name	Trade Name	Dosage and Administration
Antidopaminergic Drugs		
Chlorpromazine hydrochloride	Thorazine Largactil†	RECTAL: *Adults*—50 to 100 mg every 6 to 8 hr. *Children*—1 mg/ kg body weight every 6 to 8 hr. INTRAMUSCULAR: *Adults*—25 mg, then 25 to 50 mg every 3 to 4 hours to stop vomiting. *Children*—0.5 mg/kg body weight every 6 to 8 hr; maximum, 40 mg (up to 5 yr or 50 lb), 75 mg (5 to 12 yr or 50 to 100 lb) daily. ORAL: *Adults*—10 to 25 mg every 4 to 6 hr. *Children*—0.5 mg/ kg body weight every 4 to 6 hr.
Droperidol	Inapsine*	INTRAMUSCULAR: *Adults*—2.5 to 10 mg as premedication. Individualize according to patient condition and medications. *Children*—2-12 yrs. 1 to 1.5 mg/10 kg body weight. INTRAVENOUS: *Adults*—1.25 mg 5 min before terminating anesthesia to prevent postoperative vomiting. Can repeat dose intramuscularly if needed. 1 mg 30 to 60 min before treatment with cancer chemotherapy, followed by one intramuscular injection within 4 hrs, if requested. *Children*—1 to 15 yr. 0.005 mg/kg for postoperative vomiting. 0.01 mg/kg initially and repeated in 6 hrs. if needed to prevent vomiting in cancer chemotherapy.

Fluphenazine hydrochloride	Prolixin	INTRAMUSCULAR: *Adults*—1.25 mg every 6 to 8 hr as needed.
Haloperidol	Haldol*	INTRAMUSCULAR, ORAL: *Adults*—1, 2, or 5 mg every 12 hr as needed.
Perphenazine	Trilafon*	ORAL: *Adults*—8 to 24 mg daily in 2 or more divided doses. INTRAMUSCULAR: *Adults*—5 mg daily.
Prochlorperazine	Compazine	RECTAL: *Adults*—25 mg 2 times daily. *Children*—over 10 kg 0.4 mg/kg body weight daily divided into 3 to 4 doses.
Prochlorperazine edisylate	Compazine Stemotil†	DEEP INTRAMUSCULAR: *Adults*—5 to 10 mg every 3 to 4 hr; maximum, 40 mg daily, *Children*—over 10 kg, 0.2 mg/kg body weight daily.
Prochlorperazine maleate	Compazine	ORAL: *Adults*—5 to 10 mg every 3 to 4 hr; maximum, 40 mg daily. *Children*—over 10 kg, 0.2 mg/kg body weight daily.
Promazine hydrochloride	Sparine*	ORAL: *Adults*—25 to 50 mg every 4 to 6 hr as needed. INTRAMUSCULAR: *Adults*—50 mg.
Thiethylperazine maleate	Torecan*	ORAL, INTRAMUSCULAR, RECTAL: *Adults*—10 to 30 mg daily.
Triflupromazine hydrochloride	Vesprin	ORAL: *Adults*—20 to 30 mg daily. *Children*—0.2 mg/kg body weight divided into 3 doses; maximum daily dose, 10 mg. INTRAMUSCULAR: *Adults*—5 to 15 mg every 4 hr as needed; maximum daily dose, 60 mg. *Elderly*—2.5 to 15 mg daily. *Children*—0.2 to 0.25 mg/kg body weight; maximum daily dose, 10 mg.

cont'd. next page

*Available in U.S. and Canada
†Available in Canada only

Table 23-1 Administration of antiemetics—cont'd.

Generic Name	Trade Name	Dosage and Administration
Miscellaneous Drugs		
Benzquinamide hydrochloride	Emete-Con	INTRAMUSCULAR: *Adults*—0.5 to 1 mg/kg body weight at least 15 min before chemotherapy or emergence from anesthesia. Repeat in 1 hr, then every 3 to 4 hr as required. INTRAVENOUS: *Adults*—0.2 to 0.4 mg/kg body weight diluted in 5% dextrose, sodium chloride injection, or lactated Ringer's injection and administered over 1 to 3 min. Additional doses are given IM.
Diphenidol hydrochloride	Vontrol*	ORAL: *Adults*—25 to 50 mg 4 times daily. *Children*—over 6 mo and 12 kg, 5 mg/kg body weight daily divided into 4 doses. INTRAMUSCULAR: *Adults*—20 to 40 mg 4 times daily. *Children*—3 mg/kg body weight divided into 4 daily doses. INTRAVENOUS: *Adults*—20 mg; repeat once at 1 hr if necessary. INTRAVENOUS, INTRAMUSCULAR: *Adults*—10 mg as often as 6 times/day, maximum: 1 mg/kg daily. *Children*—0.1 to 0.2 mg/kg 3 to 6 times/day, maximum: 1 mg/kg daily. ORAL: *Adults*—10 mg 4 times/day 15 to 30 min before meals and at bedtime. *Children*—1 drop (0.3 mg)/kg of 1% solution 3 times daily 15 to 30 min before meals and at bedtime if necessary.

		Oral doses may be doubled if no improvement in two weeks. RECTAL: *Adults*—60 mg 3 to 4 times daily. *Children* 1 to 2 yr: 10 mg 1 or 2 times daily. *Children* 2 to 4 yr: 30 mg 1 or 2 times daily. *Children* 4 to 6 yr: 30 mg up to 3 times daily. *Children* 6 to 10 yr: 30 mg up to 4 times daily.
Metoclopramide	Reglan* Maxeran†	INTRAVENOUS: *Adults*—10 to 20 mg, administered over 2 min. *Children* up to 6 yr—0.1 mg/kg *Children* 6 to 14 yr—2.5 to 5 mg. ORAL: *Adults*—5 to 10 mg 3 times daily 15 to 30 min before meals. Higher doses in chemotherapy-induced nausea: 0.5 to 1mg/kg
Trimethobenzamide hydrochloride	Tigan*	INTRAMUSCULAR: *Adults*—200 mg 3 to 4 times daily. For preventing postoperative nausea and vomiting, give 1 dose before or during surgery and another 3 hr after surgery. ORAL: *Adults*—250 mg 3 to 4 times daily. *Children*—15 mg/kg body weight divided into 3 to 4 doses, or 100 to 200 mg divided into 3 to 4 doses. RECTAL: *Adults*—200 mg 3 or 4 times daily. *Children*—30 to 90 lbs—100 to 200 mg 3 or 4 times daily; under 30 lbs—100 mg 3 or 4 times daily.

*Available in U.S. and Canada
†Available in Canada only

324   Pocket Nurse Guide to Drugs

thiethlyperazine may cause hypotension and anticholinergic effects. The *antidopaminergics* occasionally cause extrapyramidal symptoms. *Diphenidol* may cause dry mouth, nausea, heartburn, tachycardia, dizziness, hallucinations, disorientation, or confusion. *Trimethobenzamide* may cause drowsiness, vertigo, diarrhea, skin rashes, extrapyramidal reactions in children or the elderly, tachycardia, and orthostatic hypotension.

Nursing Implications for Antiemetics

All Antiemetics

- Most individuals develop tolerance to the stimulus causing the motion sickness after two or three days. Taking medication one to two hours prior to travel is more effective than waiting until the individual experiences nausea or vomiting. Scopolamine is very useful for this problem, but the side effects limit the use of this drug. There is available a sustained-release form of this drug called Transderm Scop. The drug is supplied in a small adhesive disc, which can be applied behind the ear. It should not be used in children or the elderly, as they are more susceptible to the side effects of the drug. The drug is released over 3 days; only one disc should be used at a time, but if still needed after 3 days, a new one can be applied. It should be applied four hours prior to the time the drug effect is needed.

- Sucking on hard candy or chewing gum may help to relieve the dry mouth associated with some of these drugs. If the patient has vomited, assisting the patient to rinse the mouth out with water; mouthwash will help to decrease the unpleasant taste. The postoperative patient who still may not eat may find relief by sucking on ice chips; check with the physician.

- If possible, measure the emesis as a part of the fluid intake and output record.

- Keeping the environment neat and free of odors may ease the discomfort of the nauseated patient somewhat. The nauseated person may not tolerate the sight of food; keep the door closed or the curtains drawn during meal times if appropriate. Begin feeding the person who has been experiencing nausea with small amounts of clear liquids before progressing to a more complete diet.

- Intramuscularly administered antiemetics may cause pain or burning at the injection site.
- Antiemetics should be used with caution in children who may be suffering from Reye's syndrome. This syndrome is characterized by an abrupt onset of persistent severe vomiting, lethargy, irrational behavior, progressive encephalopathy, convulsions, coma, and death.

Benzquinamide Hydrochloride

- Intravenous administration has been associated with an increase in blood pressure and transient cardiac arrhythmias, including premature ventricular contractions (PVCs). The intramuscular route is preferred.
- Monitor the blood pressure and pulse.

Diphenidol

- This drug may cause hallucinations, disorientation, or confusion. If these symptoms occur, notify the physician. Assess whether the patient can be left unattended.
- Monitor the blood pressure and pulse every 4 hours.

Trimethobenzamide

- After oral administration, effectiveness may be variable. Pain at the injection site has been reported; children should not be given this drug via the intramuscular route. This drug is not recommended for intravenous administration. Rectal suppositories should not be used in infants.

Antidiarrheal Drugs

24

Opioids and related drugs
  Codeine phosphate
  Codeine sulfate
  Diphenoxylate hydrochloride
    with atropine
  Loperamide
  Opium tincture
  Paregoric

Bismuth salts
  Bismuth subsalicylate

Actions of Antidiarrheal Drugs

Opioids and related drugs decrease the tone of the small and large intestines in a manner that slows the transit of fecal material. Bismuth salts control some forms of diarrhea by binding toxins and removing the cause of diarrhea.

Indications for Antidiarrheal Drugs

Opioids are nonspecific antidiarrheal agents. Bismuth salts are often effective in the treatment of "traveller's" diarrhea.

Nurse Alert for Antidiarrheal Drugs

- The opioids are contraindicated when diarrhea is caused by poisons, infections, or bacterial toxins, because the elimination of these agents may be delayed.
- Loperamide is contraindicated in patients with liver disease.
- Antidiarrheal drugs should be used with caution in pregnancy or lactation.
- Patients taking diphenoxylate should be cautioned to avoid activities requiring mental alertness until individual effects are evaluated, because of the drowsiness; drowsiness may be pronounced in the presence of other drugs that depress the central nervous system.

Antidiarrheal Drugs 327

Table 24-1 Administration of antidiarrheal drugs

Generic Name	Trade Name	Dosage and Administration
Opioids and Related Drugs		
Codeine phosphate; codeine sulfate		ORAL: *Adults and children over 12 yr*—15 to 60 mg every 4 to 8 hr as needed. INTRAMUSCULAR: *Adults and children over 12 yr*—15 to 30 mg every 2 to 4 hr.
Diphenoxylate hydrochloride with atropine	Colonil Lomotil* Lofene Various others	ORAL: *Adults*—5 mg 3 to 4 times daily. *Children*—8 to 12 yr; 10 mg daily in 5 divided doses; 5 to 8 yr, 8 mg daily in 4 divided doses; 2 to 5 yr, 6 mg daily in 3 divided doses.
Loperamide	Imodium*	ORAL: *Adults*—4 mg initially, then 2 mg with each diarrheal episode, up to 16 mg daily.
Opium tincture		ORAL: 0.6 ml 4 times daily
Paregoric		ORAL: *Adults*—5 to 10 ml 1 to 4 times daily. *Children*—0.25 to 0.5 ml/kg 1 to 4 times daily.
Bismuth Salts		
Bismuth subsalicylate	Pepto-Bismol	ORAL: *Adults*—30 ml. *Children*—10 to 14 yr, 20 ml; 6 to 10 yr, 10 ml; 3 to 6 yr, 5 ml.

*Available in U.S. and Canada

Side Effects of Antidiarrheal Drugs

In therapeutic antidiarrheal doses the *opioids* do not cause euphoria or analgesia; toxic doses produce respiratory depression that can be reversed with a narcotic antagonist. *Diphenoxylate* in high doses may produce side effects similar to

328   Pocket Nurse Guide to Drugs

those of meperidine; overdose resembles overdose with a narcotic analgesic and is treated similarly (see Ch. 5). *Diphenoxylate* preparations contain atropine and in accumulated doses may cause the side effects of atropine (Ch. 21). Side effects of *loperamide* are rare in prescribed doses but may include abdominal pain or distention, constipation, drowsiness, nausea, vomiting, and fatigue.

Nursing Implications for Antidiarrheal Drugs

- Keep a record of the frequency of bowel movements, as the patient may become constipated from the effects of the drug.
- Fluid and electrolyte loss can be severe. Encourage patients with diarrhea to switch to a clear liquid diet. Total fluid intake should be at least 3000 ml per day, although in cases of severe diarrhea, up to 5000 to 6000 ml per day may be necessary.
- Most cases of short-term diarrhea are self-limiting, especially if a result of a viral infection. Instruct the patient to consult the physician if any of the following occur: diarrhea persists longer than 3 to 5 days; the medications are not bringing relief; the stools are particularly foul-smelling or contain flecks of blood or large amounts of mucus; or the patient is unable to take in sufficient replacement fluids. Symptoms of hypokalemia are muscle weakness, fatigue, anorexia, vomiting, drowsiness, irritability, and eventually coma and death. Symptoms of hypochloremia include hypertonic muscles, tetany, and depressed respirations.
- Question the patient carefully about recent activities that might have caused diarrhea. Examples include recent travel, especially international; recent antibiotic use; or recent cancer chemotherapy.
- Opium tincture is not used frequently now. Dilute the ordered number of drops in 15 to 30 ml of water to ensure that the patient receives the entire dose.
- Many patients find combination drugs such as Parepectolin much more palatable than paregoric alone. Note that combination drugs subject the patient to additional ingredients that may or may not be helpful or needed.

Laxatives and Cathartics

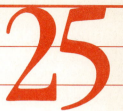

Bulk-forming laxatives
    Karaya gum
    Methylcellulose
    Carboxymethylcellulose sodium
    Plantago (psyllium) seed
    Polycarbophil
    Psyllium hydrocolloid
    Psyllium hydrophilic mucilloid
Stimulant cathartics
    Bisacodyl
    Cascara sagrada
    Castor oil
    Emulsified castor oil
    Danthron
    Glycerin suppositories
    Phenolphthalein
    Senna concentrate
    Senna pod
    Whole leaf senna
    Sennosides A & B
Saline cathartics
    Magnesium citrate
    Magnesium hydroxide
    Magnesium sulfate
    Monosodium phosphate
    Sodium phosphate
    Sodium phosphate with sodium biphosphate
Lubricants
    Mineral oil
Fecal softeners
    Docusate calcium
    Docusate sodium
Miscellaneous
    Lactulose
    Glycerin

Actions of Laxatives and Cathartics

Bulk-forming laxatives act by retaining water so that the stool remains large and soft and fills the rectum to stimulate defecation with little strain or irritation. Stimulant cathartics increase the motility of the large intestine and also inhibit the reabsorption of water. Saline cathartics attract water osmotically into the lumen of the large intestine to increase bulk and thus stimulate peristalsis. Fecal softeners, or wetting agents, inhibit the absorption of water so that the fecal mass remains large and soft. Lubricant laxatives soften the feces and ease the strain of defecation. Lactulose increases stool bulk by osmotic action.

Indications for Laxatives and Cathartics

Laxatives and cathartics are indicated for patients with constipation, caused by poor bowel habits, narcotic analgesics, drugs with anticholinergic side effects, and the loss of intestinal muscle tone caused by surgery, bedrest, or age; for patients for whom straining is painful or risky, such as with episiotomies, hemorrhoids, hernias, or aneurysms; and to empty the large intestine before surgery or examination. Lubricant laxatives are used to ease the strain of irritation of defecation.

Nurse Alert for Laxatives and Cathartics

- *Bisacodyl* should not be taken with 60 minutes of milk or antacid ingestion.
- *Cascara* and *senna* should not be used in lactation.
- *Saline cathartics* should not be used in patients with poor kidney function because the extra salt load may not be eliminated.
- *Laxatives* and *cathartics* are contraindicated with vomiting, diarrhea, severe abdominal pain, suspected intestinal obstruction, suspected appendicitis, or other possible acute abdominal processes. Pregnant and lactating women should consult the physician before self-dosing with laxatives and cathartics.
- *Sodium salt* preparations are contraindicated in patients with a history of heart disease.
- *Lactulose* should be used cautiously in diabetics because it may contribute to hyperglycemia.

Side Effects of Laxatives and Cathartics

Used at recommended doses and frequency, laxatives and cathartics cause few side effects other than increasing dependence. Mineral oil reduces the absorption of the fat-soluble vitamins and should therefore not be used reg-

Laxatives and Cathartics **331**

ularly. With continued use, the stimulant cathartics cause loss of large intestine tone and may produce severe diarrhea and dehydration. Stimulant cathartics affect urine color. Stimulant and saline cathartics may cause mild abdominal cramping. Lactulose may cause initial flatulence and abdominal cramps that subside with continued use.

Nursing Implications for Laxatives and Cathartics

- Instruct the patient to increase dietary intake of foods known to be bulk-producing or stimulating to the gastrointestinal tract.
- Advise the patient to increase the fluid intake to at least 2500 to 3000 ml per day.
- Increasing the level of activity may assist in decreasing constipation.
- Abuse of drugs to relieve constipation sometimes occurs with individuals who feel that a daily bowel movement is necessary. Try to teach patients that it may be normal to defecate only every 2 or 3 days.
- Remind patients to follow the directions on the package of over-the-counter drugs in terms of dose and frequency.
- Read the physician's order carefully. Many of these drugs have similar names or are manufactured as combination products.
- The stimulant cathartics and saline cathartics may cause some mild abdominal cramping. If cramping is excessive, it may indicate that the dose of medication was too high or that there may be some additional pathological condition present such as obstruction. In the elderly, smaller doses of these drugs may be sufficient to stimulate defecation.
- When one or more of these drugs is prescribed to prepare the patient for a diagnostic procedure, it is important to review the instructions with the patient and to emphasize the necessity of following the directions carefully.
- Changes in bowel habits, especially when no easily explainable cause can be found, should be investigated with a thorough medical examination.
- Keep a record of bowel movements on all immobilized, incapacitated, or institutionalized patients.

Text continued on p. 336

Table 25-1   Administration of laxatives and cathartics

Generic Name	Trade Name	Dosage and Administration
Bulk-forming Agents		
Karaya gum		ORAL: 5 to 10 Gm daily, taken with water.
Methylcellulose; carboxymethyl cellulose	Cologel Hydrolose	ORAL: *Adults*—15 to 60 ml daily. *Children*—over 6 yr, 10 to 15 ml daily.
Plantago (psyllium) seed		ORAL: *Adults*—2.5 to 30 Gm daily. *Children*—over 6 yr, 1.25-15 Gm daily. Add to water and drink rapidly.
Polycarbophil	Mitrolan*	ORAL: *Adults*—4 to 6 Gm daily. *Children*—6 to 12 yr, 1.5 to 3 Gm daily; 2 to 5 yr, 1 to 1.5 Gm daily; to 2 yr, 0.5 to 1 Gm daily.
Psyllium hydrocolloid Psyllium hydrophilic mucilloid	Effersyllium L.A. Formula Metamucil* Modane Bulk	ORAL: *Adults*—1 round teaspoonful (7 gm) or 1 packet. Add to a glass of water and drink rapidly and then follow with a second glass of water. Repeat 1 to 2 times daily if necessary.
Stimulant (Irritant) Cathartics		
Bisacodyl	Bisco-Lax* Dulcolax* Various others	ORAL: *Adults*—10 mg. Up to 30 mg may be given to clear gastrointestinal tract. *Children*—over 6 yr, 5 mg. RECTAL: *Adults and children over 2 yr*—10 mg. *Children under 2 yr*—5 mg.

Laxatives and Cathartics 333

Cascara sagrada	Cas-Evac	ORAL: *Adults*—200 to 400 mg of extract, 0.5 to 1.5 ml of fluid extract, or 5 ml of aromatic extract.
Castor oil		ORAL: *Adults*—15 to 60 ml. *Children*—over 2 yr, 5 to 15 ml; under 2 yr, 1 to 5 ml.
Castor oil, emulsified	Neoloid	ORAL: *Adults*—30 to 60 ml. *Children*—over 2 yr, 7.5 to 30 ml; under 2 yr, 2.5 to 7.5 ml.
Danthron	Dorbane* Modane*	ORAL: *Adults*—75 to 150 mg. *Children*—6 to 12 yr, 37 to 75 mg; 1 to 6 yr, 10 to 15 mg.
Glycerin suppositories		RECTAL: *Adults*—3 Gm. *Children*—under 6 yr, 1 to 1.5 Gm.
Phenolphthalein	Chocolax Ex-lax Feen-A-Mint Phenolax Various others	ORAL: *Adults*—30 to 270 mg daily. *Children*—over 6 yr, 30 to 60 mg daily; 2 to 6 yr, 15 to 20 mg daily.
Senna concentrate	Senokot* suppositories	RECTAL: *Adults*—1 suppository. *Children*—over 60 lb, ½ suppository.
Senna concentrate	Senokot* Various others	ORAL: *Adults*—twice daily give 1 to 2 teaspoonfuls (granules), 2 to 3 teaspoonfuls (syrup), or 2 to 4 tablets. *Children, pregnant or postpartum women, or geriatric patients*—½ adult dose. *Children*—1 mo to 1 yr, 1.25 to 2.5 ml (syrup).

cont'd. next page

*Available in U.S. and Canada
†Available in Canada only

Table 25-1 Administration of laxatives and cathartics—cont'd.

Generic Name	Trade Name	Dosage and Administration
Senna, whole leaf		ORAL: *Adults*—0.5 to 2 Gm or 2 ml of senna fluid extract. *Children*—6 to 12 yr, ½ adult dose; 2 to 5 yr, ¼ adult dose; under 2 yr, ⅛ adult dose.
Sennosides A & B	Glysennid	ORAL: *Adults*—12 to 24 mg at bedtime. *Children*—over 10 yr, same as adult; 6 to 10 yr, 12 mg at bedtime.

Saline Cathartics

Generic Name	Trade Name	Dosage and Administration
Magnesium citrate		ORAL: *Adults*—1 glassful (about 240 ml). *Children*—0.5 ml/kg.
Magnesium hydroxide	Milk of Magnesia	ORAL: *Adults*—10 to 15 ml (concentrated) or 15 to 30 ml (regular). *Children*—0.5 ml (regular)/kg.
Magnesium sulfate	Epsom salt	ORAL: *Adults*—15 Gm in a glass of water. *Children*—0.25 Gm/kg.
Monosodium phosphate	Sal Hepatica	ORAL: *Adults*—5 to 20 ml with water.
Sodium phosphate		ORAL: *Adults*—4 Gm in a glass of warm water.
Sodium phosphate with sodium biphosphate	Phospho-Soda	ORAL: *Adults*—20 to 40 ml in a glass of cold water. *Children*—5-15 ml.

Lubricants

Mineral oil	Agoral, Plain Kondremul Plain* Neo-Cultol Petrogalar Plain	ORAL: *Adults*—15 to 30 ml at bedtime. *Children*—5 to 15 ml at bedtime.

Fecal Softeners

Docusate calcium	Surfak	ORAL: *Adults*—50 to 360 mg daily. *Children*—50 to 150 mg daily.
Docusate sodium	Colace Comfolax D-S-S Various others	ORAL: *Adults*—50 to 360 mg. *Children*—6 to 12 yr, 40 to 120 mg; 3 to 6 yr, 20 to 60 mg; under 3 yr, 10 to 40 mg.

Miscellaneous

Lactulose	Cephulac* Chronulac*	ORAL: *Adults*—15 to 30 ml, increased to 60 ml per day if necessary (15 ml = 10 Gm).
Glycerin suppositories		RECTAL: *Adults*—3 Gm. *Children*—under 6 yr, 1 to 1.5 gm.

*Available in U.S. and Canada
†Available in Canada only

Bulk-forming Laxatives

- The prescribed dose should be stirred into an 8 oz glass of fluid and consumed while still suspended in solution. For best results, the dose should be followed by another full glass of water. These drugs should be taken dry because they could cause obstruction. If taken in pill form, the pill should be swallowed whole and not chewed first.
- Regular use of these agents (1 to 3 times daily) is usually needed to promote regular defecation.

Stimulant Cathartics

- Because most of these medications, when taken orally, require about 6 hours to stimulate defecation, they are often better taken at bedtime, allowing the patient to have a bowel movement the next morning.
- Enteric-coated tablets, such as bisacodyl preparations, should be swallowed whole and not chewed.
- Bisacodyl oral preparations should not be given within 60 minutes of milk or antacids. Do not administer bisacodyl suppositories before eating or at any time in which the stimulation of defecation 15 to 20 minutes later will interfere with other activities in the patient's day.
- Before administering castor oil preparations, check with the patient to see which juice the patient prefers as a diluent. Regular castor oil will not mix with a water-based diluent and sits on the top of the juice. The addition of a small amount of baking soda (less than ¼ teaspoon) immediately before administering to the patient will cause the mixture to fizz, and the castor oil will be partially suspended in the juice for a minute or two; the patient may find it easier to drink this way. In an institution, the routine use of baking soda for this purpose should be cleared by the pharmacy or physician.
- Review with patients the anticipated changes in the color of urine and/or feces.
- Suppositories should be kept in the refrigerator if they are to be kept for long periods of time. If the cold suppository is rolled between the fingers, the warmth will meet the outside part, causing it to become slippery and easily inserted.

Saline Cathartics

- Magnesium citrate is usually better tolerated if chilled first. The entire dose should be consumed at one time.
- These cathartics are helpful in eliminating parasites after antihelminthic therapy, because the trophozoites are not destroyed, and can be better examined in the laboratory.

Mineral Oil

- When mineral oil is used on a regular basis, there may be leakage of the oil and/or fecal material from the anus. Warn patients of this. The oil will stain clothing. It may be necessary for patients to wear a perianal pad to protect clothing and sheets.
- The regular use of mineral oil has been associated with an increased incidence of lipid pneumonia, especially in the elderly. Caution the patient to always sit upright when taking this medication. If the patient will be using an agent on a long-term basis to relieve constipation, a medication other than mineral oil might be a better choice.
- Mineral oil, or any oil-based substance, should never be used to lubricate around the nose because of the possibility of inhaling minute quantities that might contribute at a later time to lipid pneumonia.

Fecal Softeners

- Many patients misunderstand the function of fecal softeners, and expect defecation to occur a few hours following a dose of a fecal softener, just as it might after a stimulant-type drug.
- To be effective, fecal softeners need to be used on a daily basis or more often to keep the stools at a softer consistency regularly.

Lactulose

- Monitor serum electrolytes, especially in the elderly, when this drug is used for long periods (greater than 6 months).
- This drug is also used to treat hyperammonemia.

Digestants

Pancrelipase
Pancreatin
Glutamic acid HCl
Diluted hydrochloric acid
Dehydrocholic acid
Bile salts

Actions of Digestants

Pancrelipase and *pancreatin* are combinations of pancreatic enzymes that aid in the digestion and absorption of fats, triglycerides, and carbohydrates. *Glutamic acid HCl* and *diluted hydrochloric acid* are gastric acidifiers that help destroy or inhibit the growth of microorganisms in ingested foods and aid in digestive processes in the stomach. *Dehydrocholic acid* aids in the formation of low viscosity bile. *Bile salts* aid in the digestion of fats and increase the flow of bile.

Indications for Digestants

Pancrelipase and *pancreatin* are used in deficiencies of pancreatic secretions, such as occurs in cystic fibrosis, chronic pancreatitis, pancreatectomy, and pancreatic cancer. *Glutamic acid hydrochloride* and diluted *hydrochloric acid* are indicated for deficiencies of stomach acid such as occurs with pernicious anemia, some allergies, and gastric carcinoma. *Dehydrocholic acid* is indicated for constipation and biliary tract conditions. *Bile salts* are indicated for constipation.

Nurse Alert for Digestants

- *Pancrelipase* and *pancreatin* are contraindicated in cases of hypersensitivity to one of more of the components; both in

Digestants **339**

Table 26-1 Administration of digestants

Generic Name	Trade Names	Administration
Pancrelipase	Cotazym* Cotazym-S Ilozymes Ku-Zymes HP Pancrease	ORAL: *Adult*—1 to 3 capsules or tablets or 1 to 2 packets before or with meals and snacks; up to 8 capsules or tablets for severe deficiency.
Pancreatin	Pancreatin Enseals Pancreatin Viokase	ORAL: *Adult*—1 to 3 tablets with meals.
Hydrochloric acid		ORAL: *Adult*—2 to 8 ml well diluted in 25 to 50 ml of water.
Glutamic acid hydrochloride	Acidulin	ORAL: *Adult*—340 mg to 1 Gm (1 to 3 tablets) 3 times daily before meals.
Dehydrocholic acid	Hepahydrin Cholan-DH Decholin Neocholan Dycholium†	ORAL: *Adult*—250 to 500 mg after each meal. IV: 5 to 10 ml of 20% solution first day, 10 ml on days 2 and 3, switching to oral medication on day 4.
Bile salts	Ox Bile Extract Enseals Bilron Pulvules*	ORAL: *Adult*—150 to 600 mg with meals.

*Available in U.S. and Canada
†Available in Canada only

powdered form are irritating to nasal mucosa if inhaled and may precipitate an attack in asthmatic patients.

■ *Glutamic acid hydrochloride* and *hydrochloric acid* are contraindicated in cases of peptic ulcer or gastric hyperacidity.

Pocket Nurse Guide to Drugs

- *Dehydrocholic acid* is contraindicated in cases of severe liver disease or complete obstruction of the bile duct and in patients experiencing nausea or abdominal pain; give a skin test before using IV solution to patients with allergies or asthma.
- *Bile salts* are contraindicated in cases of complete biliary obstruction or severe jaundice.

Side Effects of Digestants

Pancrelipase and *pancreatin* in high doses may cause nausea, abdominal cramps, and diarrhea. Overdose of *glutamic acid* or *hydrochloric acid* may cause systemic acidosis. *Dehydrocholic acid* may cause diarrhea. *Bile salts* may cause loose stools and mild cramping.

Nursing Implications for Digestants

For pancrelipase and pancreatin, antacids containing calcium carbonate or magnesium hydroxide decrease the effectiveness of these enzymes. Iron absorption may also be decreased. Stomach acid inactivates these enzymes. Cimetidine decreases stomach acid and thereby keeps these enzymes active.

- Glutamic acid HCl can be used instead of hydrochloric acid to avoid damage to tooth enamel.
- Hydrochloric acid can be sipped through a nonmetallic straw to avoid damage to tooth enamel.
- Dehydrocholic acid may be given with bile salts.
- Bile salts tablets are bitter and should not be chewed.
- Bile salts are not a replacement for bile salt deficiency. Frequent use may result in dependence on laxatives; the patient should increase the intake of fluids and roughage.

PART V

RESPIRATORY SYSTEM DRUGS

Bronchodilators and Other Drugs for Asthma

27

Adrenergic bronchodilators
  Albuterol (salbutamol)
  Ephedrine sulfate
  Epinephrine
  Isoetharine hydrochloride
  Isoetharine mesylate
  Isoproterenol hydrochloride
  Isoproterenol sulfate
  Metaproterenol sulfate
  Terbutaline sulfate

Xanthines
  Aminophylline (theophylline ethylenediamine)
  Dyphylline
  Oxtriphylline (choline theophyllinate)
  Theophylline
  Theophylline monoethanolamine
  Theophylline sodium glycinate
Other drugs to treat asthma
  Beclomethasone dipropionate
  Cromolyn sodium
  Dexamethasone sodium phosphate
  Flunisolide
  Triamcinolone acetonide

Adrenergic Bronchodilators

Actions of Adrenergic Bronchodilators

The adrenergic bronchodilators are beta-adrenergic agonists that increase cyclic AMP and cause dilation of the bronchioles.

Indications for Adrenergic Bronchodilators

Bronchodilator therapy is used for patients with asthma or other respiratory diseases with bronchospasm as a component, including some cases of bronchitis and emphysema. Epineph-

Text continued on p. 348

342

Table 27-1 Administration of adrenergic bronchodilators

Generic Name	Trade Name	Dosage and Administration	Onset (min)	Duration (hr)
Albuterol (Salbutamol) sulfate	Proventil Ventolin†	INHALATION: *Adults and Children over 12 years*: One or two inhalations every 4 to 6 hours. ORAL: *Adults and Children over 12 years*: 2 to 4 mg three or four times daily. Maximum 32 mg daily.	Inhalation 30 Oral 30	4-6 4-6
Ephedrine sulfate	Ectasule Minus	ORAL: *Adults*—25 to 50 mg every 3 to 4 hr as needed. *Children*—6 to 12 yr, 6.25 to 12.5 mg every 4 to 6 hr; 2 to 6 yr, 0.3 to 0.5 mg/kg every 4 to 6 hr.	15	2-4
Epinephrine (base)	Sus-Phrine† (1:200)	SUBCUTANEOUS: *Adults*—0.1 to 0.3 ml not more often than every 6 hr, maximum test dose, 0.1 ml. *Children*—0.005 ml/kg body weight not more often than every 4 hr, maximum test dose, 0.15 ml.		
	Asmolin (1:400)	Double above volumes.		*cont'd. next page*

*Available without a prescription.
†Available in U.S. and Canada.

344 Pocket Nurse Guide to Drugs

Table 27-1 Administration of adrenergic bronchodilators—cont'd.

Generic Name	Trade Name	Dosage and Administration	Onset (min)	Duration (hr)
Epinephrine bitartrate	Asthma Meter* Medihaler-Epi*† Primatene Mist*	INHALATION: Aerosol nebulizers metered to deliver 0.2 mg epinephrine (0.1 mg for Medihaler-Epi) with each inhalation. Allow 1 to 2 min between inhalations.	3-5	1-3
Epinephrine (racemic)	Vaponefrin microNEFRIN (2.25%)	As for epinephrine bitartrate.		
Epinephrine hydrochloride	Adrenalin Chloride (1:1000)	INTRAMUSCULAR or SUBCUTANEOUS: *Adults*—0.2 to 0.5 mg every 20 min to 4 hours as needed for an acute asthma attack. *Children*—0.01 mg/kg not to exceed 0.5 mg, every 4 hr as needed for acute asthma attack. For severe attacks, may repeat initial dose every 20 min for 3 doses.	5	1-3
	Adrenalin Chloride (1:100)*	INHALATION: Solutions for nebulization. Allow 1 to 2 min between inhalations.		

Bronchodilators and Other Drugs for Asthma

Isoetharine hydrochloride	Bronkosol	INHALATION: nebulized solution; 3 to 7 inhalations, for hand nebulizer.	2	1
Isoetharine mesylate	Bronkometer	INHALATION: aerosol; 1 to 4 inhalations every 3 to 6 hr, maximum 12 inhalations daily.	2	1
Isoproterenol hydrochloride	Isuprel Hydrochloride† Norisodrine Aerotrol	SUBLINGUAL: *Adults*—10 mg initially. No more than 15 mg 4 times daily or 20 mg 3 times daily. *Children*—5 to 10 mg, not exceeding 30 mg daily.	2-5	½-2
	Isuprel Mistometer Norisodrine Aerotrol	INHALATION: (solution for nebulization, 0.5% to 1%). *Adults and Children*—5 to 15 deep inhalations of 1:200 aerosol repeated in 10 to 30 min if necessary, up to 5 times daily.	2	½-2
Isoproterenol sulfate	Medihaler-Iso† Norisodrine Sulfate	INHALATION (aerosol metered dose): *Adults*—1 or 2 deep inhalations repeated once or twice at 5 to 10 min if necessary. Repeat after 4 hr.	2-5	½-2

cont'd. next page

*Available without a prescription.
†Available in U.S. and Canada.

Table 27-1 Administration of adrenergic bronchodilators—cont'd.

Generic Name	Trade Name	Dosage and Administration	Onset (min)	Duration (hr)
Metaproterenol sulfate	Alupent† Metaprel	ORAL: *Adults*—10 mg 3 or 4 times daily initially, increased to 20 mg 3 or 4 times daily over 2 to 4 wk. *Children*—6 to 9 yr or under 60 lb, 10 mg 3 or 4 times daily.	15	3-4
		INHALATION (metered aerosol): *Adults and children over 12 yr only*— 2 to 3 inhalations every 3 to 4 hr not to exceed 12 inhalations daily.	2	2-4
Terbutaline sulfate	Brethine Bricanyl†	SUBCUTANEOUS: *Adults*—0.25 mg repeated in 15 to 30 min if necessary, with no more than 0.5 mg administered in any 4 hr period. *Children*—0.01 mg/kg body weight to a maximum of 0.25 mg.	15	2-4

		ORAL: *Adults*—initially 2.5 mg every 8 hr, increased to 5 mg every 8 hr. Dose may be lowered to 2.5 mg if side effects are too disturbing. *Children 12 yr and younger*—1.25 to 2.5 mg 3 times daily during waking hours.	10	4-7
	Brethine	INHALATION (metered aerosol): *Adults and Children over 12 yr*— 2 inhalations, 1 min apart, every 4-6 hrs.	5-30	3-4

*Available without a prescription.
†Available in U.S. and Canada.

rine is used for relief in acute asthmatic attack. Ephedrine is used prophylactically for patients with mild to moderate asthma. Albuterol is preferred for patients with angina. Isoetharine is safer for patients with cardiovascular disease, hypertension, or diabetes mellitus. Metaproterenol is used for prophylactic treatment of asthma. Terbutaline is used in prophylactic treatment of asthma or for relief of acute attacks.

Nurse Alert for Adrenergic Bronchodilators

- Monitor the vital signs, fluid intake and output, level of consciousness, blood gas levels, vital capacity, and treatment of infectious processes.
- Use these drugs with caution in the elderly and in patients with cardiovascular disease, hypertension, diabetes mellitus, or hyperthyroidism.
- Patients with cardiovascular disease may be moved to the ICU for cardiac monitoring; drugs and equipment should be available for the treatment of arrhythmias, drug responses, and acute hypertension.
- The use of adrenergic drugs is generally not recommended in pregnancy.

Side Effects of Adrenergic Bronchodilators

The side effects of these drugs are related to their alpha, beta-1, and beta-2 effects, as shown in Table 27-2.

Nursing Implications for Adrenergic Bronchodilators

- Anxiety, insomnia, fear, and other emotional responses may aggravate bronchospasm and air hunger in the patient.
- For subcutaneous or intramuscular injection, aspirate carefully before administering the dose to avoid inadvertent intravenous administration.
- For intravenous administration, the use of an infusion control device is recommended.
- Sus-Phrine is a suspension. Shake the vial or ampule thoroughly before preparing the ordered dose and administer immediately so the drug does not settle out of the suspension.

Bronchodilators and Other Drugs for Asthma 349

Table 27-2 Side effects of adrenergic bronchodilators

Drug	Alpha Effects	Beta-1 Effects	Beta-2 Effects
Albuterol/salbutamol	0	0	+
Ephedrine	+	+	+
Epinephrine	+	+	+
Isoetharine	0	0	+
Isoproterenol	0	+	+
Metaproterenol	0	(±)	+
Terbutaline	0	0	+

Alpha Effects

Vasoconstriction—
1. Systemic: increased blood pressure.
2. Inhaled: Decreased bronchial congestion, increased duration of action for co-administered beta-2 drug.

Beta-1 Effects

1. Stimulation of heart, increasing rate, force of contraction, and rate of repolarization. Overstimulation causes palpitations, arrhythmias.
2. Increased lipolysis (breakdown of fat).
3. Relaxation of gastrointestinal tract.

Beta-2 Effects

1. Bronchiole dilation.
2. Stimulation of skeletal muscle to cause a tremulous or shaky feeling.
3. Vasodilation (mainly in blood vessels supplying muscle).
4. Glycogenolysis (breakdown of stored glucose).

Central Nervous System Effects

Stimulation, causing nervousness, anxiety, insomnia, irritability, dizziness, sweating.

* 0, No stimulation; +, stimulation; (±), modest stimulation.

- The metered-dose inhaler: The patient using a metered-dose inhaler for the first time may need assistance. The patient should assemble the inhaler and shake the cannister.
- Instruct the patient to exhale deeply, then to put the mouthpiece into the mouth with the opening directed to the

350   **Pocket Nurse Guide to Drugs**

back of the throat. Grasp the mouthpiece with the teeth and lips. Some physicians recommend holding away from teeth and lips. The patient should then inhale deeply while depressing the aerosol container or activating the spray mechanism. The patient should then try to hold the breath for as long as possible before exhaling. The patient should wait at least 5 minutes before repeating the dose, depending on the physician's instructions. It may be necessary to hold the nose shut on children. If the patient is receiving two drugs via inhalation, the bronchodilator should be taken first, to allow for inhalation of the second drug (e.g., beclomethasone).

- If sublingual tablets are being used, instruct the patient to let the tablet dissolve under the tongue and not to swallow the saliva until the tablet is completely dissolved.
- Before discharging a patient on a beta receptor agonist, ascertain that the patient understands how to take the prescribed medication.
- Caution patients not to increase the frequency of taking prescribed medications or to switch to other drugs or inhalers without notifying the physician.
- Instruct patients with diabetes mellitus who are also taking beta receptor agonists to monitor their urine glucose levels closely.

Xanthines

Aminophylline (theophylline ethylenediamine)
Dyphylline
Oxtriphylline (choline theophyllinate)
Theophylline
Theophylline monoethanolamine
Theophylline sodium glycinate

Actions of Xanthines

The xanthines are thought to act by increasing cellular cyclic AMP concentrations and thereby relaxing bronchial smooth muscle and inhibiting mast cell degranulation.

Indications for Xanthines

Xanthines can be given intravenously for the control of acute bronchospasm in status asthmaticus or orally to control the bronchospasm of mild, moderate, or severe asthma.

Nurse Alert for Xanthines

- The xanthines should be used with caution in patients with cardiac or hepatic disease, hypertension, or hyperthyroidism; peptic ulcer may be aggravated.
- Monitor the vital signs.
- If hypotension occurs, keep the patient in bed until the effects of the drug wear off.
- The xanthines should be used in pregnancy only when the benefits outweigh the risks.

Side Effects of Xanthines

All of the xanthines may cause nausea, vomiting, epigastric pain, wakefulness, restlessness, irritability, exaggerated reflexes, mild muscle tremors, headache, hypotension, vertigo and dizziness. Serious toxic effects include delirium, convulsions, hyperthermia, and circulatory collapse.

Nursing Implications for Xanthines

- To decrease gastric irritation with oral preparations, the patient may be able to take the preparation with or just after meals; check with the physician, because this will alter the rate of absorption.
- Patients should be cautioned not to smoke.
- Instruct diabetic patients to monitor their urine glucose levels carefully.
- Instruct patients to avoid over-the-counter preparations unless cleared with the physician.
- Intravenous aminophylline: Too rapid infusion may cause arrhythmias, profound hypotension, and cardiac arrest. Monitor the vital signs every 5 to 15 minutes. Use an infusion control device or volume control device and a

Table 27-3 Administration of xanthines

Generic Name	Trade Name	Dosage and Administration
Xanthines		
Aminophylline (theophylline ethylenediamine)	Sold mainly under generic name	For acute asthma attack: INTRAVENOUS: Solutions should be diluted to 25 mg/ml and injected no more rapidly than 25 mg/min to avoid circulatory collapse. Loading dose, 5.6 mg/kg over 30 min. Maintenance dose, no more than 0.9 mg/kg/hr by continuous infusion. Dose is determined by age, cardiac and liver status, and smoking history. RECTAL: *Adults*—250 to 500 mg 1 to 3 times daily. *Children*—5 mg/kg not more often than every 6 hr. ORAL: *Adults*—500 mg for an acute attack. Maintenance dose, 200 to 250 mg every 6 to 8 hr. *Children*—7.5 mg/kg for an acute attack. Maintenance dose, 5 mg/kg every 6 hr.
Dyphylline	Dilin* Dilor Dyflex Emfabid Lufyllin Neothylline	ORAL: *Adults*—200 to 800 mg every 6 hr. *Children*—2 to 3 mg/lb/24 hr given in divided doses every 6 hr. Maximum dose, 15 mg/kg every 6 hr. INTRAMUSCULAR: *Adults*—250 to 500 mg.

Oxtriphylline (choline theophyllinate)	Choledyl*	ORAL: *Adults*—200 mg every 6 hr. *Children 2 to 12 yr*—100 mg/60 lb every 6 hr.
Theophylline	Many names, elixirs, syrups, tablets, capsules, timed-release preparation, suppositories	ORAL: *Adults, children*—Initial dose, 3 to 5 mg/kg every 6 hr. For maintenance: *Adults*—100 to 200 mg every 6 hr. *Children*—50 to 100 mg every 6 hr. RECTAL: *Adults*—250 to 500 mg every 8 to 12 hr. *Children*—10 to 12 mg/kg/24 hr. Administered no more frequently than every 6 hr.
Theophylline monoethanolamine	Fleet Brand Theophylline	RECTAL: *Adults*—250 to 500 mg. Do not repeat in less than 8 hr. Do not administer more than 2 times in 24 hr.
Theophylline sodium glycinate	Glynazan Panophylline Forte Synophylate Theofort	ORAL: *Adults*—330 to 660 mg every 6 to 8 hr after meals. *Children*—over 12 yr, 220 to 300 mg; 6 to 12 yr, 165 to 220 mg; 3 to 6 yr, 110 to 165 mg; 1 to 3 yr, 55 to 110 mg every 6 to 8 hr after meals.

*Available in U.S. and Canada.

354 Pocket Nurse Guide to Drugs

microdrip infusion set. Monitor intake and output. It may be advisable to have the patient attached to a cardiac monitor. This drug should not be mixed with any other in a syringe, and it is compatible with only a few other drugs for infusion; consult the pharmacy.

- Rectal aminophylline is poorly absorbed at best, but absorption is decreased if the rectum contains feces.
- The serum theophylline concentration may be measured at regular intervals to check on the rate of theophylline clearance.
- Many of these drugs are available in a regular formulation and sustained release (SR) formulation; the two cannot be interchanged. Check the original physician's order and the medication label carefully.

Other Drugs to Treat Asthma

Beclomethasone dipropionate
Cromolyn sodium
Dexamethasone sodium
Flunisolide
Triamcinolone acetonide

Actions of Other Drugs to Treat Asthma

Cromolyn acts by inhibiting mast cell degranulation and the release of bronchospastic agents caused by immunologic (antigen IgE) or nonimmunologic stimulation (exercise, hyperventilation), with no bronchodilator or antiinflammatory actions. Beclomethasone, dexamethasone sodium, flunisolide and triamcinolone acetonide are aerosol glucocorticoids.

Indications for Other Drugs to Treat Asthma

Cromolyn and the aerosol glucocorticoids are used prophylactically and are of no value in treating ongoing asthma attacks. Beclomethasone can be used daily without causing adrenal suppression or Cushing's syndrome with normal doses, although adrenal suppression has occurred in patients who were taking 1600 μg or more daily.

Table 27-4 Administration of other drugs to treat asthma

Generic Name	Trade Name	Dosage and Administration
Beclomethasone dipropionate	Beclovant* Vanceril*	INHALATION (metered dose inhaler): each dose is 50 μg. *Adults*—2 inhalations 3 to 4 times daily. *Children 6 to 12 yr*— 1 to 2 inhalations 3 to 4 times daily.
Cromolyn sodium	Intal* Rynacrom† Nasalcrom	INHALATION: *Adults and children over 5 yr*—20 mg capsule inhaled 4 times daily. Inhalation solution
Dexamethasone Sodium phosphate	Decadron phosphate Respihaler	*Adult*—3 inhalations 3 to 4 times daily.
Flunisolide	Nasalide	*Adult*—2 inhalations twice daily
Triamcinalone acetonide	Azmacort	*Adult*—2 inhalations 3 to 4 times daily.

*Available in U.S. and Canada.
†Available in Canada only.

Nurse Alert for Other Drugs to Treat Asthma

- Patients transferred from oral glucocorticoids to beclomethasone must be monitored carefully because adrenal function may be impaired, possibly for months.
- Be careful not to use either drug during acute bronchospastic episodes because the powder may cause further irritation.

Side Effects of Other Drugs to Treat Asthma

Cromolyn may cause bronchospasm or allergic reactions in sensitive individuals; other infrequent side effects include cough, nasal congestion, wheezing, dizziness, joint swelling and pain, nausea, headache, and urticaria. The side effects of the *glucocorticoids* are discussed with the steroids in Chapter 36.

Nursing Implications for Other Drugs for Asthma

- Instructions for use of the glucocorticoid inhalers are provided by the manufacturer and should be reviewed with the patient before use.
- Advise patients to take their medications only as directed by the physician, to return to the physician for problems or questions, and to report any unexpected signs or symptoms.
- Patients using glucocorticoids should gargle and rinse their mouths after each use of the inhaler to help prevent fungal infections.
- If the patient using cromolyn complains of irritation of the mouth or throat or dry mouth after use of cromolyn, instruct the patient to suck on a lozenge or drink a glass of water after each dose. If heartburn or esophageal irritation occurs, drinking a glass of milk or taking a dose of antacid before each dose of cromolyn may help. Before using antacids on a regular basis, the patient should consult with a physician.
- InspirEase and Inhal-Aid are devices developed by Key Pharmaceuticals to aid in the delivery of medication via metered-dose inhalers. Some patients, especially children, are unable to successfully coordinate the breathing and hand activities needed to use standard metered-dose inhalers.

Bronchodilators and Other Drugs for Asthma 357

This results in lost medication and inadequate dosing of the patient. The two devices mentioned were designed to alleviate some of these problems, and can be used with a variety of medication cannisters. For additional information, consult the drug company, the instructions supplied with the devices, or the May, 1984 American Journal of Nursing.

- The turbo-inhaler or Spinhaler: The patient using a turbo-inhaler for cromolyn for the first time may need assistance. Instructions are provided by the manufacturer and should be reviewed with the patient.

Nasal Decongestants 28

Ephedrine sulfate
Epinephrine hydrochloride
Naphazoline hydrochloride
Oxymetazoline hydrochloride
Phenylephrine hydrochloride
Phenylpropanolamine hydrochloride
Propylhexedrine
Pseudoephedrine hydrochloride
Pseudoephedrine sulfate
Tetrahydrozoline hydrochloride
Xylometazoline hydrochloride

Actions of Nasal Decongestants

The nasal decongestants considered here all act by stimulating alpha-adrenergic receptors thereby causing blood vessels to constrict in the nasal passage, relieving congestion.

Indications for Nasal Decongestants

Because of rebound effects, nasal decongestants are generally used for short-term treatment of congestion (3-5 days). Many of these nonprescription drugs are included in combination cold remedies. *Pseudoephedrine* is useful for relief of a runny nose and congestion leading to earache. *Xylometazoline* is considered relatively safe for children. *Propylhexedrine* causes less stimulation of the central nervous system and is therefore safer than some other nasal decongestants.

Nurse Alert for Nasal Decongestants

- Nasal decongestants are contraindicated for patients with hyperthyroidism, diabetes mellitus, hypertension, heart disease, or receiving monoamine oxidase inhibitors or tricyclic antidepressants.

- Propylhexedrine is a volatile drug whose use by children should be supervised.
- Xylometazoline should not be used excessively or for more than a few days.

Side Effects of Nasal Decongestants

The nasal decongestants may, with repeated use, cause systemic side effects including nervousness, dizziness, palpitations, and transient hypertension. Children are especially vulnerable to overdose. Sweating, drowsiness, shock, or coma may occur. Epinephrine may also cause CNS stimulation, headaches, and palpitations. Naphazoline may also cause arrhythmias and slowing of heart rate. The adverse reactions to tetrahydrozoline can be severe, including the symptoms listed for other decongestants, and high fever and coma in young children. All nasal decongestants cause rebound effects of congestion after discontinuation.

Nursing Implications for Nasal Decongestants

- Instruct patients to read the ingredients in over-the-counter preparations and to buy only formulations containing the desired drug(s), without unnecessary other drugs.
- Only preparations designed for pediatric doses should be used with children.
- For best results with topical application, instruct the patient to blow the nose before using the medication, administer as directed, and avoid blowing the nose for several minutes.
- To prevent contamination, each patient or individual family member should have a different dropper or spray applicator. Applicators should be washed or rinsed with hot water after each use.

Table 28-1 Administration of nasal decongestants

Generic Name	Trade Name	Dosage and Administration
Ephedrine sulfate	Efedron Nasal Efedsol—1% Vatronol Nose Drops	ORAL: *Adults*—25 to 50 mg every 3 to 4 hr. *Children*—3 mg/kg body weight daily in 4 to 6 divided doses. TOPICAL: *Adults and children*—2 to 3 drops of a 1% or 3% solution in each nostril 2 to 3 times daily, no more than 4 times daily. Also may apply as a pack or tampon.
Epinephrine hydrochloride	Adrenalin Chloride	TOPICAL: 0.1% aqueous solution as a spray or 1 to 2 drops every 4 to 6 hr. Not recommended for children under 6 yr.
Naphazoline hydrochloride	Privine Hydrochloride*	TOPICAL: 0.05% and 0.1% solutions. Two drops in each nostril no more than every 3 hr or 2 sprays every 4 to 6 hr.
Oxymetazoline hydrochloride	Afrin Nafrine†	TOPICAL: *Adults*—2 to 4 drops or 2 to 3 sprays of 0.05% solution in each nostril at morning and at bedtime. *Children*—over 6 yr, as for adults; 2 to 5 yr, 0.025% solution is used as above.
Phenylephrine hydrochloride	Coricidin Decongestant Nasal Mist Neo-Synephrine Hydrochloride* Super Anahist Nasal Spray	TOPICAL: *Adults*—drops of 0.25% to 1% solution in each nostril (head in lateral, head-low position) every 3 to 4 hr. Nasal spray or nasal jelly may be used. *Children over 6 yr*—as for adults. *Infants and young children*—0.125% solution is used as above.

Nasal Decongestants

Phenylpropanolamine hydrochloride	Propadrine Hydrochloride	ORAL: *Adults*—25 mg every 3 to 4 hr or 50 mg every 6 to 8 hr. *Children 8 to 12 yr*—20 to 25 mg 3 times daily. Not recommended for children under 8 yr.
Propylhexedrine	Benzedrex	TOPICAL (inhalation): 2 inhalations in each nostril as needed.
Pseudoephedrine hydrochloride	Novafed, Sudafed*, Robidrine†	ORAL: *Adults*—60 mg every 6 to 8 hr. *Children*—15 to 30 mg every 6 to 8 hours.
Pseudoephedrine sulfate	Afrinol Repetabs	As for pseudoephedrine hydrochloride
Tetrahydrozoline hydrochloride	Tyzine	TOPICAL: *Adults*—2 to 4 drops of a 0.1% solution in each nostril. Do not repeat more frequently than every 3 hr. *Children*—6 yr and over, as for adults; 2 to 6 yr, 2 to 3 drops of a 0.05% solution in each nostril every 4 to 6 hr.
Xylometazoline hydrochloride	Neo-Synephrine II, Long-acting Otrivin Spray*, Sinutab Long-lasting Sinus Spray	TOPICAL: *Adults*—2 to 3 drops of 0.1% solution or 1 to 2 inhalations of 0.1% spray in each nostril every 8 to 10 hr. *Children*—6 mo to 12 yr, 2 to 3 drops of 0.05% solution in each nostril every 4 to 6 hr. *Infants*—1 drop of 0.05% solution in each nostril every 6 hr.

*Available in U.S. and Canada
†Available in Canada only

Drugs to Treat a Cough

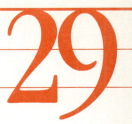

Expectorants
  Guaifenesin (glycerol guaiacolate)
  Iodinated glycerol
  Potassium iodide
  Terpin hydrate
Antitussives
  Codeine
  Hydrocodone bitartrate
  Dextromethorphan hydrobromide
  Diphenhydramine hydrochloride
  Levopropoxyphene napsylate
  Noscapine
  Chlophedianol
  Benzonatate
Mucolytic drugs
  Acetylcysteine

Actions of Anticough Drugs

The iodide expectorants are believed to stimulate the bronchial glands to secrete more fluid. Guaifenesin stimulates the secretion of respiratory tract fluid by reflex activity by irritating the stomach when swallowed. The opiate antitussives suppress a cough by inhibiting the medullary center for the cough reflex. Dextromethorphan has a similar inhibitory action but is nonnarcotic. Levopropoxyphene and noscapine are chemically related to the opiates, but do not have the common opiate side effects. Chlophedianol is a centrally acting antitussive with some local anesthetic and anticholinergic actions. Diphenhydramine is an antihistamine with an antitussive action. Benzonatate is believed to act by depressing peripheral receptors responsible for initiating a cough. Mucolytic agents break up viscous mucus so that it can be coughed up or drained; acetylcysteine breaks the disulfide bonds linking molecules in mucus.

Indications for Anticough Drugs

If a cough is not relieved by humidifying the air, increasing fluid input, and other measures, therapy may include an expectorant, antitussive, or mucolytic drug. Because of side effects, *iodide* expectorants are seldom used today. *Guaifenesin* is used for symptomatic relief of a dry, unproductive cough. *Antitussives* are used to directly or indirectly inhibit the cough reflex. *Mucolytic agents* are used to break up viscous mucus as occurs in patients with pulmonary infection or chronic obstructive lung disease when normal mechanisms for clearing the lungs are compromised.

Nurse Alert for Anticough Drugs

- Potassium iodide is contraindicated for patients with hyperkalemia, hyperthyroidism, or iodide hypersensitivity.
- Codeine and hydrocodone are opiates and are capable of causing drug dependence.
- Because antitussives may cause drowsiness, caution patients to avoid activities requiring mental alertness if possible, or adjust the medication schedule for maintained alertness during such activities.
- Patients receiving mucolytic agents should be supervised carefully to maintain patency of the airway with the increased secretions; suction equipment should be available for elderly, immobilized, nonalert, or entubated patients.
- Acetylcysteine should be used cautiously with patients with asthma because bronchospasm may occur.

Side Effects of Anticough Drugs

Iodide expectorants has a high incidence of adverse effects including rashes, hypothyroidism, and swelling of parotid glands; overdose may cause fever, skin eruptions, nausea, vomiting, and mucous membrane ulcerations. *Guaifenesin* occasionally causes nausea or vomiting. The *opiate antitussives* in normal cough-suppression doses rarely cause side effects but may include nausea, dizziness, drowsiness, and constipation. *Dextromethorphan* may occasionally cause

Table 29-1 Administration of anticough drugs

Generic Name	Trade Name	Dosage and Administration
Expectorants*		
Guaifenesin (glyceryl guaiacolate)	Anti-tuss Glycotuss Nortussin Robitussin** Various others	ORAL: *Adults*—200 to 400 mg every 3 to 4 hr. *Children*—6 to 12 yr—100 mg every 3 to 4 hr; 2 to 6 yr, 50 mg every 3 to 4 hr.
Iodinated glycerol	Organidin**	ORAL: *Adults*—20 drops of solution (50 mg) or a 60 mg tablet or 5 ml elixir (60 mg) 4 times daily. *Children*—no more than ½ adult dose daily.
Potassium iodide	Potassium Iodide SSKI Pima	ORAL: *Adults*—300 mg every 4 to 6 hr. *Children*—60 to 500 mg daily, divided in 2 to 4 doses.
Terpin hydrate		ORAL: 85 mg every 2 to 4 hr.
Antitussives		
Codeine, codeine phosphate, codeine sulfate		ORAL: *Adults*—10 to 20 mg every 4 to 6 hr, no more than 120 mg in 24 hr. *Children*—6 to 12 yr, 5 to 10 mg every 4 to 6 hr, no more than 60 mg in 24 hr; 2 to 6 yr, 2.5 to 5 mg every 4 to 6 hr, no more than 30 mg in 24 hr.

Drugs to Treat a Cough 365

Hydrocodone bitartrate	Codone Dicodid Robidone†	ORAL: *Adults*—5 to 10 mg every 6 to 8 hr. *Children*—0.6 mg/kg daily in divided doses.
Dextromethorphan hydrobromide	Coughettes Sucrets Cough Control Lozenge Romilar CF Various others	ORAL: *Adults*—10 to 20 mg every 4 hr or 30 mg every 6 to 8 hr. *Children*—6 to 12 yr, ½ adult dose; 2 to 6 yr, ¼ adult dose.
Diphenhydramine hydrochloride	Benylin Cough Syrup** Benadryl]**	ORAL: *Adults*—25 mg every 4 hr, no more than 100 mg in 24 hr. *Children*—6 to 12 yr, ½ adult dose. 2 to 5 yr, ¼ adult dose.
Levopropoxyphene napsylate	Novrad	ORAL: *Adults*—100 mg every 4 hrs. *Children*—Approximately 0.5 mg/lb every 4 hrs. Maximum daily doses: 25 lbs: 75 mg; 50 lb: 150 mg; 75-100 lb: 200 mg.
Noscapine	Tusscapine Noscattuss†	ORAL: *Adults*—15 to 30 mg every 4 to 6 hrs; maximum 120 mg in 24 hrs. *Children, 6 to 12 yrs*—15 mg, 3 or 4 times daily, maximum 60 mg in 24 hrs. *Children, 2 to 6 yrs*—7.5 to 15 mg, 3 or 4 times daily, maximum 4 doses.

cont'd. next page

*Only those exportants available by themselves have been listed. Other drugs included in cough or cold mixtures as an expectorant include potassium guaiacolsulfonate, ammonium chloride, terpin hydrate, ipecac, calcium iodide, and citric acid.

**Available in U.S. and Canada

†Available in Canada only

Table 29-1   Administration of anticough drugs—cont'd.

Generic Name	Trade Name	Dosage and Administration
Clophedianol	Ulo Ulone†	ORAL: *Adults*—25 mg, 3 or 4 times daily. *Children, 6 to 12 yrs*—12.5 to 25 mg 3 or 4 times daily. *Children, 2 to 6 yrs*—12.5 mg 3 or 4 times daily
Benzonatate	Tessalon**	ORAL: *Adults*—100 mg 3 to 6 times daily. *Children*—over 10 yr, same as adults; under 10 yr, 8 mg/kg body weight in 3 to 6 divided doses.
Mucolytics		
Acetylcysteine	Mucomyst** Airbron†	NEBULIZATION USING A FACE MASK, MOUTHPIECE, OR TRACHEOSTOMY: 1 to 10 ml of a 20% solution or 2 to 20 ml of a 10% solution every 2 to 6 hr. DIRECT INSTILLATION: 1 to 2 ml of a 10% or 20% solution as often as every hour.

*Only those expectorants available by themselves have been listed. Other drugs included in cough or cold mixtures as an expectorant include potassium guaiacolsulfonate, ammonium chloride, terpin hydrate, ipecac, calcium iodide, and citric acid.

**Available in U.S. and Canada

†Available in Canada only

drowsiness or dizziness. *Levopropoxyphene* causes sedation, dizziness, nervousness, nausea, and epigastric distress. *Chlophedianol* may cause excitement or irritability and in large doses causes sedation. *Diphenhydramine* may cause the typical antihistamine effect of drowsiness. *Benzonatate* may cause a chilly sensation, dizziness, and drowsiness. *Acetylcysteine* has the odor of rotten eggs and may cause gastrointestinal upset or nausea; other effects include stomatitis and rhinorrhea.

Nursing Implications for Anticough Drugs

- Caution patients to keep these and all medications out of the reach of children.
- Before using a mucolytic agent the first time with a patient, the patient should be informed about the purpose of the agent and instructed to cough up and expectorate loosened secretions as needed.

BODY DEFENSE SYSTEM DRUGS

PART VI

Nonnarcotic Analgesic-antipyretic Drugs

30

Salicylates
- Aspirin (acetylsalicylic acid)
- Calcium carbaspirin
- Sodium salicylate
- Salicylamide

Other analgesic-antipyretics
- Acetaminophen
- Mefenamic acid

See also Ch 32 [nonsteroidal antiinflammatory]

Actions of Analgesic-antipyretic Drugs

The analgesic action of these drugs results from a peripheral mechanism through which they interfere with local mediators released in damaged tissue to stimulate nerve endings. The antipyretic effect results from the action of reversing the effect of endogenous pyrogen in the hypothalamus. Acetaminophen has the same analgesic and antipyretic actions but unlike the other drugs has little antiinflammatory action.

Indications for Analgesic-antipyretic Drugs

Aspirin is used for analgesic, antipyretic, and antiinflammatory effects and is effective for mild to moderate headache and generalized mild muscular aches; combined with codeine, aspirin is used to treat mild to moderate pain of tooth extractions, episiotomies, cancer, bone fractures, and other conditions. Acetaminophen is used like aspirin for analgesic and antipyretic actions, particularly to avoid gastric irritation and alteration in platelet function and bleeding time. Mefenamic acid is used as an analgesic but is no more effective than aspirin for mild to moderate pain.

370

Nurse Alert for Analgesic-antipyretic Drugs

- Acetaminophen in overdoses of 10 gm or more may cause serious liver damage; 15 gm or more may result in death.
- Aspirin should not be taken when alcohol is present in the stomach because of greatly increased gastric bleeding.
- Mefenamic acid is contraindicated for patients with gastrointestinal, kidney, or liver disease; therapy for all patients should be limited to 1 week because of toxic effects.

Side Effects of Analgesic-antipyretic Drugs

Acetaminophen may cause allergic reactions, usually skin rashes, hemolytic anemia in patients with glucose-6-phosphate dehydrogenase deficiency, and methemoglobinemia (more serious in infants) in long term therapy; overdose may damage the liver; dosage over 2.6 gm in 24 hours may produce loss of appetite, nausea, vomiting, and slight jaundice. *Aspirin* commonly causes gastrointestinal upset felt as heartburn or nausea, and long-term use may cause anemia if excessive GI bleeding occurs, especially in women with heavy menses; allergic responses may cause a skin rash; mild aspirin intoxication (salicylism) may cause tinnitus, hyperventilations, and fever; toxic overdose may result in serious acid-base blood disturbances, metabolic acidosis, particularly in children, and subsequent metabolic block and hyperthermia. Children treated with aspirin may have an increased risk for developing Reye's Syndrome. *Mefenamic acid* may cause gastrointestinal upset, diarrhea, and rash, and in therapy longer than 1 week has toxic effects in the gastrointestinal, kidney, and blood-forming systems.

Nursing Implications for Analgesic-antipyretic Drugs

- Aspirin should always be administered with a full glass of milk or water to decrease gastric irritation.
- In patients taking aspirin on a long-term basis, routinely test the stool for the presence of occult blood.
- Instruct patients to read labels carefully to check dosages.
- Patients having difficulty tolerating aspirin may find that switching to a different brand will be helpful.

Table 30-1   Administration of analgesic-antipyretic drugs

Generic Name	Trade Name	Dosage and Administration
Salicylates		
Aspirin (acetylsalicylic acid)	A.S.A. Aspergum Bayer Aspirin Children's Aspirin Ecotrin* Measurin	FOR ANALGESIA OR ANTIPYRESIS: ORAL, RECTAL: *Adults*—650 mg every 4 hr, or 1.3 gm of timed-release every 8 hr. *Children*—65 mg/kg over 24 hr in divided doses, every 4 to 6 hours, OTC.**
Aspirin, buffered	Aluprin Ascriptin Bufferin Alka-Seltzer Various others	Same as for aspirin. There are no smaller dose tablets for children. OTC.**
Aspirin, aluminum		Same as for aspirin. These are chewable tablets (75 mg) for children. OTC.**
Calcium carbaspirin	Calurin	Same as for aspirin. OTC.**
Sodium salicylate	Uracel	Same as for aspirin. OTC.** An injectable form is available by prescription.

Salicylamide	Salicylamide Uromide	ORAL: *Adults and children over 12 yr*—650 mg every 6 hr. OTC.**

Other Analgesic-antipyretics

Acetaminophen	Tylenol* Datril Various others	ORAL: *Adults*—325 to 650 mg every 6 to 8 hr. No more than 2.6 Gm in 24 hr. *Children*—7 to 12 yr, ½ adult dose; 3 to 6 yr, ⅙ adult dose. OTC.**
Mefenamic acid	Ponstel Ponstan†	ORAL: *Adults and children over 14 yr*—500 mg initially, then 250 mg every 6 hr as needed. Prescription drug.

*Available in U.S. and Canada
**OTC, Over the counter; available without prescription.
†Available in Canada only

374   **Pocket Nurse Guide to Drugs**

- Patients who are allergic to aspirin, those already taking aspirin on a long-term basis, those taking oral anticoagulants, or anyone routinely using over-the-counter drugs should be cautioned to read labels carefully and to avoid inadvertent overdose with aspirin.
- Patients taking oral anticoagulants should avoid the use of aspirin; acetaminophen may ordinarily be used.
- Monitor the urine and blood sugar concentrations in patients receiving mefenamic acid.

Antihistamines for Allergic Reactions

31

Azatadine maleate
Brompheniramine maleate
Carbinoxamine maleate
Chlorpheniramine maleate
Clemastine
Cyproheptadine hydrochloride
Dexchlorpheniramine maleate
Diphenhydramine hydrochloride
Diphenylpyraline hydrochloride
Doxylamine succinate
Hydroxyzine hydrochloride

Hydroxyzine pamoate
Methdilazine hydrochloride
Promethazine hydrochloride
Pyrilamine maleate
Trimeprazine tartrate
Tripelennamine citrate or hydrochloride
Triprolidine hydrochloride
See also Ch. 23 for antihistamines for nausea and vomiting and Ch. 28 for antihistamines in cold remedies

Actions of Antihistamines for Allergic Reactions

Antihistamines act to block some actions of histamine, which may cause angioedema, anaphylaxis, asthma, eczema, purpura, rhinitis, and urticaria. The primary actions of antihistamines are in the blood vessels and the bronchioles, with a local anesthetic effect that may relieve the itching of some skin rashes.

Indications for Antihistamines for Allergic Reactions

Antihistamines are indicated primarily to decrease the discomfort of allergic reactions involving the upper respiratory system, such as hay fever, or the skin, such as hives. Antihistamines are used in many nonprescription cold and hay fever medications to dry up nasal congestion (see Ch. 28), as antitussives, or to treat motion sickness or nausea and vomiting (see Ch. 23). Diphenhydramine is used with epinephrine to treat anaphylactic reactions. Doxylamine and diphenhydramine are often included in nonprescription sleep aids. Methdilazine and trimeprazine are used to relieve skin itching.

Nurse Alert for Antihistamines for Allergic Reactions

- Antihistamines should be used with extreme caution with alcohol, hypnotics, sedatives, antipsychotics, anti-anxiety drugs, or narcotic analgesics, because of the additive central nervous system depression.
- Antihistamines must be used with caution in patients with glaucoma, hyperthyroidism, cardiovascular disease, or hypertension.
- Antihistamines are contraindicated for nursing mothers.
- An acute allergic anaphylactic reaction should be treated with epinephrine along with or followed by antihistamines—but not with antihistamines alone.
- Patients should be cautioned to avoid activities requiring mental alertness until the effects of the drug have been evaluated.
- Antihistamines should not be used in pregnant women unless the benefit clearly outweighs the risks.

Parenteral Administration of Antihistamines for Allergic Reactions

Intravenous Brompheniramine Maleate

- May be given undiluted, or may be added to infusing fluids (normal saline or 5% dextrose).
- Check with the pharmacy for compatibility with other drugs.
- Rate of infusion: A single bolus injection should be administered over at least one minute; when added to infusing fluids may be adjusted to needed rate of infusion.

Intravenous Dimenhydrinate

- Dimenhydrinate is a mixture of diphenhydramine and chlorotheophylline.

Antihistamines for Allergic Reactions

- Must be diluted for safe administration, 50 mg of drug in 10 ml of sodium chloride injection.
- Rate of administration should not exceed 25 mg per minute.

Intravenous Diphenhydramine Hydrochloride

- Can be administered slowly as direct IV push. Rate of administration should not exceed 25 mg per minute.

Intravenous Chlorpheniramine Maleate

- Can be administered slowly as direct IV push. Rate of administration should not exceed 10 mg per minute.

Intravenous Promethazine Hydrochloride

- Solutions administered should never be more concentrated than 25 mg per ml. Dilute the drug with up to 9 ml of normal saline, to make a dilution of 2.5 to 5 mg per ml.
- Rate of administration should not exceed 25 mg per minute.
- Slightly yellow solutions may be safely used. Highly discolored solutions should be discarded.

Side Effects of Antihistamines for Allergic Reactions

Drowsiness is the most common side effect, possible with all the antihistamines although less common with *carbinoxamine, chlorpheniramine, clemastine, pyrilamine,* and *triprolidine.* Possible anticholinergic effects include dry mouth, blurred vision, urinary retention, tachycardia, constipation, insomnia, tremors, nervousness, irritability, and sedation. At toxic levels, antihistamines may cause central nervous system stimulation, more commonly in children, or CNS depression, more commonly in the elderly; flushed skin, dilated pupils, and fever may occur.

Nursing Implications for Antihistamines

- Signs and symptoms of urinary retention include decreased output, palpable urinary bladder, and inability to empty the bladder during urination. Monitor the fluid intake and output. Instruct the outpatient to notify the physician if the patient suspects urinary retention.
- If blurred vision occurs, the patient should notify the physician.

Table 31-1 Administration of antihistamines for allergic reactions

Generic Name	Trade Name	Dosage and Administration
Azatadine maleate	Optimine*	ORAL: *Adults*—1 to 2 mg twice daily. *Children*—not established.
Brompheniramine maleate	Dimetane* Rolabromophen	ORAL: *Adults*—4 to 8 mg 3 to 4 times daily or 8 to 12 mg of sustained-release form 2 to 3 times daily. *Children*—over 6 yr, ½ adult dose; under 6 yr, 0.5 mg/kg daily divided into 3 to 4 doses.
Carbinoxamine maleate	Clistin	ORAL: *Adults*—4 to 8 mg 3 to 4 times daily or 8 to 12 mg of sustained-release form 2 to 3 times daily. *Children*—over 6 yr, 4 mg 3 to 4 times daily; 3 to 6 yr, 2 to 4 mg 3 to 4 times daily; 1 to 3 yr, 2 mg 3 to 4 times daily.
Chlorpheniramine maleate	Chlormene Chlortab Chlor- Trimeton‡ Ciramine Pyranistan	ORAL: *Adults*—4 mg 3 to 4 times daily or 8 to 12 mg of sustained-release form 2 to 3 times daily. *Children*—6 to 12 yr, 2 mg 3 to 4 times daily or 8 mg of sustained-release form once daily; 2 to 6 yr, 1 mg 3 to 4 times daily.
Clemastine	Tavist	ORAL: *Adults*—2.68 mg 3 times daily. Not intended for children.
Cyproheptadine hydrochloride	Periactin	ORAL: *Adults*—4 to 20 mg daily, not more than 0.5 mg/kg. Dose is started at 4 mg 3 times daily. *Children*—7 to 14 yr, 4 mg 2 to 3 times daily to a maximum of 16 mg daily; 2 to 6 yr, 2 mg 2 to 3 times daily to a maximum of 12 mg daily.

Antihistamines for Allergic Reactions

Dexchlorpheniramine maleate	Polaramine*	ORAL: *Adults*—1 to 2 mg 3 or 4 times daily or 4 to 6 mg 2 times daily or 6 mg of timed-release form 3 times daily. *Children*—under 12 yr, 0.5 to 1 mg 3 to 4 times daily.
Diphenhydramine hydrochloride	Benadryl* Hydrochloride* Bendylate Fenylhist Rohydra Valdrene	ORAL: *Adults*—25 to 50 mg 3 to 4 times daily. *Children*—over 20 lb, 2.5 to 25 mg 3 to 4 times daily; under 12 yr, 5 mg/kg in 4 divided doses each day.
Diphenylpyraline hydrochloride	Diafen Hispril	ORAL: *Adults*—2 mg every 4 hr or 5 mg of sustained-release form every 12 hr. *Children*—over 6 yr, 2 mg every 6 hr or 5 mg of sustained-release form once daily; 2 to 6 yr, 1 to 2 mg every 8 hr.
Doxylamine succinate	Decapryn‡ Unisom*	ORAL: *Adults*—12.5 to 25 mg every 4 to 6 hr. *Children*—6 to 12 yr, 75 mg divided into 4 to 6 doses daily; under 6 yr, 2 mg/kg body weight divided into 4 to 6 doses daily.
Hydroxyzine hydrochloride Hydroxyzine pamoate	Atarax	ORAL: *Adults*—25 mg 3 or 4 times daily. *Children over 6 yr*—50-100 mg daily in divided doses; *under 6 yr*—50 mg daily in divided doses.
Methdilazine hydrochloride	Dilosyn† Tacaryl	ORAL: *Adults*—8 mg 2 to 4 times daily. *Children*—over 3 yr, 4 mg 2 to 4 times daily.

cont'd. next page

*Available in U.S. and Canada
†Available in Canada only
‡Available without a prescription.

Table 31-1 Administration of antihistamines for allergic reactions—cont'd.

Generic Name	Trade Name	Dosage and Administration
Promethazine hydrochloride	Phenergan† Quadnite Remsed Zipan	ORAL: *Adults*—12.5 mg 4 times daily or 25 mg at bedtime. *Children*—½ adult dose.
Pyrilamine maleate	Allertoc‡ Zem-Histine‡	ORAL: *Adults*—25 to 50 mg 3 times daily. *Children*—6 to 12 yr, ½ adult dose.
Trimeprazine tartrate	Panectyl* Temaril	ORAL: *Adults*—2.5 mg 4 times daily or 5 mg of sustained-release form every 12 hr. *Children*—over 3 yr, 2.5 mg at bedtime or up to 3 times daily (over 6 yr can take 5 mg of sustained-release form once a day); 6 mo to 3 yr, 1.25 mg at bedtime or up to 3 times daily.
Tripelennamine citrate or hydrochloride	PBZ-SR Pyribenzamine† Ro-Hist	ORAL: *Adults*—25 to 50 mg every 4 to 6 hr or 100 mg of sustained-release form every 12 hr. *Children*—over 5 yr, 50 mg of sustained-release form every 12 hr; children and infants, 5 mg/kg daily divided into 4 to 6 doses.
Triprolidine hydrochloride	Actidil†	ORAL: *Adults*—2.5 mg 3 to 4 times daily. *Children*—over 6 yr, ½ adult dose; under 6 yr, 0.3 to 0.6 mg 3 to 4 times daily.

*Available in U.S. and Canada
†Available in Canada only
‡Available without a prescription.

Antihistamines for Allergic Reactions   **381**

- If dry mouth is a problem, the patient may find it helpful to chew gum, suck on sugarless candies or mints, use a commercially available saliva substitute, or increase fluid intake.
- Antiemetics are often ordered with a narcotic analgesic. The two drugs together potentiate the central nervous system depressant effects of the narcotic and help to reduce nausea, a side effect that often accompanies narcotic use.
- Remind the patient to keep all health care providers informed of all drugs they are taking, including over-the-counter preparations.
- Hypotension may occur. Symptoms might include dizziness, visual changes, syncope, and light-headedness. Monitor the blood pressure.
- If the hospitalized patient is unsteady or hypotensive, instruct the patient to call for assistance before ambulating; keep the side rails up.
- Gastrointestinal side effects may be relieved by taking the antihistamine with a small snack or meals.
- When used for motion sickness, antihistamines should be taken 30 minutes to 1 hour before the start of travel.
- Instruct patients to report sore throat, fever, general malaise, bruising, or unexplained bleeding.
- Instruct patients to report to the physician any unusual signs or symptoms that develop.
- Patients with allergies should be encouraged to carry medical information with them, indicating the nature of their allergies and whom to contact for additional medical information.
- Dimenhydrinate and diphenhydramine hydrochloride should be used with caution in patients receiving ototoxic drugs, since these antihistamines may mask the ototoxic symptoms of the other drugs.

Nonsteroidal Antiinflammatory Drugs

32

Aspirin and salicylates
  Aspirin
  Choline salicylate
  Diflunisal
  Magnesium salicylate
  Salsalate
  Sodium salicylate
  Sodium thiosalicylate
Phenylbutazone
Oxyphenbutazone
Indole and pyrrole derivatives of parachlorobenzoic acid
  Indomethacin
  Sulindac
  Tolmetin sodium

Phenylpropionic acid derivatives
  Fenoprofen
  Ibuprofen
  Naproxen
  Naproxen sodium
Piroxicam
Meclofenamate sodium monohydrate
See also Ch. 30 (analgesic-antipyretic)

Actions of Nonsteroidal Antiinflammatory Drugs

The nonsteroidal antiinflammatory drugs are believed to act by inhibiting the enzyme cyclooxygenase so that the prostaglandins are not synthesized.

Indications for Nonsteroidal Antiinflammatory Drugs

These drugs are also analgesic-antipyretic drugs but are used primarily to treat inflammation and its pain, for patients who cannot tolerate aspirin, and for patients with painful joint disorders, rheumatoid arthritis, osteoarthritis, ankylosing spondylitis, low back pain, gout, and menstrual cramps. Phenylbutazone and oxybutazone are prescribed only for 1 to 2 weeks to treat acute inflammatory response.

Nurse Alert for Nonsteroidal Antiinflammatory Drugs

- Magnesium salicylate is contraindicated in patients with renal failure.
- Phenylbutazone and oxybutazone should not be taken longer than 7 days by patients over 60 or longer than 14 days by younger patients.
- All antiinflammatory drugs should be used with caution in pregnancy or lactation; consult the physician.
- Because ibuprofen, naproxen, fenoprofen, piroxicam and indomethacin may cause drowsiness, caution patients to avoid activities requiring mental alertness until the effects have been evaluated.
- Do not administer ibuprofen, naproxen, fenoprofen, or piroxicam to patients who are aspirin sensitive because cross-sensitivity may occur with these drugs.

Side Effects of Nonsteroidal Antiinflammatory Drugs

Aspirin may cause gastric irritation with or without bleeding, salicylism, and decreased platelet aggregation (see also Ch. 30). The *salicylate salts* cause less gastrointestinal upset than aspirin. *Diflunisal* has a lower incidence of the same side effects as aspirin and may cause dizziness, edema, and tinnitus. *Meclofenamate* commonly causes gastrointestinal upset, sometimes with severe diarrhea. *Phenylbutazone* and *oxyphenbutazone* cause fluid retention, gastric irritation, prolonged platelet inhibition, and occasionally liver damage or bone marrow suppression. *Indomethacin* may cause nausea, vomiting, loss of appetite, diarrhea, occasionally gastrointestinal ulceration, headaches and dizziness, vertigo, insomnia, edema, weight gain, rashes, confusion, fainting, drowsiness, coma, convulsions, and behavioral changes. *Sulindac* and *tolmetin* have side effects similar to those of aspirin but with a lower incidence. *Ibuprofen, naproxen,* and *fenoprofen* may cause gastrointestinal upset, dizziness, headache, and tinnitus.

Table 32-1 Administration of nonsteroidal antiinflammatory drugs

Generic Name	Trade Name	Dosage and Administration
Aspirin and Salicylates		
Aspirin	Bayer Timed-Release, Bufferin, Arthritis strength, Measurin, Various others	ORAL: *Adults*—arthritis: 2.6 to 5.2 Gm daily in divided doses (every 8 hr for timed-release forms.) For acute rheumatic fever, up to 7.8 Gm daily in divided doses. *Children*—65 mg/kg over 24 hr in divided doses every 6 hr. OTC.‡
Choline salicylate	Arthropan	ORAL: *Adults and children over 12 yr*—870 mg (1 teaspoon) every 3 to 4 hr, up to 6 times daily. OTC.‡
Diflunisal	Dolobid	ORAL: *Adults*—500 to 1000 mg daily, taken as 2 doses. Maximum dose is 1.5 Gm daily. Prescription drug.
Magnesium salicylate	Magan, Mobidin	Same as aspirin. No pediatric forms. Prescription drug.
Salsalate	Disalcid	ORAL: *Adults only*—1 Gm 3 times daily. Prescription drug.
Sodium salicylate	Generic*	ORAL: Same as aspirin. OTC.‡ An injectable form is available by prescription.
Sodium thiosalicylate	Arthrolate, Nalate, Thiodyne	INTRAMUSCULAR: *Adults*—prescription drug. For musculoskeletal disorders, 50 to 100 mg daily or every other day. For rheumatic fever, 100 to 150 mg every 4 to 6

| | Thiolate | hr for 3 days, then 100 mg twice daily. |
| | Th-Sal | |

Phenylbutazone and Oxyphenbutazone

Phenylbutazone	Azolid	ORAL: *Adults*—300 to 600 mg daily in divided doses every 6 to 8 hr. Not for children under 14 yr.
	Butazolidin*	
	Intrabutazone†	
Oxyphenbutazone	Oxalid	ORAL: *Adults*—300 to 600 mg daily in divided doses every 6 to 8 hr. Not for children under 14 yr.
	Tandearil	

Indole and Pyrrole Derivatives of Parachlorobenzoic Acid

Indomethacin	Indocin	ORAL: *Adults*—25 mg 2 to 3 times daily. If necessary, the total daily dose can be increased 25 to 50 mg daily at weekly intervals, but the total daily dose should not exceed 150 to 200 mg. Not for children under 14 yr.
	Indocid†	
Sulindac	Clinoril	ORAL: *Adults*—initially, 150 to 200 mg twice a day. Dose is adjusted for therapeutic response. Not for children under 14 yr.
Tolmetin sodium	Tolectin*	ORAL: *Adults*—initially, 400 mg 3 times daily, then adjust. Usual maintenance dose is 0.6 to 1.8 Gm daily. *Children over 12 yr—*

cont'd. next page

*Available in U.S. and Canada
**Available without a prescription
†Available in Canada only
‡OTC, over the counter, available without prescription

Table 32-1 Administration of nonsteroidal antiinflammatory drugs—cont'd.

Generic Name	Trade Name	Dosage and Administration
Tolmetin sodium—cont'd.		initially, 20 mg/kg body weight daily in divided doses. Usual maintenance dose is 15 to 30 mg/kg daily.
Phenylpropionic Acid Derivatives		
Fenoprofen	Nalfon*	ORAL: *Adults*—300-600 mg 3 to 4 times daily.
Ibuprofen	Advil**	ORAL: *Adults*—300 to 600 mg 4 times daily. Not for children under 14 yr.
	Motrin*	
	Nuprin**	
	Rufen	
Naproxen	Naprosyn*	ORAL: *Adults*—500 to 750 mg divided in 2 doses daily. Not for children under 14 yr.
Naproxen sodium	Anaprox	
Oxicam		
Piroxicam	Feldene	ORAL: *Adults*—20 mg daily as a single or divided dose.
Fenamate		
Meclofenamate	Meclomen	ORAL: *Adults*—200 to 400 mg divided in 3 to 4 doses daily.

*Available in U.S. and Canada
**Available without a prescription

Nursing Implications for Nonsteroidal Antiinflammatory Drugs

- See also the nursing implications for analgesic-antipyretic drugs (Ch. 30).
- In the treatment of arthritis, better results will be obtained if drugs are taken routinely, as ordered, and not on an intermittent or "prn" basis. Physical activity will often be better tolerated if delayed until 30 minutes after medication is taken. Rest, application of moist heat, prescribed exercises, and other treatment modalities will also assist in the management of inflammatory diseases.
- These drugs may improve symptoms but will not alter the long-term course of the disease being treated.
- Administer these medications with food or antacids (except for fenoprofen).
- There may be a cross-sensitivity that occurs in patients allergic to aspirin or any of the other nonsteroidal antiinflammatory drugs.

Phenylbutazone and Oxyphenbutazone

- These drugs are used only on a short-term basis because of the serious side effects that can occur. Among the hematological problems that may occur are aplastic anemia, agranulocytosis, and pancytopenia. Instruct patients to report any unusual sign or symptom, including fever, rash, sore throat, stomatitis (inflammation of or sores in the mouth), and malaise.
- These drugs may cause gastric irritation, including ulceration. Instruct patients to report persistent dyspepsia, bleeding with stools, or a change in the color or consistency of stools. Monitoring stools for the presence of occult blood may be appropriate.
- Patients in whom fluid retention might be dangerous (e.g., those with cardiovascular, hypertensive, or renal disease) should be instructed to weigh themselves daily and to report weight gain in excess of 2 to 5 pounds.
- Monitor the blood pressure of the hospitalized patient at least twice a day and of the outpatient on each return visit.

Pocket Nurse Guide to Drugs

- Instruct patients to report any signs of bleeding from the gums, urinary tract, or rectum; excessive bruising; or the development of petechiae. Patients who are also receiving oral anticoagulants will probably need a dosage adjustment of the anticoagulant.

Indomethacin

- Gastrointestinal disturbances are a major problem with this drug. Monitoring stools at regular intervals for the presence of occult blood may be appropriate.
- Corneal deposits and retinal disturbances have occurred in patients receiving long-term therapy.

Sulindac and Tolmetin

- These drugs occasionally cause fluid retention and peripheral edema. Patients in whom fluid retention might be dangerous (e.g., those with cardiovascular, hypertensive, or renal disease) should be instructed to weigh themselves daily and to report weight gain in excess of 2 to 5 pounds. Monitor the blood pressure of hospitalized patients at least twice daily, and of outpatients on each return visit.
- These drugs may alter coagulation studies. Instruct patients to report any unusual bleeding, bruising, or the appearance of petechiae. There is no indication that it is necessary to change the dosage of oral anticoagulants, but patients should be observed carefully, and appropriate blood studies should be done at regular intervals.
- Because these drugs are excreted by the kidney, patients with impaired renal function should be monitored closely. Renal function studies should be performed at regular intervals.
- These drugs may cause transient abnormalities in liver function tests, especially in the alkaline phosphatase level. If abnormal values persist or continue to increase, the drug should be discontinued.
- These drugs should not be administered to patients who are hypersensitive to aspirin or other non-steroidal anti-inflammatory drugs.

Nonsteroidal Antiinflammatory Drugs **389**

- Although eye changes have not been reported with tolmetin and sulindac, the frequent eye changes seen with other non-steroidal anti-inflammatory drugs have caused the manufacturers to recommend that periodic ophthalmic examinations be performed on patients receiving these drugs on a long-term basis. Instruct the patient to report any visual changes.

Ibuprofen, Naproxen, Fenoprofen, and Piroxicam

- Blurred vision, decreased vision, changes in color vision, and other visual changes have been reported. Instruct patients to report any visual changes. Periodic ophthalmic examinations may be indicated in selected patients.
- These drugs can cause fluid retention and peripheral edema. Patients in whom fluid retention might be dangerous (e.g., those with cardiovascular, hypertensive or renal disease) should be instructed to weigh themselves daily and to report weight gain in excess of 2 to 5 pounds. Monitor the blood pressure.
- These drugs may alter coagulation studies. Instruct patients to report any unusual bleeding, bruising, or the appearance of petechiae. Monitor appropriate blood studies done at regular intervals.
- Tinnitus and decreased hearing ability have been reported. Instruct the patient to report any ear problems. If hearing loss is suspected, audiometric testing should be done at regular intervals.
- Fenoprofen may cause increases in the blood urea nitrogen (BUN), serum transaminase, lactic dehydrogenase (LDH), and alkaline phosphate levels. It is recommended that periodic liver and renal function tests be performed on patients receiving this drug on a long-term basis.
- Patients receiving phenobarbital for whom fenoprofen is prescribed may require a dosage adjustment of phenobarbital.

Antirheumatoid Drugs 33

Auranofin
Aurothioglucose
Gold sodium thiomalate
Hydroxychloroquine sulfate

Penicillamine
See also analgesic-antipyretic drugs (Ch. 30) and nonsteroidal antiinflammatory drugs (Ch. 32)

Actions of Antirheumatoid Drugs

It is not known how the gold salts aurothioglucose and gold sodium thiomalate act on the synovial tissues to suppress rheumatoid arthritis.

Indications for Antirheumatoid Drugs

Aspirin and other antiinflammatory drugs are used in treating the pain and inflammation of early rheumatoid arthritis (see Ch. 30), but these have no effect on the course of the disease. The antirheumatic drugs discussed here may be effective in altering the progression of joint erosion. The drugs are usually tried in the following order: the gold salts, auranofin, hydroxychloroquine, penicillamine, and immunosuppressive drugs. Glucocorticoids may be used for nonarticular manifestations of rheumatoid arthritis, such as vasculitis and rheumatoid lung, and occasionally for joint symptoms (see Ch. 36).

Nurse Alert for Antirheumatoid Drugs

- With hydroxychloroquine, regular ophthalmic examination is necessary because retinopathy may develop that may progress to blindness.
- Patients on penicillamine must be carefully monitored for suppression of blood cells and autoimmune responses.

Antirheumatoid Drugs **391**

- Patients receiving glucocorticoids should be warned to avoid stress on the joints because the drugs mask the normal signals of stress.
- Gold salt therapy is contraindicated in patients with renal disease, marked hypertension, cardiovascular disease, uncontrolled diabetes, hematologic diseases, eczema, colitis, and pregnancy; the elderly may not tolerate therapy well.

Side Effects of Antirheumatoid Drugs

Gold salt therapy (intramuscular) often has serious side effects requiring discontinuation: skin reactions, mouth ulcers, fever, dermatitis, stomatitis, sore throat, anorexia, malaise, excessive bruising or bleeding, petechiae, kidney damage, and blood count abnormalities. *Hydroxychloroquine* may cause retinopathy, skin rashes, peripheral neuropathy, and a depressed white count. *Penicillamine* frequently causes a loss of taste, nausea, depression of platelets and white cells, skin reactions, rashes, dermatitis, oral ulcers, hematologic side effects, tinnitus, skin wrinkling, anorexia, and proteinuria. *Auranofin* (oral gold) may cause diarrhea, abdominal pain, nausea, and a loss of appetite, most commonly in the first month of therapy.

Nursing Implications for Antirheumatoid Drugs

- See also nursing implications for nonsteroidal antiinflammatory drugs (Ch. 32)

Gold Compounds

- Review with patients aspects of good oral hygiene. If stomatitis should occur, assess the advisability of continuing the usual oral care routine. It may be necessary to discontinue flossing and/or brushing until the stomatitis clears. Oral cleansing can be done with mouthwashes or gargles and by gently swabbing the mouth. Lemon-glycerin preparations should be avoided as they are often irritating if open blisters are present. The development of a metallic taste in the mouth may be an early sign of impending stomatitis. If the patient has dentures, these should be

392 Pocket Nurse Guide to Drugs

Table 33-1   Administration of antirheumatoid drugs

Generic Name	Trade Name	Dosage and Administration
Aurothioglucose Gold sodium thiomalate	Solganal Myochrysine*	INTRAMUSCULAR (GLUTEAL): *Adults*—Weekly injections of 10 mg week 1, 25 mg week 2, 25 to 50 mg week 3, 50 mg each week thereafter until a total of 800 mg to 1 Gm has been administered. If the patient has improved and there are no toxic signs, 50 mg injections are continued every 2 wk (4 doses) then every 3 wk (4 doses), then every 3 to 4 wk. *Children*— 1 mg/kg (up to 25 mg) weekly for 20 wk, then every 2 to 4 wk if the therapy is beneficial.
Hydroxychloroquine sulfate	Plaquenil Sulfate*	ORAL: *Adults*—200 mg once or twice daily at meals, not more than 3.5 mg/lb.
Penicillamine	Cuprimine* Depen	ORAL: *Adults*— initially 125 to 250 mg daily as a single dose. May be raised every 2 to 3 mo by 250 mg daily to 500 to 750 mg daily.
Auranofin	Ridaura	ORAL: *Adults*—6 mg daily

*Available in U.S. and Canada

Antirheumatoid Drugs 393

removed from the mouth, except for mealtimes, until the stomatitis clears.

- An allergic reaction, manifested by flushing, fainting, dizziness, sweating, malaise, weakness, or even anaphylaxis, may occur after administration.

Parenteral Gold Compounds

- Patients should be observed for 15 to 30 minutes after a dose before being sent home. Instruct patients to report the development of any of these signs or symptoms. Epinephrine, corticosteroids, antihistamines, and oxygen should be readily available in any setting where gold therapy is administered. In some cases the allergic type reaction may be due to the solvent used in the gold preparation and not to the gold itself; switching to another preparation may be sufficient to eliminate the problem.
- Dermatitis may be aggravated by exposure to the sun or other sources of ultraviolet light.
- Urinalysis should be performed before each dose. If proteinuria or hematuria is present, the dose should be withheld and the patient's condition evaluated. Complete blood counts should be performed every other week.
- Inform patients that several weeks or months of therapy may be necessary before improvement is seen.
- Solganal is an oil-based suspension, and Myochrysine is an aqueous suspension. Both should be administered via deep intramuscular injection into the gluteal muscle.
- With oral compounds, monitor liver function studies and urinalysis at regular intervals.

Hydroxychloroquine

- See Chapter 49 for further discussion of this medication, which is also an antimalarial drug.

Penicillamine

- Penicillamine is a copper chelating agent and is used for this action in the treatment of Wilson's disease, a disorder of copper metabolism.
- Drug fever may occur, usually commencing about 2 to 3 weeks after the initiation of therapy. It may or may not

394 Pocket Nurse Guide to Drugs

require discontinuation of the drug. Instruct the patient to report the development of fever.

- Patients with Wilson's disease or with poor dietary intake may require pyridoxine replacement during therapy.
- Hematological side effects include bone marrow suppression, agranulocytosis, and thrombocytopenia. Frequent evaluation of the blood counts should be done. Instruct the patient to report any bleeding, bruising, sore throat, malaise, fever, or any new sign or symptom.
- Cross-sensitivity between penicillin and penicillamine does not always occur, but patients should be questioned about possible allergy to penicillin before therapy with penicillamine is begun.
- Instruct patients on this drug, especially on long-term therapy, to take the drug as ordered. If the drug is omitted for several days, then restarted, a sensitivity reaction may occur.
- Several months of therapy may be required to see improvement in the patient's condition.
- This drug is best taken on an empty stomach, one-half hour before meals, two hours after meals, or at bedtime.
- Blood urea nitrogen levels, creatinine levels, and urinalysis should be monitored at regular intervals.

Drugs for Gout

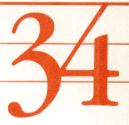

Allopurinol
Colchicine

Probenecid
Sulfinpyrazone

Actions of Drugs for Gout

Allopurinol acts by inhibiting the formation of uric acid from hypoxanthine or xanthine, which are excreted instead. Colchicine acts in an unknown manner to relieve the pain of gouty arthritis. Probenecid and sulfinpyrazone inhibit the reabsorption of uric acid by the kidney tubules and thereby promote the excretion of uric acid in the urine.

Indications for Drugs for Gout

Colchicine is used to provide relief from the pain of an acute attack of gouty arthritis and may be used prophylactically. Allopurinol is used for patients with renal uric acid crystals, impaired renal function, or gout resulting from drug therapy such as cancer therapy that increases uric acid production. Probenecid and sulfinpyrazone are used to reduce existing trophi and to prevent recurrence of a gouty attack.

Nurse Alert for Drugs for Gout

- Probenecid and sulfinpyrazone are contraindicated for patients with renal failure or a history of renal stones.
- Patients receiving probenecid or sulfinpyrazone must drink at least 8 glasses of water daily to avoid crystallization of uric acid in kidney tubules or the bladder.
- Patients receiving allopurinol should be cautioned to avoid activities requiring mental alertness until the effects of the drug have been evaluated.

396 Pocket Nurse Guide to Drugs

Table 34-1 Administration of drugs for gout

Generic Name	Trade Name	Dosage and Administration
Allopurinol	Zyloprim* Lopurin	ORAL: *Adults*—200 to 300 mg daily as a single dose; maximum, 800 mg daily. Dose is reduced if there is renal insufficiency.
Colchicine	Novocolchine† Colchicine*	ORAL: *Adults*—0.5 to 0.6 mg hourly or 1 to 1.2 mg initially and 0.5 to 0.6 mg every 2 hr. This is regimen for an acute gouty attack and is continued until the pain subsides or gastrointestinal symptoms appear. Maximum dose, 7 to 8 mg. For prophylaxis, 0.5 to 1 mg daily. INTRAVENOUS: for an acute attack, 1 to 2 mg initially, then 0.5 mg every 3 to 6 hr or 1 dose of 3 mg; maximum dose, 4 mg.
Probenecid	Benemid* Benuryl†	ORAL: *Adults*—250 mg 2 or 3 times daily the first week, then 500 mg twice daily thereafter. May increase to 2.0 Gm daily if necessary.
Sulfinpyrazone	Anturan† Anturane	ORAL: *Adults*—100 to 200 mg 2 times daily with meals or with milk at bedtime. The dosage is raised as needed to control blood urate

*Available in U.S. and Canada
†Available in Canada only

Drugs for Gout 397

Table 34-1 Administration of drugs for gout—cont'd.

Generic Name	Trade Name	Dosage and Administration
Sulfinpyrazone—cont'd.		levels (400 to 800 mg daily). The dose is then reduced to the minimum effective level, usually 300 to 400 mg daily.

*Available in U.S. and Canada
†Available in Canada only

Parenteral Administration of Colchicine

- This drug must be given intravenously; extravasation into surrounding tissues must be avoided. There is no specific antidote for extravasation. Local application of heat or cold, and administration of analgesics may be helpful.
- While it may be given undiluted, it is best diluted. Dilute the 2 ml vial to 20 ml with sterile normal sodium chloride. Solutions containing a bacteriostatic agent or solutions of 5% dextrose in water should not be used.
- Dilutions which precipitate or become turbid should not be used.
- Rate of administration should not exceed 0.5 mg per minute.

Side Effects of Drugs for Gout

Oral colchicine may cause nausea, vomiting, and diarrhea; intravenous colchicine must be diluted because it produces severe tissue inflammation. The long-term administration of colchicine may cause hematologic side effects seen as sore throat, fever, rash, malaise, excessive bruising or bleeding, and petechiae. Allopurinol rarely produces side effects, which are seen as allergic rash reactions; drowsiness may occur. Probenecid is well tolerated generally but may cause gastrointestinal upset or an allergic reaction; sulfinpyrazone is more likely to cause gastrointestinal upset.

398   Pocket Nurse Guide to Drugs

Nursing Implications for Drugs for Gout

- The patient should be instructed to stay well hydrated so that an output of at least 2000 to 3000 ml per day is maintained.
- Better relief is obtained if these drugs are used consistently, that is, as prescribed, rather than intermittently.

Colchicine

- Inform patients that nausea, vomiting, and diarrhea may occur; if they do occur, the physician should be notified. These symptoms serve as a warning that the dose being used is too high and that a lower dose is needed.

Probenecid and Sulfinpyrazone

- Patients taking either of these drugs should be taught to maintain a fluid intake of 3000 to 4000 ml per day.
- There are several preparations available that contain both probenecid and colchicine. Patients taking these combination products should be taught about each of the separate drugs.
- Gastrointestinal side effects are the most common with these drugs and may be indicative of overdosage. Taking the drugs with meals or milk may help decrease the side effects.
- Because probenecid may prolong the action of oral hypoglycemic agents, patients taking these two drugs should be alerted to the possibility that hypoglycemia may be a problem and that it should be reported if it occurs.
- Alkalinization of the urine helps prevent crystallization of the uric acid. For this reason sodium bicarbonate, potassium citrate, or other alkalinizing agents may be prescribed concurrently with probenecid or sulfinpyrazone. Once serum urate levels return to normal, it may be possible to discontinue the alkalinizing agent.
- Sulfinpyrazone may potentiate the action of oral hypoglycemic agents or insulin. Patients with diabetes mellitus should be alerted to the possibility of hypoglycemia and should report it if it occurs.

Drugs for Gout **399**

- Sulfinpyrazone may potentiate the action of oral anticoagulants. Patients receiving both drugs should be cautioned to report any excessive bleeding or bruising.
- Low doses of aspirin and other salicylates inhibit uric acid secretion. Instruct patients to avoid the use of aspirin; acetaminophen may be used.

Allopurinol

- The appearance of a rash is often the first sign of an allergic reaction and usually warrants discontinuing the drug.
- Long-term administration of this drug may be associated with elevations of alkaline phosphatase and serum transaminase levels. If these blood studies are elevated, evaluation of the patient is appropriate.
- Patients receiving mercaptopurine or azathioprine who are then started on allopurinol will require a reduction in dose of the mercaptopurine or azathioprine to one-fourth to one-half the original dose.
- Salicylates may apparently be used with this drug with no adverse interactions.
- Allopurinol prolongs the half-life of coumarin oral anticoagulants. Caution patients receiving both drugs to be alert to excessive bleeding or bruising and to report them if they occur. It may be necessary to reduce the dose of the anticoagulant.
- Hematological problems have been reported occasionally. Instruct the patient to report any sore throat, fever, malaise, rash, bruising, or bleeding.
- Patients should be reminded to maintain a high fluid intake, especially if they are also receiving a uricosuric drug.

PART VII

ENDOCRINE SYSTEM DRUGS

Drugs Affecting the Pituitary Gland

35

Neurohypophyseal hormones for diabetes insipidus
- Desmopressin acetate
- Lypressin
- Posterior pituitary extract
- Vasopressin, or antidiuretic hormone (ADH)
- Vasopressin tannate in oil
- Oxytocin
- Other drugs for diabetes insipidus
  - Chlorothiazide (see also Ch. 14)
  - Chlorpropamide (see also Ch. 37)
  - Clofibrate (see also Ch. 19)
  - Carbamazepine (see also Ch. 7)

Adenohypophyseal hormones
- Adrenocorticotropic hormone (ACTH)
- Follicle-stimulating hormone (FSH)
- Growth hormone (GH)
- Luteinizing hormone (LH), or interstitial cell-stimulating hormone (ICSH)
- Prolactin, or luteotropic hormone (LTH)
- Thyroid-stimulating hormone (TSH)

General Actions of Pituitary Hormones

The structure and function of the anterior pituitary and the posterior pituitary are different. Each section of the pituitary supplies unique hormones (neurohypophyseal hormones from the posterior pituitary and adenohypophyseal hormones from the anterior pituitary), with specific actions described separately below.

General Indications for Pituitary Hormone Administration

Neurohypophyseal hormones are used in replacement therapy (vasopressin and related drugs for diabetes insipidus) and for pharmacologic action (oxytocin to stimulate uterine muscle or

402

Drugs Affecting the Pituitary Gland **403**

promote milk letdown). Additional non-hormone drugs are included here that are used in treatment of diabetes insipidus. Oxytocics are discussed in Chapter 43.

Adenohypophyseal hormones are occasionally used in replacement therapy when other, more available steroids would be ineffective. More commonly, adenohypophyseal hormones are used diagnostically.

Neurohypophyseal Hormones for Diabetes Insipidus

Desmopressin acetate
Lypressin
Posterior pituitary extract
Vasopressin, or antidiuretic hormone (ADH)
Vasopressin tannate in oil

Other Drugs for Diabetes Insipidus

Chlorothiazide	Clofibrate
Chloropamide	Carbamazepine

Actions of Neurohypophyseal Hormones

Vasopressin increases the permeability of sections of the renal tubule to water, allowing water to be reabsorbed from the tubule and returned to the bloodstream, the normal mechanism by which the kidneys concentrate urine. Vasopressin also modulates central nervous system activity and may influence affective behavior, memory, thermoregulation, and anterior pituitary function.

Chlorpropamide, clofibrate, and carbamazepine increase the release of ADH from the posterior pituitary.

Indications for Neurohypophyseal Hormones and Related Drugs

ADH may be used in replacement therapy for diabetes insipidus for patients with traumatic head injuries or hypothalamic surgery, or for patients with chronic diabetes insipidus resulting from trauma to the hypothalamus or hypophyseal stalk.

Vasopressin is used for short-term management of unconscious patients.

Desmopressin acetate is the drug of choice for replacement therapy for chronic diabetes insipidus. Lypressin is similarly used.

Vasopressin tannate in oil has rarely been used since the introduction of lypressin and desmopressin acetate.

Chlorpropamide is used to control diuresis in diabetes insipidus and to control hyperglycemia in diabetes mellitus (p. 435).

Clofibrate is used to control diuresis in diabetes insipidus and for lipid-lowering effects (p. 285).

Carbamazepine is an anticonvulsant (pp. 92-93) occasionally used to control diuresis in diabetes insipidus.

Nurse Alert for Neurohypophyseal Hormones

- Patients with known or suspected vascular disease should be carefully monitored when therapy with vasopressin or related drugs is begun.
- Patients with angina may find that they have more heart pain while taking this drug.

Side Effects of Neurohypophyseal Hormones and Drugs for the Treatment of Diabetes Insipidus

Posterior pituitary extract is rarely used due to irritations to nasal passages and unwanted effects of proteins other than vasopressin. *Vasopressin* may cause nausea, belching, and cramps. *Clofibrate* may cause nausea or, rarely, muscle cramps or weakness. *Chlorothiazide* may cause hyponatremia or hypokalemia. *Chlorpropamide* may cause hypoglycemia. *Carbamazepine* may cause dizziness, confusion, or drowsiness.

Nursing Implications for Patients Being Treated for Diabetes Insipidus

- Diabetes insipidus may develop subsequent to traumatic head injuries or surgery to the hypothalamic region of the brain. It is therefore critically important for health personnel to monitor fluid intake, urine output, urine specific

Drugs Affecting the Pituitary Gland   405

gravity, and blood sodium levels in these patients to detect excessive diuresis and resultant dehydration. In diabetes insipidus the urine is characteristically light in color, produced in large quantities often exceeding measured fluid intake, and of low specific gravity, 1.000 to 1.005 (normal usually being 1.010 to 1.030). The diagnosis is often first made by the observant nurse.

- Excessive urine production may also occur in diabetes mellitus due to glycosuria. Careful monitoring of urine and blood glucose levels will distinguish this patient from one with diabetes insipidus.

- To administer vasopressin tannate in oil (Pitressin Tannate in oil), the following procedure is used:
  a. Heat the unopened vial in warm water for several minutes to decrease the viscosity of the peanut oil.
  b. Vigorously shake the ampule to resuspend the medication, which is usually an inconspicuous film on the side of the vial. Resuspension is adequate when no particles of medication remain on the bottom or sides of the vial. Failure to shake sufficiently will result in inaccurate dosage and erratic absorption.
  c. The correct dose should be drawn up into a syringe fitted with a large bore (19 to 21 gauge), 1½ inch needle, and administered intramuscularly immediately before the oil cools too much.
  d. Inject the medication with slow, even pressure on the plunger. Attempts to inject too rapidly can cause pressure to increase within the syringe so that the needle and syringe separate and the medication is spilled.
  e. Appropriate injection sites would include the buttocks, thigh, or ventrogluteal site. The oil base, which allows slow absorption, can produce palpable lumps at injections sites. For this reason, injection sites should be rotated and the deltoid muscle avoided.
  f. Oil-based medications should never be given intravenously.

- Because the aqueous preparation and the oil-based preparation of vasopressin have similar trade names, the nurse should clearly understand which preparation has been ordered and question an inappropriate order.

Table 35-1   Administration of neurohypophyseal hormones and drugs for the treatment of diabetes insipidus

Generic Name	Trade Name	Drug Class	Administration	Properties
Desmopressin acetate	DDAVP*	Synthetic derivative of neurohypophyseal hormone	Nasal once or twice daily	Peptide with longer serum half-life than vasopressin; increases renal reabsorption of water.
Lypressin	Diapid	Synthetic derivative of neurohypophyseal hormone	Nasal usually 4 times daily	Peptide with short serum half-life increases renal reabsorption of water.
Posterior pituitary extract	Pituitrin*	Neurohypophyseal hormone	Parenteral or nasal	Peptide with short serum half-life; contains ADH and oxytocin; increases renal reabsorption of water.
Vasopressin	Pitressin*	Neurohypophyseal hormone	Parenteral (short-term)	Peptide with short serum half-life; increases renal reabsorption of water.
Vasopressin tannate in oil	Pitressin Tannate*	Neurohypophyseal hormone	Intramuscular depot	Peptide derivative slowly absorbed; increases renal reabsorption of water.
Chlorothiazide	Diuril*	Thiazide diuretic	Oral (see p. 212)	Promotes sodium, chloride excretion.

Chlorpropamide	Diabinese*	Sulfonylurea hypoglycemic agent	Oral (see p. 436)	Increases release of ADH from posterior pituitary and increases ADH action in the kidney.
Clofibrate	Atromid S*	Hypolipidemic agent	Oral (see p. 286)	Increases release of ADH from the posterior pituitary.
Carbamazepine	Tegretol	Tricyclic antidepressant	Oral (see p. 99)	Increases release of ADH from the posterior pituitary.

*Available in U.S. and Canada

408 Pocket Nurse Guide to Drugs

- Patients with diabetes insipidus will usually find that it is not necessary to measure their urinary output to monitor the disease at home; increased frequency of urination will usually signal loss of control.
- Gastrointestinal complaints may signal too high a dose of vasopressin and weakness and fatigue in a patient receiving chlorpropamide may signal a hypoglycemic reaction to that drug.
- After pituitary surgery, even for removal of the pituitary gland, diabetes insipidus may be only temporary.
- Patients with diabetes insipidus should wear a medical identification indicating their diagnosis.
- Patients may require special help in learning to administer the nasal powders or the solutions that are snuffed into the nose. A severe cold, allergies, or nasal surgery might make the nasal mucous membrane route of administration inappropriate. These patients may require temporary control with injectable forms of vasopressin.
- Patients taking medications via the nasal route will usually find that no significant increase in drug level occurs if more than two sprays per nostril are used. It is usually of more benefit to increase the frequency of dosing rather than to increase the number of sprays per nostril.
- Patients with known or suspected vascular disease should be carefully monitored when therapy with vasopressin or related drugs is begun. Patients with angina may find that they have more heart pain while taking this drug.
- Overdoses of vasopressin may produce water intoxication characterized by hyponatremia (low blood sodium) and excessive water retention with sodium loss via the kidney. Patients should therefore be instructed not to repeat their dosage until diuresis recurs.

Adenohypophyseal Hormones

Adrenocorticotropic hormone (ACTH)
Follicle-stimulating hormone (FSH)
Growth hormone (GH)
Luteinizing hormone (LH), or interstitial cell-stimulating hormone (ICSH)

Prolactin, or luteotropic hormone (LTH)
Thyroid-stimulating hormone (TSH)

Note: These hormones are rarely used in replacement therapy. Table 35-2 summarizes the physiologic actions of adenohypophyseal hormones.

Actions of Adenohypophyseal Hormones

Growth hormone controls growth of long bones, is a potent anabolic agent in many tissues, increases the rate of amino acid transport into cells, elevates liver glycogen and blood glucose levels, and increases mobilization of fats for energy. FSH and LH regulate maturation and function of sexual organs, and in females stimulate ovarian estrogen production. ACTH stimulates the adrenal cortex to synthesize and release cortisol and glucocorticoids and minor amounts of sex steroids. Prolactin stimulates milk formation.

Indications for Adenohypophyseal Hormones

Panhypopituitarism, a syndrome resulting from insufficient hypophyseal hormones, is treated with steroids and thyroid hormones rather than by replacement adenohypophyseal hormones. Children with true pituitary dwarfism may be treated by replacement therapy with growth hormone. Treatment for deficiencies of FSH and LH generally uses steroids rather than adenohypophyseal hormones.

Side Effects of Growth Hormone

Because growth hormone actions antagonize those of insulin, prolonged treatment may precipitate diabetes mellitus in predisposed individuals.

Nursing Implications for Growth Hormone

- Treatment with growth hormone should be reserved for patients in whom growth hormone deficiency is clearly demonstrated. Growth hormone purified from human cadavers is no longer available; however, human growth hormone produced by recombinant DNA methods is expected to become available shortly.
- Growth hormone should be prescribed only when epiphyses have not yet closed and there is significant short stature.

Table 35-2 Physiologic actions of adenohypophyseal hormones

Descriptive Name	Other Names	Hypothalamic Releasing Factor	Target Tissue	Target Tissue Response
Adrenocorticotropic hormone	ACTH Corticotropin	Corticotropin-releasing factor (CRF)	Adrenal cortex Pigment cells of skin	Increased steroid synthesis Increased pigmentation
Follicle-stimulating hormone	FSH	Gonadotropin-releasing hormone (GnRH); FSH-releasing hormone (FRH or FSH-RH)	Ovary Seminiferous tubules	Increased estrogen production Maturation
Growth hormone	GH Somatropin STH	Somatropin or growth hormone-releasing factor (SRF or GRF); somatostatin or somatotropin-release inhibitory factor (SRIF)	Whole body	Increased anabolism, cell size, cell numbers
Luteinizing hormone or interstitial cell-stimulating hormone	ICSH LH	Gonadotropin-releasing hormone (GnRH); luteinizing hormone-releasing factor or hormone (LRF, LRH, LHRF, or LHRH)	Ovary Leydig cells	Ovulation; formation of corpus luteum Increased androgen synthesis
Prolactin	LTH Luteotropic hormone	Prolactin-inhibiting factor (PIF); prolactin-releasing factor (PRF)	Breast	Milk formation
Thyroid-stimulating hormone	Thyrotropin TSH	Thyrotropin-releasing hormone or factor (TRH or TRF)	Thyroid gland	Increased T_3, T_4 synthesis

Drugs Affecting the Pituitary Gland **411**

- The drug is administered intramuscularly three times a week. Injection sites should be rotated.
- Growth hormone should be used cautiously if there is progression of any underlying intracranial lesion.
- Treatment with growth hormone can precipitate hypothyroidism.
- Growth hormone has a potential diabetogenic effect. Monitor urine sugar concentration, and teach the patient or family to test the urine for sugar at home. Insulin may be required during the course of therapy.
- In diabetic adults destruction of the pituitary gland with loss of growth hormone may cause the patient to require less insulin.
- During therapy with growth hormone, parents should be instructed to keep weekly weight and height charts and to report any excessive gain in either area, according to parameters outlined by the physician.

Nursing Implications for Panhypopituitarism

- The patient who loses all or nearly all pituitary function due to trauma, surgery, or disease must be treated with replacement hormonal therapy to survive. Treatment with exogenous forms of cortisol usually substitutes for ACTH loss. Thyroid hormones usually replace TSH. Except in the child, growth hormone is not replaced. ADH may only need temporary replacement, as it is synthesized in the hypothalamus. The gonadotropic hormones, follicle-stimulating hormone, luteinizing hormone, and prolactin are rarely used in replacement therapy. More often the estrogens or androgens (Chapters 39 and 44) are used to help the patient maintain his or her own sexual identity. In the female it is difficult to recreate the monthly cyclic surges of these hormones, so this may not be attempted unless requested by the patient; thus the female is sterile. Oxytocin is not usually replaced unless the woman has been able to conceive and the hormone would be needed to assist with labor and delivery.
- Patients should wear medical identification indicating what replacement therapy they are receiving.

Adrenal Steroids and Other Drugs Affecting the Adrenal Gland

36

Adrenal steroids
  Amcinonide
  Beclomethasone
  Betamethasone
  Clocortolone
  Cortisone
  Desonide
  Desoximetasone
  Desoxycorticosterone
  Dexamethasone
  Diflorasone
  Fludrocortisone
  Flunisolide
  Flumethasone
  Fluocinolone
  Fluocinonide
  Fluorometholone
  Fluprednisolone
  Flurandrenolide
  Halcinonide
  Hydrocortisone (cortisol)
  Medrysone
  Meprednisone
  Methylprednisolone
  Paramethasone
  Prednisolone
  Prednisone
  Triamcinolone
Drugs used in diagnosis of
adrenal gland dysfunction
  Adrenocorticotropic hormone
  (ACTH)
  Cosyntropin
  Metyrapone

Actions of Adrenal Steroids

Mineralocorticoids cause the kidney to retain sodium and associated water while promoting potassium loss. Glucocorticoids have many actions, including stimulating gluconeogenesis, mobilizing amino acids from muscle protein, maintaining water diuresis by antagonizing the effects of antidiuretic

Adrenal Steroids and Other Drugs Affecting the Adrenal Gland

hormone, suppressing lymphoid tissue activity, reducing inflammatory processes, and sensitizing the arterioles to norepinephrine.

Indications for Adrenal Steroids

The *mineralocorticoids* desoxycorticosterone and fludrocortisone are used in replacement therapy in adrenal insufficiency, and as therapy for adrenal disease causing sodium loss.

The *glucocorticoids* are used in replacement therapy in adrenal insufficiency and for their antiinflammatory and immunological effects in a number of nonendocrine conditions including the following:

Table 36-1 Nonendocrine conditions effectively treated with glucocorticoids (FDA designation)

Condition	Treatment Regimen
Allergic States	
Bronchial asthma	Systemic steroids used to control acute
Serum sickness	episodes unresponsive to conventional therapy.
Contact dermatitis	Topical therapy as required. Systemic therapy rarely justified.
Collagen Diseases	
Systemic lupus erythematosus	Systemic steroids to control acute episodes or lower doses for maintenance. Topical
Acute rheumatic carditis	steroids to control dermatological manifestations of lupus erythematosus.
Dermatological Diseases	
Seborrheic dermatitis	Topical therapy as needed. Some skin lesions may require injection at the site.
Mycosis fungoides	Systemic therapy may be employed when
Pemphigus	symptoms are widespread or especially
Severe erythema multiforme	severe.
Severe psoriasis	*cont'd. next page*

414 Pocket Nurse Guide to Drugs

Table 36-1 Nonendocrine conditions effectively treated with glucocorticoids (FDA designation)—cont'd.

Condition	Treatment Regimen
Edematous States	
Nephrotic syndrome	Systemic steroids for short periods to control acute episodes; used with other treatment.
Cerebral edema	
Hematological Disorders	
Autoimmune hemolytic anemia	Systemic steroids in large doses for acute disease; lower doses for maintaining remission.
Thrombocytopenia	
Neoplastic Diseases	
Leukemias	Systemic steroids along with other antineoplastic agents produce remissions and palliation of symptoms.
Lymphomas	
Ophthalmic Diseases	
Allergic conjunctivitis	Superficial conditions may be treated with steroids applied directly to the eye. Diseases of the internal structures of the eye may require systemic therapy.
Allergic corneal marginal ulcers	
Chorioretinitis	
Iritis and iridocyclitis	
Keratitis	
Optic neuritis	
Rheumatic Disorders	
Acute and subacute bursitis	Intraarticular injection may be required for selected cases. Modest oral doses minimize side effects while providing relief for many patients.
Acute nonspecific tenosynovitis	
Acute gouty arthritis	
Ankylosing spondylitis	
Psoriatic arthritis	
Rheumatoid arthritis	

Adrenal Steroids and Other Drugs Affecting the Adrenal Gland   415

Table 36-1 Nonendocrine conditions effectively treated with glucocorticoids (FDA designation)—cont'd.

Condition	Treatment Regimen
Respiratory Diseases	
Pulmonary tuberculosis	Systemic steroids may give symptomatic relief to certain patients.
Symptomatic sarcoidosis	

Table 36-2 Nonendocrine conditions for which glucocorticoid treatment is "probably" effective (FDA designation)

Condition	Treatment Regimen
Allergic States	
Urticaria	Systemic steroids when disease not adequately controlled by conventional methods
Dental Conditions	
Postoperative inflammatory reactions	Local application
Edematous States	
Cirrhosis of the the liver with ascites	Systemic steroids in conjunction with diuretics
Congestive heart failure	
Gastrointestinal Diseases	
Ulcerative colitis	Systemic steroids may aid in short-term recovery but do not change the long-term prognosis
Regional enteritis	
Intractable sprue	
Respiratory Diseases	
Pulmonary emphysema with bronchial edema	Systemic steroids in conjunction with other therapy or after other therapy has failed
Interstitial pulmonary fibrosis	

ACTH or Cosyntropin, dexamethasone, and metyrapone are used to diagnose adrenal disorders: ACTH or cosyntropin is used to distinguish between primary adrenal insufficiency (Addison's disease) and secondary insufficiency resulting from pituitary dysfunction; dexamethasone is used diagnostically to test steroid suppression of synthesis or cortisol; metyrapone is used to test the ability of the pituitary gland to increase ACTH release.

Nurse Alert for Adrenal Steroids

- Glucocorticoids affect the actions of many other drugs, and the dose of either the steroid or the other drug may need to be modified because of interaction. Aspirin should be avoided except as prescribed.
- Patients should avoid contact with individuals with active infections.
- Steroids usually are not advised in pregnancy except in replacement therapy or life-threatening conditions.
- Bone fractures may occur very easily in patients with osteoporosis taking glucocorticoids; patients should be cautioned to report any musculoskeletal pain and to avoid strenuous activities. Immobilized patients should be moved very carefully.

Side Effects of Adrenal Steroids

Mineralocorticoids can cause edema and hypokalemia. *Glucocorticoids* may produce symptoms of Cushing's disease: increases in certain fat stores, weakness in extremities, muscle wasting, fragile and easily bruised skin, skin fungal infections, bone thinning and susceptibility to spine compression fractures, precipitation of diabetes, hypertension, atherosclerosis, and mood changes. Reactions to long-term therapy may include impaired glucose tolerance and/or hyperglycemia, peptic ulcer or intestinal perforation, muscle wasting, pancreatitis, growth inhibition, mood changes or psychoses, osteoporosis or fractures, sodium retention and potassium loss, increased susceptibility to infection, glaucoma, cataracts, menstrual irregularities, hirsutism, increased appetite,

Text continued on p. 422

Table 36-3 Administration of adrenal steroids

Generic Name	Chemical Form	Trade Name	Administration
Amcinonide	—	Cyclocort*	Topical
Beclomethasone	Dipropionate	Beconase* / Vancenase*	Nasal inhaler
Betamethasone	—	Celestone*	Oral, topical
	Benzoate	Benisone / Uticort	Topical
	Dipropionate	Diprosone	Topical
	Sodium phosphate	Celestone phosphate	Intra-articular, intradermal, IM, IV
	Sodium phosphate + acetate	Celestone soluspan	Intra-articular, intrabursal, intradermal, IM
	Valerate	Valisone	Topical
Clocortolone	Pivalate	Cloderm	Topical
Cortisone	Acetate	Cortone acetate	Oral, IM
Desonide	—	Tridesilon*	Topical
Desoximetasone	—	Topicort*	Topical
Desoxycorticosterone	Acetate	Percorten acetate	IM
	Pivalate	Percorten pivalate	IM

cont'd. next page

*Available in U.S. and Canada

Table 36-3 Administration of adrenal steroids—cont'd.

Generic Name	Chemical Form	Trade Name	Administration
Dexamethasone	—	Decadron* Dexone Hexadrol*	Oral
		Aeroseb-Dex Decaderm Decaspray	Topical
		Maxidex*	Ophthalmic
	Acetate	Decadron-LA Dexasone-LA Solurex-LA	Intra-articular, intradermal, IM
	Sodium phosphate + acetate	Decadron phosphate Hexadrol phosphate	Intra-articular, intradermal, IM
		Decadron phosphate	Topical, ophthalmic
		Turbinaire decadron phosphate	Nasal aerosol
		Decadron phosphate respihaler	Inhaler
Diflorasone	Diacetate	Florone*	Topical
Fludrocortisone	Acetate	Florinef acetate*	Oral
Flunisolide	—	Nasalide	Nasal aerosol

Adrenal Steroids and Other Drugs Affecting the Adrenal Gland

Flumethasone	Pivalate	Locorten	Topical
Fluocinolone	Acetonide	Fluonid	Topical
		Synalar*	Topical
Fluocinonide	—	Lidex*	Topical
Fluorometholone	—	Oxylone	Topical
		FML liquifilm*	Ophthalmic
Fluprednisolone	—	Alphadrol	Oral
Flurandrenolide	—	Cordran	Topical
Halcinonide	—	Halciderm	Topical
		Halog*	Topical
Hydrocortisone (also called cortisol)	—	Cortef*	Oral, IM
		Alphaderm	Topical
		Cort-Dome	
		Cortril	
		Optef	Ophthalmic
		Cortenema	Rectal
		Rectoid	
	Acetate	Cortef acetate	Intra-articular, intrabursal, intradermal
		Cortril acetate	
		Hydrocortone acetate	

cont'd. next page

*Available in U.S. and Canada

Table 36-3   Administration of adrenal steroids—cont'd.

Generic Name	Chemical Form	Trade Name	Administration
Hydrocortisone (also called cortisol) —cont'd.		Cortifoam*	Rectal form
		Hydrocortone acetate	Ophthalmic
	Cypionate	Cortef fluid	Oral
	Sodium phosphate	Hydrocortone phosphate	IV, IM, SC
	Sodium succinate	A-hydrocort	IV, IM
		Solu-Cortef*	
	Valerate	Westcort	Topical
Medrysone	—	HMS Liquifilm*	Ophthalmic
Meprednisone	—	Betapar	Oral
Methylprednisolone	—	Medrol*	Oral
	Acetate	Depo-Medrol*	Intra-articular and soft tissue, IM
		Duralone	
		Medrol acetate	Topical
		Medrol Enpak	Rectal
	Sodium succinate	A-methapred	IV, IM
		Solu-medrol*	
Paramethasone	Acetate	Haldrone	Oral
Prednisolone	—	Delta-cortef	Oral
		Meti-Derm	Topical
	Acetate	Articulose	Intra-articular and soft tissue, IM

		Meticortelone acetate*	
		Econopred	Ophthalmic
		Predulose	
	Sodium phosphate	Hydeltrasol	IV, IM, intra-articular and soft tissue
		PSP-IV	
		Solu-Predalone	
		Metreton	Ophthalmic
	Tebutate	Hydeltra-T.B.A.	Intra-articular and soft tissue
		Predcor-TBA	
Prednisone	—	Deltasone*	Oral
		Meticorten	
		Orasone	
Triamcinolone	—	Aristocort*	Oral
		Kenacort*	
	Acetonide	Kenalog*	Intra-articular, intrabursal, intradermal, IM**
		Tri-Kort	
		Aristocort	Topical
		Kenalog	
	Diacetate	Aristocort intralesional	Intra-articular, intradermal, IM
		Tracilon	
	Hexacetonide	Aristospan*	Intra-articular, intralesional

*Available in U.S. and Canada
**Not all products may be used by all the routes shown. Check the package insert or consult the pharmacist.

422 Pocket Nurse Guide to Drugs

Table 36-4 Administration of drugs to diagnose adrenal disease

Generic Name	Trade Name	Dosage and Administration
Adrenocortico-tropic hormone	ACTH* Acthar* Corticotropin*	INTRAMUSCULAR, SUBCUTANEOUS: 20 units 4 times daily. INTRAVENOUS: 25 to 40 units in 500 ml of dextrose or saline infused over 8 hr.
Adrenocortico-tropic hormone	ACTH gel Corticotropin Gel Cortigel Cortrophin Zinc H. P. Acthar Gel	INTRAMUSCULAR REPOSITORY: 40 to 80 units every 24 to 72 hr.
Cosyntropin	Cortrosyn*	INTRAMUSCULAR, INTRAVENOUS: *Adults*—0.25 mg single dose. *Children under 2 yr*—0.125 mg single dose.
Metyrapone	Metopirone*	ORAL: 750 mg every 4 hr for 6 doses.

*Available in U.S. and Canada

euphoria or depression, allergic reactions, and acne. The side effects of *ACTH* used to diagnose adrenal gland insufficiency are those expected of other adrenal steroids. *Metyrapone* may induce adrenal insufficiency in some patients.

Nursing Implications for Mineralocorticoids

■ The major mineralocorticoid-related problems are associated with sodium retention and electrolyte imbalance. Monitor and record the weight daily or every other day; monitor the blood pressure daily initially, tapering to less often after therapy is adjusted. Patients may need to learn to keep these measurements themselves after discharge. Monitor carefully any patient in whom sodium retention or fluid overload might be a problem, including those with cardio-

Adrenal Steroids and Other Drugs Affecting the Adrenal Gland 423

vascular disease, hypertension, seizures, peripheral vascular disease, and arteriosclerosis.

- Consult with the physician, patient, and dietitian, determine an appropriately restricted low sodium diet, and teach the patient about the diet and its importance.
- Potassium deficit often accompanies sodium retention. Symptoms include anorexia, drowsiness, muscle weakness and cramping, nausea, polyuria, postural hypotension, and mental depression. The patient may require potassium replacement therapy and should also be instructed to increase the intake of potassium-rich foods.
- Teach the patient to report any signs of potassium depletion.
- The patient should wear medical identification.
- Instruct the patient to keep other physicians and dentists informed regarding drug therapy.

Nursing Implications for Glucocorticoids

- Most side effects of glucocorticoid administration will not be a problem when the course of therapy is less than 7 to 10 days.
- Monitor the urine sugar levels of patients receiving steroids. Even in previously nondiabetic individuals, insulin may be required to reduce hyperglycemia. The need for insulin will decrease as the dose of steroids is reduced. Known diabetics will need specific guidelines regarding changes in insulin dosage based on urine sugar levels.
- To decrease the possibility of peptic ulceration:
  a. Suggest that the patient take oral steroids with meals.
  b. Some physicians prescribe four to six daily doses of antacids when patients are receiving steroids, with or without concomitant use of cimetidine or ranitidine.
  c. Small, more frequent meals during the day may reduce gastric irritation.
  d. Monitor stools for occult blood.
  e. Instruct the patient to inspect stools and report any change or the formation of dark, tarry stools.
  f. Monitor the vomitus of the hospitalized patient for occult blood. Teach the outpatient to report bloody vomitus or the appearance of coffee-ground-like emesis.

424   Pocket Nurse Guide to Drugs

- Caution the arthritic patient not to overuse joints that may feel better after systemic or intraarticular steroids.
- Monitor blood pressure regularly.
- Weigh the patient regularly.
- Patients receiving steroids on a long-term basis, especially those who might also be receiving other immunosuppressive drugs, should be taught the importance of reporting immediately any fever, cough, sore throat, chest congestion, signs of urinary tract infection, or any other infection so that treatment can be started at once. Any delay in healing should be reported to a physician.
- In addition to regular medical follow-up, the patient receiving steroids on a long-term basis should have regular follow-up every 3 to 6 months with an ophthalmologist to help detect increased intraocular pressure and cataract formation.
- The patient should be taught the importance of taking the prescribed steroid every day, as ordered. If the patient is sick and unable to take the medication, the physician should be notified. For some patients, especially those with known adrenal insufficiency, it may be appropriate to teach self-administration of parenteral steroids for those times when the patient cannot take an oral dose. Consult with the physician.
- Explain to the patient why it is necessary to taper the dose of steroids when the decision has been made to reduce or stop long-term therapy.
- The patient receiving long-term steroid therapy should wear medical identification.
- For patients with a history of previous tuberculosis or positive TB test, isoniazid or other antituberculosis drug may be prescribed while they are receiving steroids.
- Instruct patients to advise other physicians and dentists providing treatment that they are receiving steroid therapy. Allergy skin testing while the patient is receiving steroids may not be accurate. Smallpox vaccination should be avoided.
- Various dietary adjustments may be necessary or helpful: increased intake of potassium-rich foods, decreased intake of sodium, and increased protein intake.

Adrenal Steroids and Other Drugs Affecting the Adrenal Gland   425

- Increased stress may result in a need for an increased dose in steroids. Instruct the patient to report any feeling of increased malaise, weakness, or other unusual signs during or following periods of intense stress.
- Read vials carefully; there are a limited number of steroids safe for intravenous administration.
- Patients receiving glucocorticoids as replacement therapy for adrenal insufficiency should be reassured that the doses of medication they are receiving are not expected to cause symptoms like those of Cushing's syndrome.
- Be careful if patients are switched from one glucocorticoid preparation to another, as doses vary significantly.

Antidiabetic Agents 37

Insulin preparations
   Insulin injection
   Prompt insulin zinc suspension
   Isophane insulin suspension
   Insulin zinc suspension
   Protamine zinc insulin suspension
   Extended insulin zinc suspension

Oral hypoglycemic agents
   Tolbutamide
   Acetohexamide
   Tolazamide
   Glipizide
   Glyburide
   Chlorpropamide

Insulin Preparations

Actions of Insulin Preparations

Insulin use constitutes replacement therapy, restoring the ability of cells to utilize glucose as energy source and to correct the many metabolic derangements of diabetes mellitus.

Indications for Insulin Preparations

Insulin preparations are used to treat diabetes mellitus when presumably there are no functional B cells in the islets of the pancreas left to respond to glucose levels, as occurs in juvenile onset diabetes (Type I diabetes, insulin-dependent diabetes).

Nurse Alert for Insulin Preparations

- Insulin overdosage may cause coma from a hypoglycemic reaction, and insulin underdosage may cause ketoacidosis or hyperosmolar coma—it is crucial for the nurse to be able to differentiate between these two conditions.

Table 37-1 Administration of insulin preparations

Generic Name	Trade Name	Concentration	Pharmacokinetic Properties		
			Onset of Action	Peak Action	Duration of Action
Insulin injection	Regular Iletin I	40 or 100 units/ml	Within 1 hr	2 to 4 hr	6 to 8 hr
	Beef Regular Iletin	100 units/ml			
	Beef Regular Iletin II	100 units/ml			
	Regular Purified Pork	100 units/ml			
	Pork Regular Iletin II	100 units/ml			
	Regular Concentrated Iletin II, purified pork	500 units/ml			
	Velosulin	100 units/ml			
	Novolin R Human	100 units/ml			
	Humulin R	100 units/ml			
Prompt insulin zinc suspension	Semilente Iletin	40 or 100 units/ml	1.5 to 2 hr	4 to 7 hr	12 to 16 hr
	Semilente Insulin	40 or 100 units/ml			
	Semilente Purified Pork, Prompt Insulin	100 units/ml			

cont'd. next page

Antidiabetic Agents

427

428   Pocket Nurse Guide to Drugs

Table 37-1 Administration of insulin preparations—cont'd.

Generic Name	Trade Name	Concentration	Onset of Action	Peak Action	Duration of Action
			Pharmacokinetic Properties		
Isophane insulin suspension (NPH)	NPH Iletin I	40 or 100 units/ml	1 to 2 hr	10 to 16 hr	18 to 30 hr
	NPH Insulin	40 or 100 units/ml			
	Beef NPH Iletin II	100 units/ml			
	Purified NPH	100 units/ml			
	Pork NPH Iletin II	100 units/ml			
	Insulatard NPH	100 units/ml			
	NPH Purified Pork	100 units/ml			
	Humulin N Human NPH	100 units/ml			
	Novolin N Human NPH	100 units/ml			
	Mixtard	100 units/ml	Within 1 hr	4 to 8 hr	Up to 24 hr
Insulin zinc suspension	Lente Iletin I	40 or 100 units/ml	1 to 2 hr	10 to 16 hr	18 to 30 hr
	Lentard	100 units/ml			
	Lente Insulin	40 or 100 units/ml			
	Beef Lente Iletin II	100 units/ml			
	Purified Lente	100 units/ml			
	Pork Lente Iletin II	100 units/ml			

	Lente Purified Pork	100 units/ml			
	Novolin L Lente	100 units/ml			
Protamine zinc insulin suspension	Protamine, Zinc & Iletin I	40 or 100 units/ml	6 to 8 hr	14 to 24 hr	24 to 36 hr or longer
	Protamine Zinc Insulin	100 units/ml			
	Protamine, Zinc & Iletin II	100 units/ml			
Extended insulin zinc suspension	Ultralente Iletin I	40 or 100 units/ml	5 to 8 hr	16 to 18 hr	24 to 36 hr or longer
	Ultralente Insulin	100 units/ml			
	Ultralente Purified Beef	100 units/ml			

430 Pocket Nurse Guide to Drugs

- Systemic allergic responses to insulin preparations may occur, which should be prevented in a sensitive patient by use of a more highly purified insulin preparation.
- Careful rotation of injection sites minimizes lipoatrophy occasionally caused by insulin injections.
- Insulin requirements change in pregnancy, usually decreasing in first trimester and increasing in the second and third trimesters.
- Alcohol should be avoided or used in moderation, with consideration of caloric content.
- Discharge planning is crucial for the teaching of the insulin-dependent patient and should be continuous throughout hospitalization.

Administration of Insulin Preparations

Insulin dosage may be individualized in many different ways for different patients but always follows the same principle: doses are timed to avoid hyperglycemia and to prevent hypoglycemia during peak periods of insulin action, with dose effects monitored by urine testing.

Side Effects of Insulin Preparations

See Nurse Alert section above for effects of overdosage and underdosage. Local allergic reactions may also occur, which generally do not require treatment. Atrophy of subcutaneous fat near injection sites (lipoatrophy) may occur. Systemic reactions are rare and can be prevented by use of a different form of insulin preparation.

Nursing Implications for Insulin Preparations

- Human insulin has a somewhat shorter duration of action than pork insulin and should not be exchanged for pork insulin except under a doctor's supervision.
- Insulin can be safely stored for about 1 month at room temperature, but for longer periods of time it should be refrigerated. Insulin should not be frozen.
- Insulin should not be administered cold but allowed to warm to room temperature. Cold insulin alters anticipated

Antidiabetic Agents 431

rates of absorption, causes more local reaction, and is thought to promote lipodystrophy at injection sites.

- Inspect each vial of insulin before using. Note that regular insulin should be crystal clear; all other forms of insulin will be cloudy.
- Gently rotate each vial of insulin for at least 1 minute between both hands before drawing up the dose. This helps to resuspend the modified insulin preparations and will help to warm the medication. Vigorous shaking will promote foaming and bubbles in the solution and should be avoided.
- Accurate measuring of the ordered dose is essential.
- Syringes designed for insulin should be used. These customarily are 1 ml in volume for use with U100 insulin (U100 insulin contains 100 units of insulin/ml). For patients taking very small amounts of insulin, usually less than 35 units, there are syringes available that have clearer, more accurate markings for small doses of insulin. There are also available 2 ml insulin syringes for patients requiring greater than 100 units of insulin. Tuberculin syringes are not recommended for use with insulin.
- Caution patients to use only the insulin prescribed, and to check carefully each time insulin is purchased that the correct form, brand and strength of insulin have been supplied.
- Two kinds of insulin can be mixed in the same syringe within the following guidelines: Regular insulin can be mixed with any other kind of insulin. The lente insulins can be mixed with each other but should not be mixed with other insulins except regular insulin. A single form of insulin in a syringe is stable for weeks to months. Mixtures of insulins are generally not stable, and should be administered within 5 minutes of mixing. The product Mixtard, which is 70% NPH and 30% regular insulin, is stable for weeks to months in a syringe.
- The procedure for mixing two insulins in the same syringe is as follows:
  a. With the syringe, inject air, in the amount equivalent to the dose to be drawn up, into the vial of modified, or longer-acting, insulin. Remove syringe.

432 Pocket Nurse Guide to Drugs

    b. Inject the correct amount of air into the vial of insulin injection; then withdraw the correct dose. Eliminate any air bubbles in the syringe.

    c. Return to the vial of modified insulin and withdraw the correct dose. If an error occurs, discard the syringe and begin again.

Remember: The insulin injection (unmodified, i.e., the rapid-acting form) is always aspirated into the syringe first. Instruct patients who mix insulins at home to always use the same technique for mixing insulins, and the same brand of syringe, to avoid inadvertent incorrect dosage.

- Only regular insulin is ever administered intravenously. All other insulins are administered subcutaneously. Acceptable sites for insulin injection include the upper arms, back, outer thighs, abdomen (avoiding the navel and midline tissue), and buttocks, although some experts feel the buttocks contain too much fatty tissue.

- The following method results in best absorption with fewest side effects:

    a. Clean skin with alcohol. Let alcohol evaporate.

    b. Pinch up the skin at the injection site.

    c. Insert the needle at a 20- to 45-degree angle at the base of the pinched skin. Aspirate for blood.

    d. Inject the insulin into the "space" between the fat and the muscle.

    e. Withdraw the needle. Apply pressure to the site if needed to stop bleeding. Do not rub the area. Note that the obese individual may require a needle longer than the 5/8-inch needle supplied with the insulin syringe. Rarely would an individual require a needle shorter than 5/8 inch.

    f. There are variations in acceptable technique. For example, not all experts require aspiration for blood prior to administering the dose. Institutional policy should be followed.

- Local reactions to insulin injection are not uncommon and may include itching, a reddened area, or excessive discomfort at the injection site. The reactions usually will clear on

Antidiabetic Agents   **433**

their own in 2 to 3 weeks, although some individuals may require oral antihistamines to decrease discomfort. Sometimes the irritation is due to not allowing the alcohol to dry before giving the injection; reevaluate the patient's injection technique.

- Systemic reactions to insulin are rare, but when they occur they often result from reaction to the animal source of the insulin: beef, pork, or mixed beef and pork. The reaction should be treated symptomatically and an alternate source of insulin tried.

- Hypertrophy (thickening) of the skin and lipodystrophy (dimpling) at injection sites were once thought to be unavoidable complications of insulin use. Today it is thought that these two problems often represent careless injection technique, repeated use of the same injection site, or an immune response that occurs when less pure insulin preparations are used. From the time the first insulin injection is given to a patient, a record of site use should be kept and sites rotated. No individual injection site should be used more often than every 6 or 7 weeks.

- Intravenous insulin is one of the drugs used in the treatment of diabetic coma. Note that only regular insulin injection is safe for intravenous administration. (Note that Mixtard contains NPH insulin in addition to regular insulin; it should NOT be administered intravenously.) Intravenous insulin is incompatible with many other intravenous solutions and is unstable at a pH range outside 3.0 to 3.5. Check with the pharmacy before administering if questions occur.

- Glucagon may be given to counteract an overdose of insulin, but the action of glucagon depends on the patient having sufficient glycogen stored in the liver to break down to glucose. Some physicians prefer to use glucose directly.

- If the problem at the injection site is one of atrophy (lipoatrophy), injection of a purified pork preparation directly into the atrophied area over two to four weeks may cause the subcutaneous tissue to increase. The site should then be used every two to four weeks regularly. The use of a less purified preparation may cause the atrophy to recur.

434   Pocket Nurse Guide to Drugs

- Many times the insulin dose is calculated on the basis of the urine test. Whenever possible, a double-voided specimen should be used, since this type specimen more accurately reflects blood glucose values near the time when insulin dosage is due.
- Many drugs can influence the result of the urine test, producing false positive or false negative results. If there is any question about the influence of a drug on the urine test, try another test, consult with the pharmacy, or notify the physician.
- The presence of ketones in the urine is an important indicator of the diabetic's degree of control. During hospitalization the urine should always be tested for ketones when tested for sugar. At the time of discharge, the physician may indicate that the patient need only test for ketones at home if the urine sugar exceeds a certain level. The diabetic patient needs to be able to perform this test accurately and to identify when to test for ketones if not with each specimen. In addition, patients should know what to do if they begin to spill ketones (e.g., increase the insulin, notify the physician); clarify with the physician before discharge.
- It is appropriate for insulin-dependent diabetics to have their insulin technique and rotation schedule reevaluated on each admission to the hospital.
- Relatively inexpensive machines are now available for measuring blood glucose at home. Many patients use home glucose monitoring for adjusting insulin requirements. The patient and a family member (especially for a minor patient) should be carefully instructed on the proper techniques for obtaining accurate results with the particular machine chosen.
- In addition to information about their medications, diabetics should be well-informed about diet, foot care, prevention of complications, and all other aspects of the disease.
- At least one family member should also receive training in recognizing the complications of diabetes and know the proper action to take.

Oral Hypoglycemic Agents

Acetohexamide
Chlorpropamide
Glipizide
Glyburide
Tolazamide
Tolbutamide

Actions of Oral Hypoglycemic Agents

The oral hypoglycemic agents, sulfonylureas, act by stimulating insulin release from the pancreas, and the newer agents may also diminish hepatic glucose production and directly increase tissue responsiveness to insulin. These actions tend to diminish fasting glucose concentrations and improve glucose utilization by fat and muscle cells.

Indications for Oral Hypoglycemic Agents

The oral hypoglycemic agents are used only for patients able to produce some insulin on their own—patients with Type II diabetes (non-insulin dependent diabetes mellitus [NIDDM] or adult-onset diabetes).

Nurse Alert for Oral Hypoglycemic Agents

- Patients receiving oral hypoglycemic agents should routinely avoid alcohol because of the many possible interactions with the drugs.
- Risk of hypoglycemia is increased when these drugs are used with the antiinflammatory agent phenylbutazone, salicylates, and sulfonamide antibiotics.
- Oral hypoglycemic agents are contraindicated in pregnancy.
- Oral hypoglycemic agents are contraindicated with inadequate renal or liver function.

Side Effects of Oral Hypoglycemic Agents

Sulfonylurea therapy may cause gastrointestinal distress, neurological symptoms such as muscle weakness and paresthesias, altered liver function tests, mild hematopoietic toxicity, and allergic skin responses. Hypoglycemia may occur with drug overdose, drug interactions, altered drug metabolism, or failure to eat.

Table 37-2   Administration of oral hypoglycemic agents

Generic Name	Trade Name	Dosage Range	Duration of Action
Tolbutamide	Orinase*	0.5 to 3 Gm daily, divided doses.	6 to 12 hr
Acetohexamide	Dymelor*	0.25 to 1.5 Gm daily, as a single or divided dose.	12 to 24 hr
Tolazamide	Tolinase	0.1 to 0.75 Gm daily; single dose for lower range, divided dose for higher range.	12 to 24 hr
Glipizide	Glucotrol	2.5 to 40 mg daily. Doses above 15 mg should be divided.	12 to 24 hr
Glyburide	Diabeta* Micronase	1.25 to 20 mg daily.	16 to 24 hr
Chlorpropamide	Diabinese*	0.1 to 0.5 Gm daily, single dose.	Up to 60 hr

*Available in U.S. and Canada

Nursing Implications for Oral Hypoglycemic Agents

- It is essential that diabetics requiring only oral hypoglycemic agents for control be helped to understand the importance of adherence to their prescribed diet.
- The major side effect of oral hypoglycemic agents is hypoglycemia, and this is frequently a problem with elderly patients. Nausea, vomiting, and skin rashes are usually transient. In rare cases, agranulocytosis is seen, so patients should be cautioned to report to their physician any sore throat, fever, or whenever they do not feel well.
- There are numerous drug interactions with the oral hypoglycemic agents. Caution patients to avoid taking any medications without prior approval of the physician, and to keep all health care providers informed of all medications being taken.
- Patients should be taught to take their oral hypoglycemic agents as prescribed and not to "catch up" with missed doses. In addition, oral agents should not be taken at bedtime.
- Patients being switched from insulin to oral agents or the reverse need to be carefully watched for hypoglycemia.
- Individuals who can usually be managed on oral agents may require insulin during times of illness, infection, hospitalization, or surgery.

Drugs Affecting the Thyroid and Parathyroid Glands

38

Drugs for hypothyroidism
    Thyroid U.S.P.
    Thyroglobulin
    Levothyroxine sodium (T_4)
    Liothyronine sodium (T_3)
    Liotrix
    Thyroid-stimulating hormone (TSH)
    Protirelin, thyrotropin-releasing hormone (TRH)
Drugs for hyperthyroidism
    Propylthiouracil
    Methimazole
    Propranolol hydrochloride
    Potassium or sodium iodide
    Radioactive iodine

Drugs to alter calcium metabolism
    Calcitonin
    Parathyroid hormone
    Vitamin D
    Calcifediol
    Calcitriol
    Dihydrotachysterol
    Ergocalaferol

Drugs for Hypothyroidism

    Thyroid U.S.P.
    Thyroglobulin
    Levothyroxine sodium (T_4)
    Liothyronine sodium (T_3)
    Liotrix
    Thyroid-stimulating hormone (TSH)
    Protirelin, thyrotropin-stimulating hormone (TRH)

Actions of Drugs for Hypothyroidism

Drugs for hypothyroidism supply the body with thyroid hormones when the natural hormones are produced in insufficient quantities. The actions are the same as natural hormones. Thyroid U.S.P. and thyroglobulin contain T_4 and T_3. Levothyroxine sodium is a synthetic form of thyroxine and has the properties of T_4. Liothyronine sodium is a synthetic form of triiodothyronine and has the properties of T_3. Liotrix is a preparation containing both T_3 and T_4.

Indications for Drugs for Hypothyroidism

All the natural and synthetic thyroid hormones are used in replacement therapy for thyroid deficiencies, and occasionally for individuals with normal thyroid hormone levels but with enlarged thyroid glands, to permit the gland to return to normal size. These hormones should never be used to treat obesity.

Thyroid-stimulating Hormone

(TSH) is used to diagnose hypothyroidism. *Protirelin* is used diagnostically to differentiate pituitary-induced hypothyroidism from other types of hypothyroidism.

Nurse Alert for Drugs for Hypothyroidism

- One common and dangerous problem observed occasionally even with low doses is the production of angina pectoris, coronary occlusion, or stroke in elderly or predisposed patients. Another difficulty some patients may experience is a relative adrenal insufficiency. This latter difficulty arises primarily in patients with inadequate pituitary function who suffer from both secondary hypothyroidism and secondary adrenal insufficiency. If thyroid hormone therapy is begun in these patients without also restoring adequate glucocorticoid levels, the patients may suffer a dangerous adrenal crisis.

Administration of Drugs for Hypothyroidism

In a newly diagnosed hypothyroid patient, thyroid medications are begun at very low doses and increased at varying intervals until the euthyroid state is achieved. Thyroid U.S.P. and levothyroxine doses are doubled roughly every 2 weeks,

Table 38-1 Administration of drugs for hypothyroidism

Generic Name	Trade Name	Dosage and Administration	Properties
Natural Thyroid Hormones			
Thyroid U.S.P.	Thyrar Thyrocrine Thyro-Teric	ORAL: *Adults*—60 to 180 mg daily is usual for maintenance. Initial doses 15 mg daily. Double the dose every 2 wk until effective maintenance dose is reached.	Impure mixture of thyroid components that includes T_3 and T_4.
Thyroglobulin	Proloid*	ORAL: *Adults*—32 to 180 mg daily for maintenance. Initial doses are small and are gradually increased to maintenance levels.	Contains T_3 and T_4, as well as other iodine-containing compounds.
Synthetic Thyroid Hormones			
Levothyroxine sodium	Eltroxin† Levothroid Synthroid*	ORAL: *Adults*—150 to 200 μg daily for maintenance. Initial doses are small and are gradually increased to maintenance levels. *Children over 1 yr*—3 to 5 μg/kg daily. INTRAVENOUS: *Adults*—0.5 mg with mannitol (Synthroid) or	Chemically pure form of T_4.

Drugs Affecting the Thyroid and Parathyroid Glands

Drug	Brand names	Dosage	Remarks
		without (Levothroid).	
Liothyronine sodium	Cytomel* Cytomine	ORAL: *Adults*—25 to 75 μg daily for maintenance. Initial doses should be low and gradually increased to maintenance levels.	Chemically pure form of T_3.
Liotrix	Euthroid Thyrolar*	ORAL: *Adults*—30 μg T_4 with 7.5 μg T_3 or 25 μg T_4 with 6.25 μg T_3. Doses may be gradually increased as needed.	Chemically pure T_4 and T_3 combined in a ratio of 4:1.
Adenohypophyseal Hormones			
Thyroid-stimulating hormone (TSH)	Thytropar*	INTRAMUSCULAR, SUBCUTANEOUS: 10 IU once or twice daily.	Extract of bovine anterior pituitary contains natural peptide, TSH.
Protirelin (thyrotropin-releasing hormone, TRH)	Relefact TRH* Thypinone*	INTRAVENOUS: *Adults*—400 to 500 μg.	Synthetic preparation of natural hypothalamic tripeptide hormone.

*Available in U.S. and Canada
†Available in Canada only

442 Pocket Nurse Guide to Drugs

but liothyronine doses are doubled weekly until adequate control is achieved. In terms of biological activity, 60 mg of thyroid U.S.P. = 60 mg thyroglobulin = 1 mg or less of levothyroxine = 0.025 mg of liothyronine = liotrix tablets containing 0.06 mg T_4 + 0.015 mg T_3 or 0.05 mg T_4 + 0.0125 mg T_3. A wide range of tablet sizes is available in each of these preparations so that a dosage may be easily adjusted to the patient's particular need.

Side Effects of Drugs for Hypothyroidism

Overdose of the natural thyroid hormones produces symptoms of hyperthyroidism. Too large a dose at onset of therapy may cause vascular occlusion, especially in patients with arteriosclerosis. Thyroid medications may enhance the toxic effects of digitalis preparations. Thyroid drugs can produce hyperglycemia; diabetics may need to increase their dose of insulin or hypoglycemic agents. TSH may cause cardiovascular symptoms and, rarely allergic reactions. TRH may transiently produce nausea, flushing, changes in blood pressure, and an urge to urinate.

Nursing Implications for Drugs for Hypothyroidism

- Signs and symptoms of excessive thyroid medication are the same as for hyperthyroidism. The easiest way to monitor the effect of thyroid medication is to take the pulse. A pulse rate greater than 100 beats per minute in an adult may indicate overdosage with thyroid medication.
- It may be appropriate to teach the patient to take the pulse and to report rates over a certain limit determined after consultation with the physician. Parents of a hypothyroid child should also be taught to measure the child's height and to take the child's pulse regularly, although the upper limits of a normal pulse rate vary depending on the child's age.
- The patient needs to understand that thyroid medication may need to be continued for life; it should not be discontinued once the patient feels better.
- Occasionally what appears to be a treatment failure may result from the use of old thyroid medication that has lost potency because of lengthy or improper shelf storage. The

Drugs Affecting the Thyroid and Parathyroid Glands **443**

medication should be kept dry and remain in a light-resistant container if so supplied.

- Treatment of congenital hypothyroidism (cretinism) should be begun and maintained as soon as the diagnosis is made. Treatment will not, however, reverse any mental retardation that has already occurred.
- Many states now require that newborns be tested for adequate thyroid hormone levels.
- Thyroid medications increase the action of anticoagulants; patients receiving both may need their dose of anticoagulants reduced.
- Adrenal insufficiency should be corrected before beginning thyroid medication. Patients already taking adrenal steroids may need their dosages readjusted.
- Patients undergoing neurosurgery for pituitary tumors or destruction of the pituitary gland for pain control or other reasons, will be evaluated 2 to 3 weeks after surgery for thyroid function, and may require thyroid replacement therapy if pituitary thyroid stimulating hormone (TSH) is lost.
- Patients on long-term thyroid medication should wear medical identification.

Drugs for Hyperthyroidism

Propylthiouracil
Methimazole
Propranolol hydrochloride
Potassium or sodium iodide
Radioactive iodine

Actions of Drugs for Hyperthyroidism

The drugs to treat hyperthyroidism fall into 2 categories: drugs to control the symptoms of hyperthyroidism and drugs to lower the production of T_3 and T_4 by the thyroid. *Propranolol* blocks the beta adrenergic receptors to treat the symptoms of palpitation, tremor, sweating, proximal muscle weakness, mental agitation, and cardiac arrhythmias. The *thioamides* inhibit the synthesis of thyroid hormones at each step in the synthesis except iodine uptake. *Lithium carbonate* inhibits thyroid hormone synthesis and release. *Iodine* inhibits the uptake of iodine and the synthesis of thyroid hormones and also reduces the vascularization of the gland. *Radioactive iodine* destroys thyroid gland tissue.

Indications for Drugs for Hyperthyroidism

Propranolol is used to control symptoms and to prepare a hyperthyroid patient for surgery. *Thioamides* are used in maintenance doses to control hyperthyroidism, but clinical improvement is delayed. *Iodine* is used as presurgical medication to reduce the vascularization and the size of the thyroid gland after thioamide therapy. Iodine may also be used intravenously after thioamides for emergency therapy for hyperthyroid crisis. *Radioactive iodine* is used to destroy thyroid tissue without surgery for the control of Graves' disease or thyroid carcinoma; it may also be used for diagnostic testing.

Nurse Alert for Drugs for Hyperthyroidism

- With propranolol, bronchospasm may occur in asthmatics, or may precipitate heart failure in patients with heart function maintained by sympathetic tone.
- The thioamides can be cautiously given to a pregnant woman, although as a woman approaches term the physician will monitor her closely and may discontinue the medication or add a thyroid preparation to prevent hypothyroidism in the infant. The drugs are excreted in breast milk so mothers taking one of the thioamides should not breast-feed.
- To prevent damage to the infant, radioactive iodine should not be taken by pregnant women or nursing mothers.
- Sodium iodide is contraindicated in persons with known iodine sensitivity. There is no specific antidote; treatment of a sensitivity reaction is supportive.

Side Effects of Drugs for Hyperthyroidism

With *thioamides*, agranulocytosis may occur in 1.4% of patients during first 2 months of therapy; skin rashes occur in

Drugs Affecting the Thyroid and Parathyroid Glands **445**

about 3%. *Iodine* may produce iodism. *Radioactive iodine* generally eventually leads to hypothyroidism. Signs of overdosage with the thioamides are those of hypothyroidism. The easily monitored signs include the pulse rate, weight changes, and facial edema. Signs develop slowly.

Propylthiouracil can produce hypoprothrombinemia. Caution the patient to report excessive bruising, purpura, or unexplained or excessive bleeding. Signs of iodism (excessive iodide) include metallic taste in the mouth, sneezing, swollen and tender thyroid gland, vomiting, and bloody diarrhea. Concomitant excessive use of over-the-counter preparations containing iodine (e.g., asthma or cough preparations) may contribute to iodism. Side effects (other than eventual hypothyroidism) are rare with *radioactive iodine* but include soreness over the thyroid gland and in rare cases difficulty swallowing and breathing because of gland enlargement. *Propranolol* may cause bronchospasm, hypoglycemia, bradycardia, dizziness, and other symptoms.

Nursing Implications for Drugs for Hyperthyroidism

- Although the radiation dose of radioactive iodine is not high, those preparing the preparation should be careful not to spill the mixture on themselves or countertops. Rubber gloves should be worn.
- Patients taking thioamides should be taught to report to their physician any sore throat, fever, or rash, signs of agranulocytosis. Other reported side effects of these drugs include nausea, vomiting, dizziness, and drowsiness.
- Long-standing exophthalmus may not improve in appearance even after treatment for hyperthyroidism has begun.
- Oral anticoagulants may be potentiated by propylthiouracil, necessitating a reduction in the dosage of anticoagulant.
- Lugol's solution or any iodide solution is foul tasting and should be well diluted in juice, milk, or beverage of the patient's preference. It may stain teeth, so it should be taken through a straw.
- Thyroid surgery carries with the possible side effect of accidental removal or destruction of the parathyroid glands. Signs of hypoparathyroidism include hypocalcemia, muscle twitching, muscle spasm, numbness and tingling of fingers

Table 38-2   Administration and dosage of drugs for hyperthyroidism

Generic Name	Trade Name	Dosage and Administration	Properties
Thioamides			
Propylthiouracil (PTU)		ORAL: *Adults*—50 to 300 mg daily in 3 doses. Initially 300 to 600 mg daily, is given in 3 or 4 doses. *Children over 10*—half the adult dose. *Children 6 to 10*—one quarter the adult dose.	Inhibits thyroid hormone synthesis but not release.
Methimazole	Tapazole*	ORAL: *Adults*—5 to 20 mg daily in 2 or 3 doses. Initially 30 to 60 mg daily is given in 3 or 4 doses. *Children 6 to 10*—0.4 mg/kg daily in 3 or 4 doses.	Inhibits thyroid hormone synthesis but not release.
Beta Adrenergic Blocker			
Propranolol hydrochloride	Inderal*	ORAL: *Adults*—40 to 240 mg daily in divided doses. INTRAVENOUS: *Adults*—5 mg or less administered at 1 mg/min or more slowly.	Controls symptoms of hyperthyroidism but does not lower T_3 and T_4 release from the thyroid.

Drugs Affecting the Thyroid and Parathyroid Glands 447

Iodine			
Potassium or sodium iodide	Strong Iodine Solution Lugol's Solution	ORAL: *Adults*—0.1 to 0.3 ml 3 times daily. INTRAVENOUS: *Adults*—250 to 500 mg daily for thyrotoxic crisis.	Produces short-term inhibition of thyroid hormone synthesis by direct action on the thyroid.
Radioactive Iodine			
^{131}I as NaI		ORAL: *Adults*—4 to 10 mCi as a single dose for Graves' disease. For thyroid carcinoma, single doses of up to 150 mCi may be used. Smaller doses are used for diagnostic purposes.	These radionuclides are concentrated in the thyroid and release radiation, which destroys thyroid tissue.

*Available in U.S. and Canada

448 Pocket Nurse Guide to Drugs

and toes, and tetany; Chvostek's and Trousseau's signs are positive. Treatment for acute hypocalcemia is usually with a 10% solution of calcium gluconate intravenously. The drug can be given diluted or undiluted but should be given slowly because of potential cardiac effects; it will also increase digitalis toxicity. Calcium gluconate should be readily available to those caring for patients undergoing thyroid surgery.

■ Emergency treatment of thyroid crisis might include intravenous sodium iodide, which is given after an antithyroid drug has been administered. The ordered dose of iodine (usually 1 to 2 Gm) should be diluted in at least 100 ml of normal saline solution, 5% dextrose in saline solution or water, or Ringer's solution. Administer slowly over 30 minutes. Discard any cloudy or colored solution or one containing particulate matter.

Drugs to Alter Calcium Metabolism

Calcitonin
Parathyroid hormone
Vitamin D
Calcifediol

Calcitriol
Dihydrotachysterol
Ergocalciferol

Actions of Drugs Affecting Calcium Metabolism

Calcitonin prevents the loss of calcium from bone, augments the urinary excretion of calcium and phosphate, and blocks the absorption of calcium from the small intestine. Parathyroid hormone in many ways acts in the exact opposite manner: increases calcium reabsorption from bones, lowers renal excretion of calcium and phosphate, and with vitamin D increases calcium absorption from the intestine. Parathyroid hormone, calcitonin, and vitamin D interact to maintain blood calcium levels in a very narrow range.

Indications for Drugs Affecting Calcium Metabolism

Therapy for hyperparathyroidism is primarily surgical rather than pharmacologic. *Calcitonin* may temporarily be used to control hypercalcemia in hyperparathyroidism. *Vitamin D* with or without calcium is the preferred treatment for hypoparathyroidism; *parathyroid hormone* can theoretically be used also.

Calcitonin can also be used to lower hypercalcemia in vitamin D intoxication or to control Paget's disease. *Parathyroid hormone* is used in the diagnosis of pseudohypoparathyroidism. *Calcifediol* is used to treat metabolic bone disease in patients on dialysis for chronic renal failure. *Calcitriol* is used to treat rickets and pseudohypoparathyroidism. *Dihydrotachysterol* is used to treat hypoparathyroidism. *Ergocalciferol* is used to treat rickets and hypoparathyroidism.

Nurse Alert for Drugs Affecting Calcium Metabolism

- *Calcitonin* is protein in nature and may cause an allergic response. Epinephrine, antihistamines, glucocorticoids, and equipment for possible resuscitation should be available in settings where calcitonin is used.
- *Parathyroid hormone* may also cause an allergic reaction; keep epinephrine and other emergency treatment drugs available.
- Prior to administering parathyroid hormones, test the patient for sensitivity reaction with a skin test.

Side Effects of Drugs Affecting Calcium Metabolism

An excess or deficiency of *vitamin D* produces symptoms expected of high or low blood calcium concentrations. Vitamin D intoxication may cause weakness, headache, somnolence, vomiting, dry mouth, constipation, muscle pain, bone pain, polyuria, polydipsia, anorexia, elevated BUN, SGOT, hypertension, and cardiac arrhythmias. *Calcitonin* may cause an allergic response or nausea and local irritation resulting from the injection. The side effects of *parathyroid hormone* include anorexia, diarrhea, vomiting, and weakness; allergic reactions may also occur. Overdose with parathyroid hormone cause symptoms of hypercalcemia: muscular weakness, anorexia, nausea, vomiting, constipation, polyuria, thirst, and altered levels of consciousness.

450 **Pocket Nurse Guide to Drugs**

Table 38-3   Administration of drugs affecting calcium metabolism

Generic Name	Trade Name	Dosage and Administration
Calcitonin	Calcimar*	INTRAMUSCULAR, SUBCUTANEOUS: 100 units daily or higher if required.
Parathyroid hormone		INTRAVENOUS: 200 units.
Vitamin D Products		
Calcifediol	Calderol	ORAL: 50 to 100 μg daily or 100 to 200 μg on alternate days.
Calcitriol	Rocaltrol*	ORAL: 0.25 to 1 μg daily.
Dihydrotachysterol	Hytakerol*	ORAL: doses range from 0.1 to 2.5 mg daily, as needed to maintain normal serum calcium concentration.
Ergocalciferol	Deltalin Drisdol* Ostoforte†	ORAL: 400 units daily is normal replacement; therapy of rickets or hypoparathyroidism may require 50,000 to 500,000 units daily.

*Available in U.S. and Canada
†Available in Canada only

Nursing Implications for Drugs Affecting Calcium Metabolism

Calcitonin

- Monitor the serum calcium and serum alkaline phosphotase levels to chart progress of the underlying condition.
- Calcitonin is administered via subcutaneous or intramuscular routes. For outpatient therapy, the subcutaneous route is

Drugs Affecting the Thyroid and Parathyroid Glands **451**

preferred. In preparation for discharge, the patient should be able to demonstrate sterile technique in preparing and administering the dose and should be able to explain the need for rotation of sites.

Parathyroid Hormone

- Monitor the calcium and phosphate levels, intake and output, vital signs. Serum calcium levels should rise within 4 hours, but the effect will wear off in 20 to 24 hours.
- The drug may be given undiluted. The rate of administration should not exceed 20 units per minute.

Vitamin D

- Monitor the serum calcium, phosphorus, magnesium, alkaline phosphatase, and the 24 hour urinary calcium and phosphorus at regular intervals.
- Aluminum carbonate or hydroxide gels should be used to control serum phosphate levels in patients undergoing dialysis.
- The serum calcium times phosphate (Ca $\times$ P) product should not be allowed to exceed 70.
- Renal dialysis patients taking calcitriol should not use magnesium-containing antacids concomitantly, as this may contribute to the development of hypermagnesemia.
- Review with patients the need to take vitamin D as prescribed, to adhere to any prescribed dietary restrictions, to avoid the use of non-prescription drugs unless approved by the physician, and to report the development of the side effects of vitamin D intoxication.

PART VIII

FEMALE REPRODUCTIVE SYSTEM DRUGS

Estrogens

Chlorotrianisene
Dienestrol
Diethylstilbestrol (DES)
Estradiol
Estradiol cypionate
Estradiol valerate
Estrogens
Conjugated estrogens
Esterified estrogens
Estrogenic substance
Estrone
Estropipate
Ethinyl estradiol
Quinestrol
See also Ch. 42 for estrogens in oral contraceptives

Actions of Estrogens

Estrogens promote the development of the female reproductive system during early puberty. In the breast, estrogen promotes proliferation of stromal and ductile tissues to allow milk formation. Secondary sexual characteristics also depend on estrogen, along with the growth spurt of puberty. Ovulation and endometrial function in the uterus also depend on estrogen.

Indications for Estrogens

Estrogens as used in oral contraceptives are described in Chapter 42.

Estrogen is used most commonly in replacement therapy for conditions resulting from estrogen deficiency, including endocrine disorders, amenorrhea, symptoms occurring after menopause, dysfunctional uterine bleeding, and pelvic endometriosis. Estrogens may also be used to treat certain metastatic breast carcinomas.

Estrogens may also be used to treat prostate and some breast cancers in men.

Nurse Alert for Estrogens

- Estrogens are contraindicated during pregnancy. A woman who misses two consecutive periods while taking estrogens should stop the medication until pregnancy is ruled out.
- Because of the increased incidence of thrombophlebitis associated with estrogens and progestins, women with a history of thromboembolic disorders should not take these drugs. In addition, patients should be instructed to report leg pain, sudden onset of chest pain, shortness of breath, coughing up blood, headache, dizziness, changes in vision or speech, or weakness or numbness of an arm or leg.

Side Effects of Estrogens

Side effects of estrogens include overreactions of certain reproductive tissues to the hormones. Breast tenderness is reported by many women receiving estrogens. The endometrium is stimulated to proliferate by estrogens, and there is some evidence that estrogens may increase the risk of endometrial cancer. There is no firm evidence that estrogens increase the risk for breast cancer.

Estrogens are frequently associated with acute adverse reactions such as nausea, vomiting, anorexia, and mild diarrhea. Malaise, depression, or excessive irritability are also related to estrogen therapy in some women. Estrogens promote salt and water retention and may therefore produce edema in some patients. Atherosclerosis is a definite risk for patients receiving estrogens, especially if they have other high-risk factors, such as smoking. Hypertension has been associated with estrogen use.

In the male, estrogen therapy may produce gynecomastia, reduced libido, cessation of spermatogenesis, and testicular atrophy. Reassure the male that female characteristics will usually disappear after therapy is stopped.

The cancer patient with metastasis to bone may develop severe hypercalcemia after starting estrogen therapy. Instruct the patient to report the appearance of the following symptoms: thirst, polyuria, anorexia, nausea, vomiting, constipation, and lethargy. Coma may eventually develop. In some

Text continued on p. 460

Table 39-1   Administration of estrogen*

Generic Name	Chemical Form	Trade Name	Administration
Chlorotrianisene	Nonsteroid	TACE**	Capsules for oral use, primarily for prostatic carcinoma.
Dienestrol	Nonsteroid	Dienestrol DV**	Vaginal creams and suppositories.
Diethylstilbestrol (DES)	Nonsteroid	Stilbestrol Honvol†	Tablets for oral use.
	Nonsteroid diphosphate	Stilphostrol Stilbilium†	Tablets for oral use or solution for injection; used primarily as antineoplastic agent.
Estradiol	—	Estrace**	Tablets for oral use.
	Cypionate	Depo-estradiol cypionate Depogen Dura-estrin	Oil solution for intramuscular injection.
	Valerate	Delestrogen** Estate Valergen	Oil solution for intramuscular injection.
Estrogens	—	Hormonin	Oral tablets contain estriol, estrone and estradiol.
Estrogens, conjugated	Sulfate esters	Premarin	Tablets for oral use or vaginal cream.

Estrogens, esterified	Sulfate ester, primarily estrone	Amnestrogen Estratab Evex Menest	Tablets for oral use.
Estrogenic substance	—	Gynogen Kestrin Unigen	Water suspension or oil solution for intramuscular injection.
Estrone	—	Theelin Femogen**	Aqueous suspension for intramuscular injection. Intravaginal cream.
	Estrone + potassium estrone	Mer-estrone Spanestrin P	Aqueous suspension for injection intramuscularly.
Estropipate	Estrone piperazine sulfate	Ogen**	Tablets for oral use, or vaginal cream.
Ethinyl estradiol		Estinyl** Feminone	Tablets for oral use.
Quinestrol		Estrovis	Tablets for oral use.

*Estrogen doses used in the clinical setting vary depending on the nature of the condition being treated. When used in replacement therapy, estrogen doses tend to be low. Higher doses are used to treat conditions such as advanced breast cancer.
**Available in U.S. and Canada
†Available in Canada only

Table 39-2 Estrogens in combinations*

Estrogen	Other Active Ingredients	Trade Name	Administration
Conjugated estrogens	Meprobamate (antidepressant)	Milprem PMB	Tablets for oral use.
	Methyltestosterone, methamphetamine, vitamin, and mineral supplements (androgen, central nervous system stimulant)	Mediatric	Tablets, capsules, or liquid for oral use.
Diethylstilbestrol	Methyltestosterone (androgen)	Tylosterone	Tablets for oral use.
Esterified estrogens	Chlordiazepoxide (antidepressant)	Menrium	Tablets for oral use.
	Methyltestosterone (androgen)	Estratest	Tablets for oral use.
Estradiol cypionate	Testosterone cypionate (androgen)	Depo-Testadiol Duratestrin Spenduo	Oil solution for intramuscular injection.
Estradiol valerate	Testosterone enanthate (androgen)	Deladumone Testradiol-90/4	Oil solution for intramuscular injection.

Estrone	Testosterone (androgen)	Andesterone	Aqueous suspension for intramuscular injection.
	Testosterone, B vitamins (androgen)	Android-G Geriamic	Aqueous suspension for intramuscular injection.
Ethinyl estradiol	Fluoxymesterone (androgen)	Halodrin	Tablets for oral use.

*For other fixed combinations of estrogens and progestins, see Chapter 42, Oral Contraceptives.

460 **Pocket Nurse Guide to Drugs**

instances it may be necessary to stop estrogen therapy, at least temporarily, to lower the concentration of calcium in the blood.

Nursing Implications for Estrogens

- Encourage patients receiving these drugs to continue with regular health care follow-up, to take their medications only as ordered, and to report any unexplained signs or symptoms.
- Question women carefully for family or patient history of obesity, cardiovascular disease, thromboembolic disease, hypertension, and diabetes. Patients should stop smoking when taking estrogens, progestins, or combinations of these two.
- Monitor the patient's weight weekly and blood pressure at regular intervals. Patients with conditions that can be aggravated by fluid retention should be especially careful when taking these medications.
- Use of diuretics and/or a sodium-restricted diet may help. Patients with a history of seizures may find that fluid restriction increases the incidence of seizures.
- Patients with diabetes mellitus may find that their glucose balance is altered while taking these drugs; they may require changes in insulin dosage. Side effects may include nausea or vomiting, but these often subside after 1 to 2 months of therapy.
- Taking the medication at bedtime, followed by a light, bland snack may lessen the nausea.
- Visual changes can occur. Teach the patient to report immediately any headaches, blurring, diplopia, loss of vision, or other visual problems.
- Teach the patient to report any change in skin color or color of sclera, because these may indicate liver damage.
- The effects of these hormonal agents on the body continue for several months, even after therapy has been discontinued. Teach patients to report to all physicians, pathologists, and dentists that they are or have been on some form of hormonal therapy or birth control pills.

Estrogens **461**

- Taking estrogens, progestins, or birth control pills predisposes to candidal vaginal infections.
- Overdosage with vaginal creams and suppositories is possible
- Taking estrogen, whether alone or in combination, will usually result in clearing of acne, although initially the acne may worsen. In rare individuals, estrogens will cause acne to worsen. After discontinuing estrogen therapy, some women may experience several months of rebound worsening of acne.
- The effects of estrogen may be reduced when the patient is also taking rifampin, barbiturates, phenylbutazone, phenytoin, or ampicillin.
- Estrogen therapy, like birth control pills, is often cyclic to prevent continuous hormonal stimulation of the body. The schedule is frequently to take the medication for 3 weeks and stop for 1 week, or to take the estrogen for the first 21 days of the month and to omit the medication for the rest of the month, then resume the estrogen on the first of each month. Before discharging the patient, ascertain that she can correctly repeat her dosage schedule.
- Estrogen therapy has been associated with a reported increased incidence of gallbladder disease and benign liver tumors.
- Some estrogen preparations are available as pellets for subcutaneous implantation. When administered via this route, they are effective for about 3 months.
- Oil-based solutions may be cloudy if they have been stored in the refrigerator. Let the preparation warm to room temperature before administering; it should then be clear.
- Roll vials of aqueous suspensions between both hands for several minutes before administering, to resuspend the medication.
- Estradurin may cause pain when administered intramuscularly; concomitant use of a local anesthetic may be indicated. See literature supplied by the manufacturer and check with the physician.
- Teach female patients how to perform regular self examinations of the breasts.

Progestins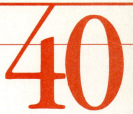

Hydroxyprogesterone
Medroxyprogesterone
Megestrol
Norethindrone

Progesterone
See also combinations with estrogen in Ch. 42, Oral Contraceptives

Actions of Progestins

Progestins stimulate the uterine lining, reducing the activity of the myometrium and preventing muscular contractions and promoting the development of the secretory capacity of the endometrium. Progesterone prevents sloughing of the endometrium in early pregnancy and prevents uterine contractions until levels normally fall at the end of pregnancy.

Indications for Progestins

Progestins combined with estrogens may be used to treat amenorrhea (see also Ch. 39), to treat infertility resulting from luteal phase defect, and to treat some metastatic breast carcinomas and metastatic endometrial carcinomas. High doses are used to suppress bleeding of the endometrium.

 ## Nurse Alert for Progestins

- Progestins are contraindicated during pregnancy. A woman who misses two consecutive periods should stop the drug until pregnancy is ruled out.
- Because progestins are associated with thrombophlebitis, progestins are contraindicated for women with a history of thromboembolic disorders. Patients should be instructed to report symptoms such as leg pain, sudden onset chest pain, shortness of breath, coughing of blood, headache, dizziness, vision or speech changes, or weakness or numbness in extremities.

Table 40-1 Administration of progestins

Generic Name	Chemical Form	Trade Name	Administration
Hydroxyprogesterone	Caproate	Delalutin* Gesterol L.A. Hyproval-P.A.	Oil solution for intramuscular injection; action persists 9 to 17 days.
Medroxyprogesterone	Acetate	Depo-provera* Amen Curretab Provera*	Aqueous suspension for intramuscular injection. Tablets for oral use.
Megestrol	Acetate	Megace*	Tablets for oral use in treating endometrial carcinoma.
Norethindrone		Micronor† Norlutin	Tablets for oral use.
	Acetate	Norlutate*	Tablets for oral use.
Progesterone		Profac-O Progelan Progestilin†	Aqueous suspension or oil solution for intramuscular injection.

*Available in U.S. and Canada
†Available in Canada only

Pocket Nurse Guide to Drugs

Side Effects of Progestins

Some side effects are similar to those seen with estrogens: edema, breast tenderness and swelling, gastrointestinal disturbances, depression, and weight change. Other effects include changes in menstrual blood flow, midcycle spotting or breakthrough bleeding, cholestatic jaundice, and rashes. Many of the progestins have some androgenic activity and may cause masculinization of female fetuses. Because of this danger, the use of progestins as a test for pregnancy is no longer recommended. Patients with a history of thromboembolic disorders or thrombophlebitis should not be treated with progestins.

Nursing Implications for Progestins

- Many of the nursing implications for patients on progestins are similar to those with estrogens; see pp. 460-461 for additional nursing implications.
- The effects of progestins may be reduced when the patient is taking phenobarbital or phenylbutazone or increased when the patient is also taking phenothiazines.
- Some progestins are prescribed to treat hormonal imbalance and not to prevent ovulation. Instruct the patient that conception can occur. It is possible to accurately monitor basal body temperature to help determine ovulation in cases of amenorrhea being treated with progestins.

Fertility Agents

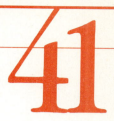

Bromocriptine mesylate
Clomiphene citrate

Human chorionic gonadotropin (HCG)
Menotropins

Actions of and Indications for Fertility Agents

These agents have different mechanisms of action and are used to treat infertility resulting from different causes. *Bromocriptine mesylate* suppresses secretion of prolactin, which in high levels interferes with pituitary and/or ovarian function to cause infertility. *Clomiphene citrate* activates the pituitary and stimulates ovulation, probably by hypothalamic mechanisms. *HCG* stimulates ovulation by an action resembling that of LH. *Menotropins* consist of FSH and LH and stimulate the ovary in women whose pituitary is not supplying sufficient gonadotropins.

Bromocriptine may also be indicated for galactorrhea or postpartum breast engorgement, by suppressing prolactin release and preventing the excessive stimulation of breast secretory tissue. It is also used to treat Parkinson's disease.

Nurse Alert for Fertility Agents

- Bromocriptine mesylate is contraindicated in pregnancy. Because hypotension may occur as a side effect, in the postpartum patient vital signs should be stable before bromocriptine is administered. Monitor blood pressure of all patients beginning therapy. Caution patients who feel lightheaded, or show other signs of hypotension, to sit or lie down.
- The usual dilution of HCG is 1000 units/ml; the average dose is 5000 to 10,000 units IM. Divide the dose so that no volume larger than 5 ml is administered per injection site. The drug should be given intramuscularly.

Table 41-1 Administration of fertility agents

Generic Name	Trade Name*	Classification	Administration
Bromocriptine mesylate	Parlodel*	Inhibitor of prolactin release	Tablets for oral use.
Clomiphene citrate	Clomid* Serophene	Nonsteroid stimulator of ovulation	Tablets for oral use.
Human chorionic gonadotropin (HCG)	A.P.L. Secules* Follutein	Placental hormone related to LH	Intramuscular injection.
Menotropins	Pergonal*	Human menopausal gonadotropins (urinary)	Intramuscular injection.

*Available in U.S. and Canada

- The dose of clomiphene is individualized for the patient. The usual starting dose is 25 to 50 mg per day, starting on the third day of the menstrual cycle and continuing for 5 days. The basal body temperature and other parameters are monitored to ascertain if ovulation occurs during that cycle. If ovulation has not occurred and the patient has suffered no serious side effects, the dose is increased monthly. The usual daily dose rarely exceeds 100 mg, although some patients require doses as high as 150 to 200 mg per day.
- When menotropins are administered, monitoring of urinary estrogen secretion is often done. If the 24-hour level of urinary estrogen exceeds 150 μg, the drug is withheld. The actual dose is based on individual response. For additional information see the leaflet supplied by the manufacturer.
- To administer menotropins, dissolve the contents of one ampule of the drug in 1 to 2 ml of sterile saline, and administer intramuscularly. Discard any unused solution.

Side Effects of Fertility Agents

Human Chorionic Gonadotropin (HCG)

Side effects include headache, depression, edema, gynecomastia, irritability, precocious puberty in young males, and pain at the injection site. Severe ovarian hyperstimulation can require hospitalization.

Clomiphene

Side effects include hot flashes, breast tenderness and engorgement, cyclic ovarian pain, and nausea, but these rarely require cessation of therapy and subside after the drug is discontinued. If visual problems occur, they should be reported immediately; the drug will usually be discontinued.

Menotropins

Side effects caused by ovarian stimulation result in ovarian enlargement, abdominal discomfort, flatulence, nausea, vomiting, and diarrhea. Severe ovarian stimulation can result in increased weight, ascites, pleural effusion, oliguria, and hypotension, and may require hospitalization. If significant ovarian stimulation occurs, the couple should refrain from intercourse during that cycle and contact the physician.

468 **Pocket Nurse Guide to Drugs**

Bromocriptine Mesylate

Nausea, vomiting, and constipation may occur with this drug. In the higher doses sometimes used to treat Parkinson's Disease, additional side effects may be seen, including mental disturbances, dyskinesias, and erythromelalgia.

Erythromelalgia is characterized by red, tender, warm, edematous lower extremities.

While many of the side effects are dose related, there is also significant individual variation in response. Instruct the patient to report the development of any unusual sign or symptom. Side effects usually disappear when the drug is discontinued.

Nursing Implications for Fertility Agents

- When a couple is using HCG for ovulatory stimulation, they should be instructed to monitor the woman's basal body temperature, character of vaginal secretions, or collect 24-hour urine specimens for urinary estrogen excretion. The couple should have sexual intercourse daily or every other day, beginning on the day before HCG is administered until one or more of the parameters just listed indicates that ovulation has occurred.
- HCG is used to treat cryptorchidism in boys; if there is no anatomical obstruction, administration of HCG will cause the testes to descend.
- Menotropins are rarely given alone because they stimulate only follicular growth and maturation; usually HCG is also administered. The couple should be informed that the incidence of multiple births may be as high as 20%. An increased incidence of abortion has also been reported.
- Taking bromocriptine with meals is recommended to reduce gastric side effects.
- Drowsiness and dizziness may occur with bromocriptine, independent of hypotension. Caution patients to avoid driving or operating dangerous equipment until the effects of the medication can be evaluated.
- Abnormalities in blood tests may occur with bromocriptine, including elevations in BUN, SGOT, SGPT, GGPT, CPK, alkaline phosphatase, and uric acid.

Oral Contraceptives 42

Ethynodiol diacetate
Levonorgestrel
Norethindrone
Norethindrone acetate
Norethynodrel

Norgestrel
Norethindrone
Mestranol
Ethinylestradiol

Actions of Oral Contraceptives

Oral contraceptives contain estrogen and progestins, which together suppress the hypothalamus and pituitary so that no LH is released at the time ovulation would normally occur; ovulation is thereby suppressed.

Indications for Oral Contraceptives

In addition to preventing pregnancy, oral contraceptives may be used for symptomatic relief in dysmenorrhea.

Nurse Alert for Oral Contraceptives

- Because oral contraceptives are contraindicated during pregnancy, women who miss two consecutive periods should stop the pills and see a physician to rule out the possibility of pregnancy.
- As with any medication, the oral contraceptives must be considered in terms of the risk-to-benefit ratio. Of first importance may be how much value the patient places on almost complete protection against unwanted pregnancy. Women who desire this high level of control should next consider the safety factors of the medication. Many of the dangerous complications, such as stroke and thromboembolitic diseases, are rare even among oral contraceptive

470   Pocket Nurse Guide to Drugs

users. The risk of these complications is greater than the risk among nonusers of oral contraceptives, but much lower than the risk of these complications during pregnancy. Also to be considered are the other predisposing risk factors, such as smoking, obesity, and hypertension. The combination of oral contraceptives with these conditions leads to unacceptable risk for many patients. All women receiving oral contraceptives should be urged to stop smoking.

■ Current medical information suggests that oral contraceptives are safe drugs when used in relatively young women in whom other risk factors are minimized. The most prudent course of action seems to be to carefully select patients before administering oral contraceptives. Women with a history of hypertension or thromboembolitic diseases probably should not receive the drugs. Women who elect to receive oral contraceptives should be given thorough physical examinations yearly. The dose of estrogen and progestin should be the lowest dose that achieves contraception and prevents unwanted side effects such as breakthrough bleeding.

■ Careful history taking may reveal symptoms that the patient has not linked to oral contraceptive use. Migraine headaches, dizziness, and visual disturbances are frequently not related by the patient to oral contraceptive use and may not be mentioned spontaneously. However, breakthrough bleeding, excessive cervical mucus formation, breast tenderness, and other changes in the reproductive tract are usually quickly connected to oral contraceptive use by the patient. These latter symptoms are usually more annoying than serious. However, severe headaches or visual disturbances are frequently early signs of impending stroke, and such symptoms may be sufficient cause to discontinue the medications.

Administration of Oral Contraceptives

Oral contraceptives are formulated to contain the correct daily dosage of estrogen and progestin. They are usually taken for 20 or 21 consecutive days, then withdrawn for 7 or 8 days. Table 42-1 indicates the amount of progestin and estrogen in the various oral contraceptives.

Side Effects of Oral Contraceptives

An excess of either estrogen or progestin in an oral contraceptive may cause side effects. Estrogen excess in a patient may be associated with nausea, bloating, breast fullness, edema, hypertension, and cervical discharges. These symptoms may suggest that the patient be tried on a preparation with less estrogen. Progestin excess in a patient taking oral contraceptives may produce hair loss, hirsutism, oily scalp, acne, increased appetite and weight gain, tiredness and depression, breast regression, and reduced menstrual blood flow.

Other potential adverse reactions are listed in Table 42-2.

Some medical conditions are actually improved or the symptoms are ameliorated by oral contraceptives. Many patients report a reduction in menstrual disorders and especially in dysmenorrhea. Menstrual blood flow is usually reduced, and anemia is prevented or lessened in many women. Benign breast tumors are improved in a time-dependent fashion by oral contraceptive therapy.

Nursing Implications for Oral Contraceptives

- The nursing implications for patients receiving oral contraceptives include many of the same nursing implications for estrogen therapy; in addition to the implications listed below, see also pp. 460-461.
- If a single birth control pill is missed, the patient should take the missed dose as soon as she remembers. If 2 consecutive pills are missed, the patient should double up on each of the next 2 days, then resume her regular schedule but use additional birth control measures until she completes that cycle. If 3 or more consecutive tablets are missed, the patient should stop the pills for 7 days after the first missed tablet, then begin a new cycle of tablets. She should also use additional contraceptive measures from the time the missed tablets are noticed until 7 days after the new course of therapy is started.
- Anovulation and amenorrhea may persist for as long as 6 months after birth control therapy has been discontinued.

Text continued on p. 477

Table 42-1 Oral contraceptives: amounts of progestin and estrogen

Progestin	Estrogen	Trade Name	Progestin/Estrogen Ratio
Ethynodiol diacetate	Mestranol	Ovulen*	1.0 mg:100 μg
	Ethinyl estradiol	Demulen*	1.0 mg:50 μg
		Demulen 1/35	1.0 mg:35 μg
Levonorgestrel	Ethinyl estradiol	Nordette	0.15 mg:30 μg
		Triphasil**	0.05 mg:30 μg, 0.075 mg:40 μg, 0.125 mg:30 μg
Norethindrone	Mestranol	Norinyl 2 mg* or Ortho-Novum 2 mg*	2.0 mg: 100 μg
		Norinyl 1 + 80* or Ortho-Novum 1/80	1.0 mg:80 μg
		Norinyl 1 + 50* or Ortho-Novum 1/50*	1.0 mg:50 μg
	Ethinyl estradiol	Ovcon-50	1.0 mg:50 μg
		Brevicon* or Modicon	0.5 mg:35 μg
		Ovcon-35	0.4 mg:35 μg
		Ortho-Novum 7/7/7†	0.5 mg, 0.75 mg and 1.0 mg:35 μg
		Tri-Norinyl‡	0.5 mg and 1.0 mg:35 μg
Norethindrone acetate	Ethinyl estradiol	Norlestrin 2.5/50*	2.5 mg:50 μg
		Loestrin 1.5/30*	1.5 mg:30 μg

		Norlestrin 1/50*	1.0 mg:50 μg
		Loestrin 1/20	1.0 mg:20 μg
Norethynodrel	Mestranol	Enovid 5 mg	5.0 mg:75 μg
		Enovid-E	2.5 mg:100 μg
Norgestrel	Ethinyl estradiol	Ovral*	0.5 mg:50 μg
		Lo/Ovral	0.3 mg:30 μg
Norethindrone	None	Micronor*	0.35 mg
		Nor-QD	
Norgestrel	None	Ovrette	0.075mg

*Available in U.S. and Canada

**This preparation is designed so that 0.05 mg:30 μg pills are taken for the first 6 days of the cycle, 0.075 mg:40 μg pills for the next 5 days, and 0.125 mg:30 μg pills for the last 10 days of the cycle, followed by a week of no medication.

†This preparation is designed so that 0.05 mg:35 μg pills are taken for the first 7 days of the menstrual period, the 0.75 mg:35 μg pills for the second 7 days and 1.0 mg:35 μg pills for the third week, followed by a week of no medication.

‡This preparation is designed so that 0.5 mg:35 μg pills are taken for the first 7 days of the menstrual period, the 1.0 mg:35 μg pills for the next 9 days, and 0.5 mg:35 μg pills again for the last 5 days, followed by a week of no medication.

Table 42-2 Potential adverse reactions of oral contraceptives

Adverse Reaction	Relation to Oral Contraceptives	Comments
Thromboembolitic diseases	Risk increased 2- to 7-fold in users over nonusers. Incidence about 100/100,000 woman years; fatalities 2/100,000 woman years.	Obesity, family history of thromboembolitic disorders, immobility, and/or group A blood type may increase risk. Group O blood type women have lower risk. May be related to estrogen dosage.
Thrombotic stroke	Risk increased 3.1 to 6-fold. Incidence about 25/100,000 woman years; fatalities 0.5/100,000 woman years.	Hypertension increases the risk.
Hemorrhagic stroke	Risk increased at least 2-fold. Incidence about 10/100,000 woman years.	Hypertension and heavy smoking are strong risk factors.
Myocardial infarction	Risk increased about 2-fold over non-users.	Synergistic increase in risk if oral contraceptives are used by heavy smokers.
Hypertension	Between 1% and 5% of patients show an increase in blood pressure. Clinical hypertension is more rare.	Risk is increased by age, obesity, and parity.
Gallbladder disease	Risk increased an estimated 2-fold.	Risk may be related to the dose of progestin.

Liver disease	20% to 50% of patients show reduced liver function. Incidence 10/100,000 woman years for jaundice. Tumors are exceedingly rare.	Reversible. Dangerous for patients with preexisting liver disease (hepatitis, cholestasis). Liver tumors may be related specifically to mestranol.
Carbohydrate metabolism	Most patients show reduced glucose tolerance.	Important only in prediabetics who may become insulin dependent.
Lipid metabolism	Most patients have increased serum triglyceride levels.	Reversible effect; relationship to coronary artery disease in these patients is unknown.
Chloasma	3% to 4% of patients treated.	Increased sensitivity to sunlight also occurs. Reversible.
Headaches	Variable reports with no clear conclusion.	Appearance of chronic headache may presage stroke.
Visual disturbances	Often mentioned but not yet causally linked to oral contraceptive use.	Temporary blindness, blind spots, and changes in field of vision have been mentioned.
Emotional state	Variable reports with no clear conclusion.	No evidence that oral contraceptives significantly increase depression.
Endometrial cancer	No increased risk when combined estrogen-progestin agents used.	Risk is increased by estrogens alone but reduced by progestins.
Cervical cancer	No relationship established.	Frequency of coitus and number of sexual partners more important risk factors.

cont'd. next page

Table 42-2 Potential adverse reactions of oral contraceptives—cont'd.

Adverse Reaction	Relation to Oral Contraceptives	Comments
Breast cancer	No relationship established.	Benign breast tumors are actually improved.
Permanent infertility	No relationship established.	Most patients quickly return to fertility when oral contraceptives are discontinued.
Outcome of later pregnancies	No increased risk to mother or fetus has been demonstrated.	Data are for pregnancies begun after oral contraceptives have been discontinued.

Oral Contraceptives **477**

- If a woman discontinues birth control tablets for the purpose of becoming pregnant, it has been recommended that she use an alternate form of birth control for 2 months after stopping the pills to ensure more complete excretion of the hormonal agents before conceiving and thus reduce the potential effects of the medications on the fetus.
- The "mini-pill," the oral contraceptive containing only progestins, should be taken daily, all year long, even if the patient is menstruating.
- If elective surgery is planned, it may be desirable to stop birth control pills at least a month before surgery. Check with the physician.
- Many of the side effects related to birth control pills are dose-related. Switching patients to different dose combinations may relieve many side effects.

Oxytocic Drugs 43

Oxytocin
Ergonovine maleate
Methylergonovine maleate

Carboprost tromethamine
Dinoprost tromethamine
Dinoprostone

Actions of Oxytocic Drugs

The prostaglandins *carboprost tromethamine*, *dinoprost tromethamine*, and *dinoprostone* are similar to the natural hormone that stimulates uterine contractions when progesterone levels fall at the end of pregnancy. *Oxytocin* stimulates uterine contractions, while allowing the uterus to relax between contractions, and acts on breast tissue to stimulate the myoepithelium and promote milk letdown.

Indications for Oxytocic Drugs

Oxytocin is the drug of choice to induce or stimulate labor; the other oxytocic drugs have a greater risk of causing fetal anoxia. Oxytocin's effects on uterine contractions after delivery have the advantages of expelling the afterbirth and cleansing the uterus and controlling postpartum bleeding by clamping ruptured vessels. Oxytocin may also be indicated to stimulate milk letdown to aid in breast feeding.

Ergonovine maleate and *methylergonovine maleate* may be indicated for the control of postpartum bleeding because their action is longer lasting than oxytocin.

Dinoprost tromethamine, *carboprost tromethamine*, and *dinoprostone* stimulate uterine contractions to lead to abortion in the second trimester.

478

Nurse Alert for Oxytocic Drugs

- Induction of labor with one of the oxytocic drugs carries with it the risk of producing prolonged fetal anoxia. Therefore all patients in whom labor is being induced should receive continuous care, and fetal monitoring should be done where possible.
- Oxytocic drugs should be used only in the hospital or where a physician is immediately available.
- Oxytocic drugs are contraindicated any time that hyperstimulation of the uterus would be dangerous, or when hypertension is contraindicated.

Table 43-1 Administration of oxytocic drugs

Generic Name	Trade Name	Dosage and Administration
Posterior Pituitary Hormone		
Oxytocin	Pitocin Syntocinon*	INTRAVENOUS: 10 milliunits/ml infused at 1 to 2 milliunits/min, gradually increased up to about 10 milliunits/min for induction of labor. 20 to 40 milliunits/ml infused at 40 milliunits/min to control uterine atony postpartum. INTRAMUSCULAR: 3 to 10 units (0.3 to 1 ml) postpartum.
	Syntocinon*	NASAL: 1 spray of 40 units/ml solution before nursing. Onset of action is within 2 or 3 min, and duration of action is short.

cont'd. next page

*Available in U.S. and Canada

480   Pocket Nurse Guide to Drugs

Table 43-1   Administration of oxytocic drugs—cont'd.

Generic Name	Trade Name	Dosage and Administration
Ergot Alkaloids		
Ergonovine maleate	Ergotrate maleate*	ORAL: 0.2 to 0.4 mg 2 to 4 times daily for 2 days. INTRAMUSCULAR: 0.2 mg repeated in 2 to 4 hr if needed. INTRAVENOUS: 0.2 mg as emergency medication.
Methylergonovine maleate	Methergine	ORAL, INTRAMUSCULAR, INTRAVENOUS: As for ergonovine maleate.
Prostaglandins		
Carboprost tromethamine	Prostin/15M	INTRAMUSCULAR: 250 μg initially, repeated at 1.5 to 3.5 hr intervals as needed.
Dinoprost tromethamine	Prostin F2 alpha	INTRAUTERINE: 40 mg slowly infused. Second dose of 10 or 20 mg may be given 6 hr later if needed.
Dinoprostone	Prostin E2*	VAGINAL: 20 mg suppositories inserted every 3 to 5 hr until abortion ensues.

*Available in U.S. and Canada

■ Monitor the mother's blood pressure and the fetal pulse rate, and carry out electronic fetal monitoring when possible during intravenous oxytocic administration. Have available drugs to counteract a hypertensive crisis.

Side Effects of Oxytocic Drugs

Oxytocin may cause fetal or maternal cardiac arrhythmias, acute hypertension, nausea, and water intoxication; overdose may produce uterine hypertonicity with fetal and/or maternal injury. The *ergot alkaloids* may cause nausea and vomiting, hypertension (more likely with vasopressors or spinal anesthesia), headache, dizziness, palpitation, or chest pain. *Carboprost tromethamine* commonly causes vomiting, diarrhea, and fever. *Dinoprost tromethamine* may cause vasomotor disturbances, cardiac arrhythmias, hyperventilation, and chest pain. *Dinoprostone* commonly causes gastrointestinal symptoms; cardiovascular symptoms are possible.

Nursing Implications for Oxytocic Drugs

- See earlier section on contraindications and precautions.
- The nasal spray Syntocinon also causes nasal vasoconstriction.

MALE REPRO-DUCTIVE SYSTEM DRUGS

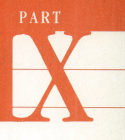

Androgens

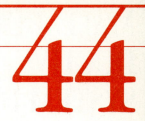

Testosterone
Testosterone cypionate
Testosterone enanthate
Testosterone propionate
Fluoxymesterone
Methyltestosterone

Actions of Androgens

Androgens stimulate the growth and maturation of the male reproductive organs, including the penis, scrotum, seminal vesicles, prostate gland, and other accessory tissues. Testosterone is also the major hormone responsible for development of secondary male sexual characteristics. Androgens are also anabolic (see Chapter 45 for anabolic steroids) and stimulate synthetic processes, increasing nitrogen retention and protein formation, and increasing overall metabolic rate. Calcium retention and red blood cell production are also increased.

Indications for Androgens

Androgens are primarily used in replacement therapy when endogenous androgen production is reduced (resulting in male climacteric, eunuchoidism, and certain types of impotence). Androgens may also be used in females for certain types of breast carcinomas.

Nurse Alert for Androgens

- Androgens are contraindicated in males with cancer of the breast or prostate gland and used with caution in males with benign prostatic hypertrophy.
- Androgens are contraindicated in females in pregnancy and lactation and used with caution in women of childbearing age.

Androgens **485**

- Androgens should be used with caution with all patients with existing medical conditions aggravated by fluid retention: hypertension, cardiovascular disease, and renal disease.

Side Effects of Androgens

Methyltestosterone and *fluoxymesterone* are associated with liver toxicity of various types, including cholestatic jaundice. These two androgens may also cause nausea and vomiting, diarrhea, and peptic ulcer-like symptoms and may increase sensitivity to anticoagulants.

All the testosterone androgens may cause precocious sexual development and premature epiphyseal closure in children, masculinization in females, and short-term increased libido or long-term inhibition of testicular function in males.

Potentially serious hypercalcemia may occur in immobilized patients and women treated for breast cancer, with symptoms of thirst, polyuria, anorexia, nausea, vomiting, constipation, lethargy, and eventually coma.

Nursing Implications for Androgens

- Monitor fluid retention with daily weights tapered to weekly, and monitor blood pressure. Diuretics and/or sodium-restricted diet may help reduce fluid retention.
- Oily skin and acne may occur; teach patient to maintain good hygiene.
- Gastric irritation may be reduced by taking oral medications with meals.
- Since women treated for breast cancer may experience a rise in serum calcium levels, review the symptoms with the patient and instruct her to report symptoms.
- Androgens can enhance the effects of anticoagulants; teach patients using both drugs to report signs of bruising, petechiae, or unexplained bleeding.
- Virilization in females can be particularly upsetting. Older women in particular may find an increased libido to be disconcerting. Teach patients to report changes in menses, hirsutism, balding, voice changes, clitoral enlargement, or any other unusual sign or symptom. Some changes may

Table 44-1 Administration of androgens

Generic Name	Trade Name	Drug Form and Dosage	Duration of Action
Natural Hormones			
Testosterone	Android T Andronaq Histerone Testaqua Oreton	INTRAMUSCULAR: *Adults*— aqueous suspension for intramuscular use only. Doses range from 10 to 100 mg.	Relatively short. Doses must be repeated 2 or 3 times per week.
		SUBCUTANEOUS: *Adults*—pellet for implantation, 150 to 450 mg.	3 to 4 months due to slow absorption.
Testosterone Esters			
Testosterone cypionate	Depo-Testosterone* Duratest Malogen CYP	INTRAMUSCULAR: *Adults*—oil solution for deep injection into gluteal muscle, 100 to 400 mg.	3 to 4 weeks.
Testosterone enanthate	Delatestryl* Span-Test Testate	INTRAMUSCULAR: *Adults*—oil solution for deep injection into gluteal muscle, 100-400 mg.	3 to 4 weeks.
Testosterone propionate		INTRAMUSCULAR: *Adults*—oil suspension for intramuscular use only. Doses range from 10 to 100 mg.	Relatively short. Doses must be repeated 2 or 3 times per week.

Oral Androgens

Fluoxymesterone	Halotestin* Ora-Testryl	ORAL: *Adults*—tablets for oral administration. 2 to 10 mg (male); 10 to 30 mg (female).	Short. Doses must be repeated daily.
Methyltestosterone	Android Metandren* Oreton Methyl Testred	ORAL: *Adults*—tablets or capsules. 10 to 40 mg (male); 80 to 200 mg (female).	Short. Doses must be repeated daily.

Buccal Agents

Methyltestosterone	Metandren linguets* Oreton Methyl	ORAL: *Adults*—tablets for buccal administration. 5 to 20 mg (male); 40 to 100 mg (female).	Short. Doses must be repeated daily.
Testosterone propionate		ORAL: *Adults*—tablets for buccal administration. 5 to 20 mg (male); 40 to 100 mg (female).	Short. Doses must be repeated daily.

*Available in U.S. and Canada

Pocket Nurse Guide to Drugs

reverse after discontinuing the drug. Virilization is usually dose related.

- Teach patients receiving oral androgens to report pruritus, jaundice, changes in skin color or color of sclera. These may be signs of liver dysfunction, an occasional side effect.
- Androgens have a sustained effect on the body and may produce alterations in laboratory studies up to several weeks after the drug is discontinued. Instruct patients to report to their physicians that they have been taking androgens even if they are not presently taking them.
- Androgens may decrease the fasting blood sugar concentration or predispose to hypoglycemia. In the diabetic this may necessitate a reduction in insulin dose.
- Androgens can cause increased circulating levels of oxyphenbutazone or phenylbutazone; reduction in the dosage of these two drugs may be necessary.
- Buccal tablets should be placed in the mouth between the upper or lower gum and the cheek and allowed to dissolve. While the tablet is in place, the patient should refrain from eating, drinking, chewing, or smoking. The patient should rotate sides with each administration. The patient should be encouraged to maintain good oral hygiene and to report any oral irritation.
- Pellets for subcutaneous implantation can be inserted surgically or with a specially designed injector. Aseptic technique must be maintained. Usual sites of insertion are the infrascapular area or along the posterior axillary line. Two or more pellets may be inserted at one time, although not necessarily into the same subcutaneous pouch. The drug will be slowly absorbed from the pellets for up to 4 to 6 months. Sloughing of the pellet can occur and should be reported to the physician. Because the dosage of subcutaneous pellets cannot be easily regulated, proper dosage for the patient is usually determined by oral medication before a switch is made to subcutaneous.

Anabolic Steroids

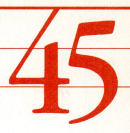

Ethylestrenol
Methandrostenolone
Methandriol
Nandrolone decanoate
Nandrolone phenpropionate
Oxandrolone
Oxymetholone
Stanozolol

Actions of Anabolic Steroids

Like other androgens, anabolic steroids stimulate synthetic processes, increasing nitrogen retention and protein formation and increasing overall metabolic rate. Calcium retention and red blood cell production are also increased.

Indications for Anabolic Steroids

Anabolic steroids are generally used for conditions in which nitrogen retention and protein formation are desirable (to alleviate the catabolic state of corticosteroid therapy, for extensive burns), for bone loss, and for the treatment of some forms of anemia.

Ethylestrenol and *methandrostenolone* are used for weight gain after traumatic injury, chronic disease, or long-term corticosteroid therapy, and to control symptoms of osteoporosis and certain anemias. Methandrostenolone is also used for growth stimulation in children and pituitary dwarves. *Methandriol* is used for osteoporosis. *Nandrolone decanoate* and *nandrolone phenpropionate* are used for refractory anemias, metastatic breast cancer, weight gain, and osteoporosis. *Oxandrolone* is used for weight gain or relief of bone pain in osteoporosis. *Oxymetholone* is used for osteoporosis and anemias. *Stanozolol* is used for aplastic anemia and osteoporosis. Anabolic steroids are *not* indicated for use in athletes seeking to increase bone or muscle mass.

Table 45-1 Administration of anabolic steroids

Generic Name	Trade Name	Drug Form and Dosage	Duration of Action
Ethylestrenol	Maxibolin*	ORAL: *Adults*—tablets or elixir, 4 to 16 mg daily. *Children*—2 mg daily.	Short. Doses must be repeated daily.
Methandriol	Anabol Methabolic Probolik Steribolic	INTRAMUSCULAR: *Adults*—aqueous suspension (Anabol) or oil solution for intramuscular injection.	Relatively long. 50 to 100 mg once or twice weekly (oil); 10 to 40 mg daily (aqueous).
Nandrolone decanoate	Deca-Durabolin* Nandrolate	INTRAMUSCULAR: *Adults*—oil solution for deep intramuscular injection, 50 to 100 mg.	Long. Repeat doses every 3 to 4 weeks.
Nandrolone phenpropionate	Durabolin* Nandrolin	INTRAMUSCULAR: *Adults*—oil solution for deep intramuscular injection, 25 to 50 mg.	Long. Repeat doses every 1 to 4 weeks.
Oxandrolone	Anavar	ORAL: *Adults*—tablets, 5 to 10 mg daily; *Children*—0.25 mg/kg intermittently.	Short. Repeat doses daily.

| Oxymetholone | Adroyd
Anadrol | ORAL: *Adults*—tablets, 5 to 10 mg daily, for osteoporosis; 1 to 5 mg/kg/day, up to 100 mg total daily dose, for anemias. | Short. Repeat doses daily. |
| Stanozolol | Winstrol* | ORAL: *Adults*—tablets, 6 mg daily. *Children*—1 mg twice daily. | Short. Doses are taken with meals. |

*Available in U.S. and Canada

Nurse Alert for Anabolic Steroids

- Anabolic steroids are contraindicated in pregnancy and lactation and should be used with caution in women of childbearing age because of the potential danger of masculinizing the fetus.
- Anabolic steroids are contraindicated in males with cancer of the breast or prostate gland and should be used with caution in men with benign prostatic hypertrophy.
- Anabolic steroids should be used with caution in patients with existing medical conditions that could be aggravated by fluid retention: hypertension, cardiovascular disease, and renal disease.

Side Effects of Anabolic Steroids

Side effects for women include androgenic effects such as increased libido, inappropriate hair development, voice changes, and personality alterations. Children may experience precocious sexual development and premature fusion of the epiphyses. Men may experience priapism (continuous erection). Additional potentially serious side effects include hepatotoxicity, hypercalcemia, reduced gonadotropin levels, lowered testosterone synthesis, and depressed spermatogenesis.

Nursing Implications for Anabolic Steroids

- To monitor fluid retention, weigh patients daily; then taper to weighing patients weekly; monitor blood pressure. A sodium-restricted diet and/or diuretics may help reduce fluid retention.
- Oily skin and acne can be a distressing side effect, especially for teenagers. Teach the patient to maintain good hygiene.
- Gastric irritation can be reduced by taking the medication with meals.
- The effectiveness of anabolic steroids in burned, traumatized, or immobilized patients will be enhanced by the concomitant use of a diet high in calories, protein,

Anabolic Steroids 493

vitamins, and minerals. Regular physical therapy should be continued to help reduce demineralization of bone.

- Because anabolic steroids can enhance the effect of anticoagulants, teach patients taking both drugs to report any signs of bruising, petechiae, or unexplained bleeding.
- Virilization in females can be particularly upsetting. Teach patients to report changes in menses, hirsutism, balding, voice changes, clitoral enlargement, or any other unusual sign or symptom. Some changes may reverse after discontinuing the drug. Virilization is usually dose related. If the androgen therapy for breast cancer is felt to be producing positive results, the physician may not want to discontinue the therapy even if some virilization is occurring.
- Teach patients to report pruritus, jaundice, changes in skin color or color of sclera. These may be signs of liver dysfunction, an occasional side effect.
- Anabolic steroids have a sustained effect on the body and may produce alterations in laboratory studies up to several weeks after the drug is discontinued. Instruct patients to report to their physicians that they have been taking androgens even if they are not presently taking them.
- Anabolic steroids may decrease the fasting blood sugar concentration or predispose to hypoglycemia. In the diabetic this may necessitate a reduction in insulin dose.
- Anabolic steroids can cause increased circulating levels of oxyphenbutazone or phenylbutazone; reduction in the dosage of these two drugs may be necessary.
- In children anabolic steroids may be used to treat pituitary dwarfism when growth hormone is not available. This therapy is not without risk, since many times the children are prepubertal. In addition to regular x-ray films, drug therapy will usually be on an intermittent basis, to prevent too early bone maturation. It is especially important to question young children tactfully about side effects: priapism, erections, clitoral enlargement, and other signs of precocious puberty.

ANTIINFECTIVE AGENTS

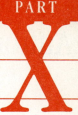

PART X

Antibiotics 46

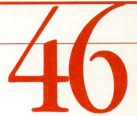

Penicillins
  Biosynthesized penicillins
    Penicillin G
    Penicillin V
  Repository penicillins
    Benzathine penicillin G
    Procaine penicillin G
  Penicillinase-resistant penicillins
    Cloxacillin sodium
    Dicloxacillin sodium
    Methicillin sodium
    Nafcillin sodium
    Oxacillin sodium
  Broad spectrum penicillins
    Amoxicillin
    Amoxicillin and K clavulanate
    Ampicillin
  Antipseudomonas penicillins
    Azlocillin sodium
    Carbenicillin disodium
    Carbenicillin indanyl sodium
    Mezlocillin sodium
    Piperacillin sodium
    Ticarcillin disodium

Cephalosporins
  First-generation
    Cefadroxil monohydrate
    Cefazolin sodium
    Cephalexin
    Cephalothin sodium
    Cephapirin sodium
    Cephradine
  Second-generation
    Cefaclor
    Cefamandole nafate
    Cefonicid sodium
    Ceforanide
    Cefoxitin sodium
    Cefuroxime sodium
  Third-generation
    Cefoperazone sodium
    Cefotaxime sodium
    Ceftizoxime sodium
    Moxalactam disodium
Penicillin substitutes
  Bacitracin
  Clindamycin
  Clindamycin palmitate
  Clindamycin phosphate
  Erythromycins
    Erythromycin base
    Erythromycin estolate
    Erythromycin ethylsuccinate

Antibiotics 497

Erythromycin gluceptate
Erythromycin
lactobionate
Erythromycin stearate
Lincomycin
Novobiocin
Spectinomycin
Vancomycin
Tetracyclines
Demeclocycline HCl
Doxycycline
Methacycline HCl
Minocycline HCl
Oxytetracycline HCl
Tetracycline HCl
Chloramphenicol
Chloramphenicol
Chloramphenicol palmitate
Chloramphenicol sodium
succinate
Aminoglycosides
Amikacin
Gentamicin
Kanamycin
Neomycin
Netilmicin
Streptomycin
Tobramycin
Polymyxins
Colistin sulfate
Colistimethate sodium
(colistin methane
sulfonate)
Polymyxin B sulfate
Sulfonamides
Single component
formulations
Sulfacytine
Sulfadiazine
Sulfamethizole
Sulfamethoxazole
Sulfasalazine
Sulfisoxazole

Fixed oral combinations
Sulfamethoxazole and
trimethoprim
Sulfamerazine and
sulfadiazine
Sulfamerazine,
sulfadiazine,
and sulfamethazine
Sulfamethizole and
phenazopyridine
Sulfamethoxazole and
phenazopyridine
Sulfisoxazole and
phenazopyridine
Topical agents
Mafenide acetate
Silver sulfadiazine
Sulfacetamide
Sulfisoxazole
Other drugs for urinary tract
infections
Nitrofurantoin
Nalidixic acid
Cinoxacin
Trimethoprim
Antituberculosis drugs
Aminosalicylate acid
sodium salt
Capreomycin
Cycloserine
Ethambutol
Ethionamide
Isoniazid, or isonicotinic
acid hydrazide (INH)
Para-aminosalicylic acid
(PAS)
Pyrazinamide
Rifampin
Streptomycin
Antileprosy drugs
Dapsone
Clofazimine
Rifampin
Sulfoxone sodium

498 Pocket Nurse Guide to Drugs

Penicillins

Biosynthesized penicillins
Penicillin G
Penicillin V
Repository penicillins
Benzathine penicillin G
Procaine penicillin G
Penicillinase-resistant penicillins
Cloxacillin sodium
Dicloxacillin sodium
Methicillin sodium
Nafcillin sodium
Oxacillin sodium
Broad spectrum penicillins
Amoxicillin
Ampicillin
Antipseudomonas penicillins
Azlocillin sodium
Carbenicillin disodium
Carbenicillin indanyl sodium
Mezlocillin sodium
Piperacillin sodium
Ticarcillin disodium

Actions of Penicillins

The penicillins are irreversible inhibitors of the bacterial enzyme transpeptidase, preventing formation of a new intact cell wall in the bacteria.

Indications for Penicillins

Penicillin G is effective against gram-positive bacteria such as *Streptococcus pneumonia*, and selected strains of *Staphylococcus aureus*, *Bacillus anthracis*, *Corynebacterium diphtherium*, *Clostridium tetani*, and *Cl. perfringens* (gas gangrene); the gram-negative bacteria *Neisseria gonorrhoea* and *N. meningitis*; and the spirochete *Treponema pallidum* (syphillis).

The repository penicillins are used to maintain modest serum levels for relatively long periods of time, for moderate or mild infections or for prophylaxis.

Penicillin V is used in oral penicillin therapy for mild to moderate infections or for prophylaxis.

The penicillinase-resistant penicillin methicillin is used only in treatment of infections in which penicillinase is produced by the pathogenic organism. The acid-stable penicillinase-resistant penicillins nafcillin, oxacillin, cloxacillin, and dicloxacillin are used in initial therapy when a penicillinase-resistant organism is suspected.

The broad-spectrum penicillins are used with gram-negative bacteria known to be sensitive to the drugs.

The anti-pseudomonas penicillins are effective against *Pseudomonas aeruginosa* and other pseudomonas infections.

Nurse Alert for Penicillins

- Dangerous anaphylactic reactions to penicillin occur in 0.04–0.2% of treated patients; patients should be asked about allergies, a skin test may be performed to identify allergic patients, or the patient may be observed after the injection for allergic response. Allergic reactions other than anaphylaxis occur in up to 10% of treated patients.
- The repository penicillins are intended only for deep muscular injections; avoid accidental injection into blood vessels, which may result in occlusion of the vessel.

Side Effects of Penicillins

Allergic responses may include skin rashes or urticaria in addition to serious anaphylactic reactions. Intrathecal injection or high doses given intramuscularly or intravenously may cause convulsions. Oral preparations may cause irritation and inflammation of the upper gastrointestinal tract, nausea, vomiting, and diarrhea. Some commercial preparations may include sodium or potassium sufficient to cause electrolyte imbalances in some patients. Methicillin may cause significant blood dyscrasias and interstitial nephritis.

Nursing Implications for Penicillins

- Monitor renal, hepatic, and hematopoietic function on patients receiving penicillin.

Text continued on p. 505

Table 46-1   Administration of penicillins

Generic Name	Trade Name	Dosage and Administration
Biosynthesized Penicillins		
Penicillin G	Pentids Pfizerpen	ORAL: *Adults*—200,000 to 500,000 units every 6 to 8 hr administered $\frac{1}{2}$ hr before or 2 hr after meals. *Children*—25,000 to 90,000 units/kg daily in 3 to 6 doses. INTRAMUSCULAR: *Adults*—300,000 to 1.2 million units daily in divided doses. *Children*—50,000 to 250,000 units/kg daily divided among 6 doses. INTRAVENOUS: *Adults and children*— As for intramuscular. Higher doses have been used for severe infections.
Penicillin V	Pen-Vee-K* V-Cillin K* Veetids	ORAL: *Adults*—125 to 500 mg every 4 to 6 hr. *Children*—25 to 50 mg/kg daily in divided doses.
Repository Penicillins		
Benzathine penicillin G	Bicillin*	INTRAMUSCULAR: *Adults*—600,000 to 1.2 million units every 2 to 4 weeks. *Children*—50,000 units/kg once.
Procaine penicillin G	Crysticillin Duracillin A.S. Wycillin*	INTRAMUSCULAR: *Adults and children*—300,000 to 1.2 million units every 12 to 24 hr. For uncomplicated gonorrhea, 4.8 million units in 1dose divided between two sites. *Infants*—50,000 units/kg once daily.

Penicillinase-Resistant Penicillins

Cloxacillin sodium	Cloxapen Tegopen*	ORAL: *Adults*—0.25 to 1 Gm every 4 to 6 hr. *Infants*—50 to 100 mg/kg daily divided into 4 doses. Administer 1 hr before or 2 hrs after meals.
Dicloxacillin sodium	Dycill Dynapen*	ORAL: *Adults*—0.125 to 1 Gm every 4 to 6 hr. *Children*—25 to 100 mg/kg daily divided into 4 doses. Administer 1 hr before or 2 hrs after meals.
Methicillin sodium	Celbenin Staphcillin*	INTRAMUSCULAR: *Adults*—1 Gm every 4 to 6 hr. *Children*—100 to 200 mg/kg daily divided into 4 to 6 doses. INTRAVENOUS: *Adults*—1 to 2 Gm diluted into 50 ml of Sodium Chloride Injection USP injected at a rate of 10 ml/min every 4 to 6 hr. *Children*—As for intramuscular.
Nafcillin sodium	Nafcil Unipen*	ORAL: *Adults*—0.25 to 1 Gm every 4 to 6 hr. *Children*—50 to 100 mg/kg daily divided into 4 doses. *Neonates*—30 to 40 mg/kg daily divided into 3 or 4 doses. INTRAMUSCULAR: *Adults*—500 mg every 4 to 6 hr. *Children*—150 mg/kg daily divided into 4 doses. INTRAVENOUS: *Adults*—0.5 to 1 Gm every 4 hr. *Children*—150 mg/kg daily divided into 4 doses.
Oxacillin sodium	Bactocill Prostaphlin*	ORAL: *Adults*—0.5 to 1 Gm every 4 to 6 hr. *Children*—50 to 100 mg/kg daily divided into 4 doses. Administer 1 hr before or 2 hr after meals.

cont'd. next page

*Available in U.S. and Canada

Pocket Nurse Guide to Drugs

Table 46-1 Administration of penicillins—cont'd.

Generic Name	Trade Name	Dosage and Administration
Oxacillin sodium—cont'd.		INTRAMUSCULAR: *Adults*—0.25 to 2 Gm every 4 to 6 hr. *Children*—50 to 100 mg/kg daily divided into 4 to 6 doses. INTRAVENOUS: *Adults*—As for intramuscular. The drug should be diluted to 20 mg/ml or less before injection.
Broad Spectrum Penicillins		
Amoxicillin	Amoxil* Larotid Polymox* Trimox	ORAL: *Adults*—250 to 500 mg every 8 hr. *Infants*—20 to 40 mg/kg daily divided into 3 doses.
Amoxicillin and K clavulanate	Augmentin	ORAL: *Adults*—250 or 500 mg amoxicillin and 125 mg K clavulanate every 8 hr. *Infants*—20 to 40 mg/kg amoxicillin and 5 to 10 mg/kg clavulanate daily, divided into 3 doses.
Ampicillin	Amcill* Omnipen Polycillin Principen	ORAL: *Adults*—250 to 500 mg every 6 hr. *Infants*—50 to 100 mg/kg daily divided into 4 doses. INTRAMUSCULAR: *Adults*—as for oral. *Infants*—100 to 200 mg/kg daily divided into 4 doses. INTRAVENOUS: *Adults*—as for oral. *Infants*—as for intramuscular. Higher doses have been administered for serious infections.

Antibiotics 503

Anti-pseudomonas Penicillins

Azlocillin sodium	Azlin	INTRAVENOUS: *Adults*—2 to 3 Gm by slow injection every 6 hr. Up to 24 Gm may be given daily for life-threatening infections.
Carbenicillin disodium	Geopen* Pyopen*	INTRAMUSCULAR: *Adults*—1 to 2 Gm every 6 hr. *Children*—50 to 200 mg/kg daily divided into 4 to 6 doses. INTRAVENOUS: *Adults*—Up to 40 Gm per day in 4 to 6 doses. *Children*—Up to 400 to 600 mg/kg daily in 4 to 6 doses.
Carbenicillin indanyl sodium	Geocillin	ORAL: *Adults*—1 or 2 tablets every 6 hr.
Mezlocillin sodium	Mezlin	INTRAMUSCULAR: *Adults*—1.5 to 2 Gm every 6 hr. INTRAVENOUS: *Adults*—1.5 to 3 Gm every 6 hr. Severe infections may be treated with up to 24 Gm daily in equally divided doses.
Piperacillin sodium	Pipracil*	INTRAMUSCULAR: *Adults*—2 to 4 Gm every 6 to 12 hr. INTRAVENOUS: *Adults*—2 to 4 Gm by slow injection every 6 to 12 hr. Up to 24 Gm may be given daily for life-threatening infections.
Ticarcillin disodium	Ticar*	INTRAMUSCULAR: *Adults*—1 Gm every 6 hr. *Children*—50 to 100 mg/kg daily divided into 3 or 4 doses. INTRAVENOUS: *Adults and children*—200 to 300 mg/kg daily in 4 to 6 doses. Drug should be infused over 10 to 20 min.

*Available in U.S. and Canada

Table 46-2 Parenteral administration of penicillins

Drug	Recommended Dilution	Rate of Administration
Ampicillin	500 mg in at least 5 ml diluent	500 mg per 5 min
Azlocillin	1 Gm/10 ml diluent	1 ml per min
Carbenicillin	Dilute as directed on vial, then further dilute each gram in at least 10 ml diluent	1 Gm per 5 min
Methicillin	500 mg reconstituted drug in at least 25 ml diluent	10 ml per min
Mezlocillin	1 Gm at least 10 ml diluent	1 Gm per 3 min
Nafcillin	Desired amount of drug in 15 to 30 ml diluent	500 mg per 5 to 10 min
Ticarcillin	1 Gm in at least 4 ml diluent, then further diluted to 1 Gm/10 ml	1 Gm per 5 min
Oxacillin	1 Gm/10 ml diluent	1 ml per min

Antibiotics 505

- Penicillins vary considerably in the amount of sodium or potassium contained in individual products. Although this may cause no problem in most patients, it can be of concern in patients with renal or cardiovascular problems or in those receiving high doses. Monitor the patient's electrolyte levels.
- The penicillins, with the exception of amoxicillin, should be taken 1 hour before meals or 2 hours after meals.
- Penicillin products containing procaine, benzathine, or a combination of these should never be given intravenously. Administer intramuscularly using the dorsogluteal site or thigh muscles in the adult, and the vastus lateralis muscle of the thigh in infants and small children. Occasionally patients are sensitive to procaine; symptoms include anxiety, confusion, agitation, fear of impending death, and convulsions.
- Many intramuscular preparations of penicillin are thick and require steady, even pressure on the plunger to prevent the needle from clogging.
- Platelet dysfunction with resulting bleeding tendencies has been reported with several of the penicillins. While excessive bleeding is uncommon, the reaction may be more common in uremic patients.
- For instructions about reconstitution of penicillins for parenteral use, refer to the medication vials and the manufacturer's accompanying literature. Note that too rapid direct infusion of penicillins may contribute to the development of seizures.

Cephalosporins

First-generation cephalosporins
    Cefadroxil monohydrate
    Cefazolin sodium
    Cephalexin
    Cephalothin sodium
    Cephapirin sodium
    Cephradine
Second-generation cephalosporins
    Cefaclor

Table 46-3 Administration of cephalosporins

Generic Name	Trade Name	Dosage and Administration
First Generation		
Cefadroxil monohydrate	Duricef* Ultracef	ORAL: *Adults*—1 to 2 Gm daily in divided doses. *Children*—30 mg/kg daily divided into 2 equal doses.
Cefazolin sodium	Ancef* Kefzol*	INTRAMUSCULAR, INTRAVENOUS: *Adults*—250 mg every 8 hr up to 2 Gm every 6 hr. *Children*—25 to 50 mg/kg total daily dose in 3 or 4 divided doses.
Cephalexin	Keflex*	ORAL: *Adults*—1 to 4 Gm daily. *Children*—25 to 50 mg/kg total daily dose divided into 4 doses.
Cephalothin sodium	Keflin*	INTRAMUSCULAR, INTRAVENOUS: *Adults*—1 to 2 Gm every 4 to 6 hr. *Children*—80 to 160 mg/kg total daily dose.
Cephapirin sodium	Cefadyl*	INTRAMUSCULAR, INTRAVENOUS: *Adults*—500 mg to 2 Gm every 4 to 6 hr. *Children*—40 to 80 mg/kg total daily dose.
Cephradine	Anspor Velosef*	ORAL, INTRAMUSCULAR, INTRAVENOUS: *Adults*—1 to 4 Gm total daily dose. *Children*—50 to 100 mg/kg divided into 4 daily doses.
Second Generation		
Cefaclor	Ceclor*	ORAL: *Adults*—1 to 4 Gm daily. *Children*—20 to 40 mg/kg not to exceed 1 Gm daily.

Cefamandole nafate	Mandol*	INTRAMUSCULAR, INTRAVENOUS: *Adults*—500 mg to 2 Gm every 4 to 6 hr. *Children*—50 to 100 mg/kg daily divided into 4 to 6 doses.
Cefonicid sodium	Monocid	INTRAMUSCULAR, INTRAVENOUS: *Adults*—1 to 2 Gm once daily. No more than 1 Gm should be given at a single intramuscular site. *Children*—Safety and effectiveness in children have not been established.
Ceforanide	Precef	INTRAMUSCULAR, INTRAVENOUS: *Adults*—0.5 to 1 Gm twice daily. *Children*—20 to 40 mg/kg daily in 2 equally divided doses.
Cefoxitin sodium	Mefoxin*	INTRAMUSCULAR, INTRAVENOUS: *Adults*—3 to 12 Gm daily in 3 or 4 equal doses. *Children*—50 to 150 mg/kg daily divided into 4 to 6 doses.
Cefuroxime sodium	Zinacef*	INTRAMUSCULAR, INTRAVENOUS: *Adults*—0.75 to 1.5 Gm every 8 hr. *Children older than 3 months*—50 to 100 mg/kg daily divided into 3 or 4 equal doses.

Third Generation

Cefoperazone sodium	Cefobid	INTRAMUSCULAR, INTRAVENOUS: *Adults*—2 to 4 Gm daily divided into 2 equal doses. More severe infections may require up to 12 Gm daily divided into 3 or 4 doses. *Children*—Safe use in children is not yet established.

cont'd. next page

*Available in U.S. and Canada

Table 46-3   Administration of cephalosporins—cont'd.

Generic Name	Trade Name	Dosage and Administration
Cefotaxime sodium	Claforan*	INTRAMUSCULAR, INTRAVENOUS: *Adults*—3 to 4 Gm daily divided into 3 or 4 equal doses. More severe infections may require up to 12 Gm daily. *Children*—50 to 180 mg/kg doses have been used.
Ceftizoxime sodium	Cefizox	INTRAMUSCULAR, INTRAVENOUS: *Adults*—3 Gm daily divided into 2 equal doses. Severe infections may require up to 12 Gm daily, divided into 6 doses. *Children*—Safety and effectiveness in children is not yet established.
Moxalactam disodium	Moxam*	INTRAMUSCULAR, INTRAVENOUS: *Adults*—2 to 6 Gm daily divided into 3 equal doses. More severe infections may require up to 12 Gm daily. *Children*—50 mg/kg every 6 to 8 hr.

*Available in U.S. and Canada

Cefamandole nafate
Cefonicid sodium
Ceforanide
Cefoxitin sodium
Cefuroxime sodium
Third-generation cephalosporins
Cefoperazone sodium
Cefotaxime sodium
Ceftizoxime sodium
Moxalactam disodium

Actions of Cephalosporins

The cephalosporins are irreversible inhibitors of the bacterial enzyme transpeptidase, preventing formation of a new intact cell wall in the bacteria.

Indications for Cephalosporins

First-generation cephalosporins are generally used as alternative therapy for infections caused by gram-positive bacteria. Second- and third-generation cephalosporins are used for specific serious infections caused by gram-negative bacteria; the second-generation drugs are used against enterobacter and Hemophilus; third-generation drugs are used for extended coverage of gram-negative organisms and central nervous system infections.

Nurse Alert for Cephalosporins

- Cephalosporins like penicillins may cause allergic reactions; most patients allergic to one are also allergic to the other.

Side Effects of Cephalosporins

Cephalosporins may cause allergic reactions, most commonly skin rashes. Oral preparations may cause gastric irritation, nausea, and vomiting. Commercial preparations that contain sodium or potassium may cause electrolyte imbalances. Intravenous cephalosporins may cause pain at the injection site and phlebitis or thrombophlebitis along the affected vein.

510   **Pocket Nurse Guide to Drugs**

Table 46-4   Parenteral administration of cephalosporins

Drug	Recommended Dilution	Rate of Administration
Cefamandole	1 Gm/10 ml diluent	1 Gm per 3 to 5 min
Cefazolin	1 Gm/10 ml diluent	1 Gm per min
Cefoperazone	2 to 25 mg/ml diluent	1 to 2 ml per min
Cefotaxime	1 to 2 Gm/10 ml diluent	10 ml per 3 to 5 min
Cefoxitin	1 Gm/10 ml diluent	1 Gm per 3 to 5 min
Ceftizoxime	Dilute as directed, then further dilute in 50 to 100 ml diluent	5 to 10 ml per min
Cefuroxime	Dilute as directed on vial, resulting in concentration of 100 mg/ml	3 ml per min
Cephalothin	1 Gm/10 ml diluent	1 Gm per 3 to 5 min
Cephapirin	1 Gm/10 ml diluent	1 Gm per 5 min
Cephradine	500 mg/5 ml diluent	1 Gm per 3 to 5 min
Moxalactam	1 Gm/10 ml diluent	1 Gm per 3 to 5 min

Nursing Implications for Cephalosporins

- Routine laboratory work to monitor renal, hepatic, and hematopoietic function should be done on patients receiving cephalosporins.
- Cephalosporins vary considerably in the amount of sodium or potassium contained in individual products; thus it can be concern in patients with renal or cardiovascular problems or in those receiving high doses. Monitor the patient's electrolyte levels.
- The cephalosporins can be taken with meals, although absorption may be faster if taken on an empty stomach.
- The cephalosporins cause pain at intramuscular injection sites and frequently contribute to thrombophlebitis when given intravenously. This latter problem can be lessened by administering the drug slowly, diluting it well, and rotating injection sites every 24 to 48 hours.
- For instructions about reconstitution of cephalosporins for parenteral use, refer to the medication vials and the manufacturer's accompanying literature.

Penicillin Substitutes

Erythromycins
  Erythromycin base
  Erythromycin stearate
  Erythromycin estolate
  Erythromycin ethylsuccinate
  Erythromycin lactobionate
  Erythromycin gluceptate
Clindamycin
Clindamycin palmitate
Clindamycin phosphate
Lincomycin
Vancomycin
Bacitracin
Novobiocin
Spectinomycin

Actions of Penicillin Substitutes

Erythromycin, clindamycin, and lincomycin bind to bacterial ribosomes and thereby prevent bacterial protein synthesis; the effect is bacteriostatic at low concentrations and bactericidal at high concentrations. Vancomycin prevents synthesis of bacterial cell walls by blocking peptidoglycan strand formation. Bacitracin blocks the regeneration of a lipid carrier that transports cell wall material through the bacterial cell membrane and interferes with bacterial cell membrane function. Novobiocin has unique actions that inhibit several bacterial processes. Spectinomycin inhibits bacterial protein synthesis.

Indications for Penicillin Substitutes

In general these drugs may be used when the patient is allergic to the penicillins or the infectious agent is resistant to penicillin. Erythromycin is the drug of choice for: atypical pneumonias such as Legionnaire's disease or those diseases caused by mycoplasma; diphtheria; and infections caused by Chlamydia. Clindamycin is most often used against anaerobic organisms such as *Bacteroides fragilis*. Vancomycin is effective primarily against gram-positive bacteria, is used most commonly with staphylococcal or streptococcal infections, and is useful for antibiotic-induced colitis caused by *Clostridium difficile*. Bacitracin is used primarily for staphylococcal infections in infants that cannot be treated with less toxic agents because of allergies or resistance. Novobiocin is used only for *Staphylococcus aureus* infections shown to be sensitive to novobiocin and resistant to other drugs. Spec-

Table 46-5 Administration of penicillin substitutes

Generic Name	Trade Name	Drug Form	Dosage and Administration
Erythromycin base	E-Mycin* Ilotycin Robimycin RP-Mycin	Enteric or film-coated tablets	ORAL: *Adults*—250 mg 4 times per day (15 to 20 mg/kg per day). *Children*—30 to 50 mg/kg per day in 3 or 4 doses. *Patients with very severe infections*—up to 4 Gm per day.
Erythromycin stearate	Erypar Erythrocin Stearate Ethril	Film-coated tablets	ORAL: *Adults and children*—as for erythromycin base.
Erythromycin estolate	Ilosone*	Tablets, capsules, suspension, chewable tablets	ORAL: *Adults and children*—as for erythromycin base.
Erythromycin ethylsuccinate	E.E.S.* Pediamycin	Drops, suspension, chewable tablets, film-coated tablets	ORAL: *Adults*—400 mg 4 times per day. *Children*—as for erythromycin base
Erythromycin lactobionate Erythromycin gluceptate	Erythrocin Lactobionate-IV Ilotycin Gluceptate-IV*	Powder stabilized with benzyl alcohol; to be reconstituted with diluent suggested by manufacturer.	INTRAVENOUS: *Adults and children*—15 to 20 mg/kg per day, preferably by continuous infusion; intervals between doses for intermittent therapy should be 6 hr or less. Doses of up to 4 Gm per day may be used for very severe infections.

Vancomycin	Vancocin	Powder	ORAL: As for intravenous. Note this route is for intestinal infections only.
		Powder to be reconstituted with sterile water	INTRAVENOUS: *Adults*—500 mg 4 times daily. *Children*—40 mg/kg per day in divided doses.
Bacitracin		Solution	INTRAMUSCULAR: *Infants*—over 2.5 kg, 1000 units/kg per day in 2 or 3 doses; infants below 2.5 kg, 900 units/kg per day in 2 or 3 doses.
		Ointment for ophthalmic or skin application	TOPICAL: *Adults and children*—ointments contain 500 units of antibiotic/Gm. Application may be every 3 hr or less frequently, depending on the infection.
Novobiocin	Albamycin	Capsules, syrup	ORAL: *Adults*—250 to 500 mg 4 times daily. *Children*—15 to 45 mg/kg per day. *Infants*—Not recommended.
Spectinomycin	Trobicin	Powder to be reconstituted with diluent.	INTRAMUSCULAR: *Adults*—2 to 4 Gm in a single dose.
Clindamycin	Cleocin HCl	Capsules (hydrochloride hydrate)	ORAL: *Adults*—150 to 450 mg 4 times daily. *cont'd. next page*

*Available in U.S. and Canada

Table 46-5   Administration of penicillin substitutes—cont'd.

Generic Name	Trade Name	Drug Form	Dosage and Administration
Clindamycin palmitate	Cleocin Pediatric	Granules in suspension	ORAL: *Children*—8 to 25 mg/kg per day in 3 or 4 doses for children over 10 kg. Smaller children should receive no more than 37.5 mg 3 times daily.
Clindamycin phosphate	Cleocin Phosphate	Solution with benzyl alcohol, disodium edetate, and/or hydrochloric acid or sodium hydroxide.	INTRAMUSCULAR, INTRAVENOUS: *Adults*—0.6 Gm to 4.8 Gm max. per day (no more than 0.6 Gm per injection site IM). *Children over 1 month*—15 to 40 mg/kg daily in 3 or 4 doses.
Lincomycin	Lincocin	Capsules, syrup	ORAL: *Adults*—500 mg 3 or 4 times daily. *Children over 1 month*—30 to 60 mg/kg per day in 3 or 4 divided doses.
		Solution with 0.9% benzyl alcohol	INTRAMUSCULAR: *Adults*—600 mg once or twice daily. *Children over 1 month*—10 mg/kg once or twice daily.
		Solution with 0.9% benzyl alcohol	INTRAVENOUS: *Adults*—600 mg to 1 Gm 2 or 3 times daily; 8 Gm is the upper limit for daily doses. *Children over 1 month*—10 mg/kg once or twice daily.

*Available in U.S. and Canada

tinomycin is used primarily with *N. gonorrhoeae* as a penicillin substitute.

Nurse Alert for Penicillin Substitutes

- Erythromycin lactobionate and gluceptate must be infused slowly into the vein to avoid pain.
- Intramuscular injections of erythromycin are very painful and should be avoided.
- Erythromycin is generally not recommended during pregnancy because it accumulates in the fetal liver.

Parenteral Administration of Penicillin Substitutes

- Parenteral erythromycin: Both the lactobionate and gluceptate forms should be reconstituted with Sterile Water for Injection (without preservatives), then diluted further with solutions of appropriate pH and compatibility (see manufacturer's literature) to a concentration of 1 Gm per 100 ml. Administer the diluted solution at a rate of 1 Gm over a period of 20 to 60 minutes. The rate should be slow enough to prevent pain in the vein.
- Parenteral lincomycin:
  a. The drug is supplied in solution form, 300 mg/ml. The usual dose for adults is 600 mg (2 ml) intramuscularly. Pain at injection site is common.
  b. For intravenous use, the solution of medication should be further diluted in compatible solutions to a concentration not stronger than 1 Gm/100 ml (see literature). The rate of administration should not exceed 1 Gm per hour.
  c. Hypotension has occurred following parenteral administration. Caution the patient to remain lying down for a while after receiving the medication or supervise ambulation.
  d. Too rapid intravenous administration has caused cardiac arrest. The use of a microdrop infusion set may be appropriate; establish the rate of infusion carefully. Check the patient frequently.
- Parenteral clindamycin:
  a. The drug is supplied in a solution containing 150 mg/ml.

516   Pocket Nurse Guide to Drugs

A single intramuscular injection greater than 600 mg (4 ml) is not recommended.

b. Pain, induration, and sterile abscesses at injection sites have occurred.

c. For intravenous administration, further dilute the drug to a dilution of 300 mg in 50 or more ml of diluent (see literature) and administer at a rate not more rapid than 50 ml in 10 minutes or longer. Administration of greater than 1200 mg over a period of 1 hour is not recommended.

d. Hypotension has occurred following parenteral administration. Caution the patient to remain lying down for a while after receiving the medication or supervise ambulation.

- Parenteral vancomycin: Dilute the 500 mg of dry powder with 10 ml Sterile Water for Injection. Further dilute this solution with sodium chloride solution or 5% dextrose in water to make a final volume of 500 mg in 100 to 200 ml. Administer 500 mg over a period of 30 minutes. This drug is incompatible with many other drugs. For further information, consult the pharmacist or check the manufacturer's literature.

- The parenteral route of administration is rarely used with bacitracin. Side effects from this route can include nausea, vomiting, rashes, pain at the injection site, and allergic reactions. In addition, the drug is very nephrotoxic; monitor the fluid intake and output, and force fluids during the course of therapy. See the manufacturer's literature for guides to proper dilution.

- The diluent for spectinomycin is provided by the manufacturer, and the drug should be reconstituted as indicated on the vial. The manufacturer recommends the use of a 20-gauge needle for administration.

Side Effects of Penicillin Substitutes

Oral erythromycins commonly cause gastrointestinal side effects including abdominal discomfort and cramping; normal doses may cause nausea, vomiting, and diarrhea. *Erythromy-*

cin may rarely cause allergic reactions ranging from urticaria to anaphylaxis. *Erythromycin lactobionate* on rare occasions may cause hearing loss. *Erythromycin estolate* may cause cholestatic hepatitis with symptoms of severe abdominal pain, liver enlargement, fever, and jaundice. *Lincomycin* or *clindamycin* may cause colitis with symptoms of diarrhea or life-threatening pseudomembranous colitis; other side effects may include rashes, anaphylaxis, nausea and vomiting, anorexia, glossitis or stomatitis, hypotension, and possibly blood dyscrasias and liver dysfunction; *lincomycin* may also cause tinnitus and vertigo. *Vancomycin* may cause tinnitus leading to deafness, fever, nephrotoxicity, nausea, and flushing and itching of the skin. *Bacitracin* is highly nephrotoxic, causing glomerular and tubular necrosis and permanent kidney damage. *Novobiocin* causes allergic skin reactions, blood dyscrasias, nausea, diarrhea, and occasionally bloody stools. *Spectinomycin* may cause nausea, chills, dizziness, fever, pain at the injection site, insomnia, oliguria, altered laboratory results, and urticaria.

Nursing Implications for Penicillin Substitutes

- Oral erythromycin preparations should be taken on an empty stomach, either 1 hour before or 2 hours after eating. The exceptions are the estolate preparations, which can be taken with meals. Sometimes patients are instructed to take erythromycin preparations with meals to decrease gastric irritation and side effects, but this will result in reduced absorption.
- Lincomycin should be taken on an empty stomach, either 1 hour before or 2 hours after eating. Clindamycin can safely be taken with meals.
- Bacitracin is used almost exclusively via the topical route and has very few side effects via this route. Caution the patient to apply only as directed and to report a rash or any other unexplained symptom.
- Bacitracin ointment requires no prescription for purchase.
- Evaluate patients receiving vancomycin frequently for hearing loss because it sometimes progresses even after the

518 Pocket Nurse Guide to Drugs

drug is discontinued. Nephrotoxicity may occur; evaluate the fluid intake and output, tell patients to report any changes in the appearance of urine, and monitor the blood urea nitrogen (BUN).

Tetracyclines

Tetracycline HCl
Oxytetracycline HCl
Methacycline HCl

Demeclocycline HCl
Doxycycline
Minocycline HCl

Table 46-6 Administration of tetracyclines

Generic Name	Trade Name	Dosage and Administration
Tetracycline HCl	Achromycin* Bristacycline Cyclopar Panmycin Sumycin Tetracyn*	ORAL: *Adults*—1 to 2 Gm per day in 2 to 4 doses. *Children over 8 yr*—25 to 50 mg/kg per day in 2 to 4 doses.
	Achromycin IM Tetracyn IM	INTRAMUSCULAR: *Adults*—300 mg to 800 mg per day in divided doses. *Children over 8 yr*—15 to 25 mg/kg not to exceed 250 mg per dose.
	Achromycin IV Tetracyn IV	INTRAVENOUS: *Adults*—250 to 500 mg every 12 hrs. *Children over 8 yr*—15 to 25 mg/kg per day in 2 doses.
Oxytetracycline HCl	Oxlopar Terramycin*	ORAL: As for tetracycline.
	Terramycin IM	INTRAMUSCULAR: As for tetracycline.
	Terramycin IV	INTRAVENOUS: As for tetracycline.

*Available in U.S. and Canada

Actions of Tetracyclines

The tetracyclines block bacterial growth by preventing ribosomes from binding messenger RNA, thereby preventing the initiation of protein synthesis.

Indications for Tetracyclines

Tetracyclines are used for infections caused by both gram-postive and gram-negative bacteria, spirochetes, chlamydia, amebic dysentery, and other infections if penicillin is contraindicated.

Table 46-6 Administration of tetracyclines—cont'd.

Generic Name	Trade Name	Dosage and Administration
Methacycline HCl	Rondomycin	ORAL: *Adults*—600 mg per day in 2 to 4 doses. *Children over 8 yr*—10 mg/kg per day in 4 doses.
Demeclocycline HCl	Declomycin*	ORAL: *Adults*—600 mg to 1 Gm per day in 4 doses. *Children over 8 yr*—6 to 12 mg/kg per day in 2 to 4 doses.
Doxycycline	Doxycycline hyclate Vibramycin*	ORAL: *Adults*—100 to 200 mg per day in 2 doses. *Children over 8 yr*—2 to 4 mg/kg per day in 2 doses.
	Vibramycin IV	INTRAVENOUS: As for oral.
Minocycline HCl	Minocin*	ORAL: 200 mg initially, then 100 mg every 12 hrs.
	Minocin IV	INTRAVENOUS: As for oral route.

*Available in U.S. and Canada

Nurse Alert for Tetracyclines

- Tetracyclines generally should not be given in pregnancy because of possible toxic effects to the fetus as well as danger of hepatotoxicity in the mother.
- Elderly or debilitated patients may suffer metabolic derangement when given tetracyclines.
- Because minocycline may cause vertigo, patients should be instructed to avoid activities that could be dangerous if vertigo occurs.
- Tetracyclines should not be used in the last half of pregnancy, or in children under age 8 because permanent staining of the teeth may occur, as well as possible depressed bone growth.

Parenteral Administration of Tetracyclines

- Intravenous doxycycline: Refer to the manufacturer's literature for instructions about dilution. The recommended minimum infusion time for 100 mg of a solution containing 0.5 mg/ml is 1 hour. Concentrations below 0.1 mg/ml or greater than 1.0 mg/ml are not recommended.
- Intravenous minocycline: The drug should be initially dissolved and then further diluted in appropriate fluids (see literature) to make a concentration of 100 to 200 mg/500 to 1000 ml. Administer at the ordered infusion rate.

Side Effects of Tetracyclines

Oral tetracyclines may cause nausea, vomiting, abdominal pain, anorexia, and enterocolitis; urticaria, rashes, dermatitis, and more rarely more serious allergic reactions such as asthma, angioedema, and anaphylaxis; delayed blood coagulation; irreversible staining of teeth in children under age 8; enamel hypoplasia; and photosensitivity.

Nursing Implications for Tetracyclines

- Kidney, liver, and hematopoietic function should be routinely monitored during tetracycline use.
- Patients receiving anticoagulants for whom tetracyclines are also prescribed may require a reduction in anticoagulant dose during tetracycline therapy.

Antibiotics **521**

- Minocycline and doxycycline may be given with food to minimize gastric irritation. All other tetracyclines should be taken on an empty stomach, at least 1 hour before or 2 hours after meals. Antacids, milk products, or vitamin and mineral products containing iron should not be administered simultaneously with tetracyclines, since these agents prevent absorption of the tetracyclines.
- Patients should be cautioned to store tetracycline preparations properly in the container provided away from heat and light. Most preparations should be stored between 15 and 30°C (59 and 86°F). Consult manufacturer's instructions for information on specific products. The course of therapy should be completed as directed, and unused portions of medications should be discarded. Health care personnel should check for the expiration date before administering tetracyclines.
- Intramuscular tetracycline can cause pain at the injection site. The is a rarely-used route of administration. Follow directions for reconstitution in the manufacturer's literature.
- Intravenous administration of the tetracyclines can cause thrombophlebitis. Proper dilution and slow administration minimize patient discomfort.
- Intravenous tetracycline and oxytetracycline: Dilute as instructed in the literature with appropriate fluids to a concentration not greater than 5 mg/ml. The rate of administration should not exceed 2 ml per minute.

Chloramphenicols

Chloramphenicol	Chloramphenicol sodium
Chloramphenicol palmitate	succinate

Actions of Chloramphenicol

Chloramphenicol inhibits bacterial protein synthesis and is bacteriostatic rather than bactericidal.

Indications for Chloramphenicol

Chloramphenicol is used only for serious infections, for typhoid fever, life-threatening bacteremias and meningitis, and gram-negative bacteria, rickettsiae, and chlamydia.

Table 46-7 Administration of chloramphenicol

Generic Name	Trade Name	Dosage and Administration
Chloramphenicol	Chloromycetin Mychel	ORAL: *Adults*—50 to 100 mg/kg per day in 4 doses. *Children*—25 mg/kg per day *or less*, depending on liver function.
Chloramphenicol palmitate		ORAL: *Children*—as for other oral forms.
Chloramphenicol succinate		INTRAVENOUS: As for oral.

Nurse Alert for Chloramphenicol

- Because aplastic anemia is more likely to occur in patients who have received chloramphenicol in the past, patients should be asked about past medication history.

Parenteral Administration of Chloramphenicol

- Intravenous chloramphenicol: Dissolve the dry powder as directed; then further dilute in Sterile Water for Injection or 5% Dextrose in Water to make a 10% concentration (100 mg/ml). Rate of administration should not exceed 100 mg per minute. If desired, the drug may be further diluted and administered over a period of 30 to 60 minutes as an intermittent infusion. For additional information see the manufacturer's literature or consult the pharmacist.

Side Effects of Chloramphenicol

Chloramphenicol may cause reversible or irreversible bone marrow depression, the latter leading to aplastic anemia; gastrointestinal irritation, allergic responses, optic neuritis, headache, confusion, depression, delirium, and severe toxic reactions in patients with reduced liver function.

Nursing Implications for Chloramphenicol

- Because of the possibility of bone marrow depression, which may occur as a result of chloramphenicol therapy, blood work should be done prior to the initiation of therapy

Antibiotics   **523**

and at regular intervals during therapy. Studies should include hematocrit, differential, reticulocyte count, and leukocyte count. Since bone marrow depression often is not seen until several weeks or months after therapy, patients should also be taught to report any fever, sore throat, fatigue, bruising, or any unusual symptoms that might occur even after completion of therapy. Note that the bone marrow depression is a possible side effect with any route of administration.

- The incidence of aplastic anemia seems to be higher among patients who have been exposed to the drug on more than one occasion.

- Health care personnel working in newborn nurseries should be alert to the development of grey syndrome, a result of chloramphenicol therapy, which is seen in newborn infants up to 3 months old. Symptoms include abdominal distention, progressive pallid cyanosis, hypothermia, irregular respirations, and acute circulatory failure. It can be rapidly fatal. The syndrome usually occurs after 3 or 4 days of therapy. Note that chloramphenicol taken during labor or the last few days of pregnancy can also precipitate grey syndrome in the newborn infant.

- Patients taking chloramphenicol who are also receiving phenytoin, tolbutamide, or coumarin anticoagulants are at risk for side effects due to increased serum concentrations of those three groups of drugs. It may be necessary to reduce the dose of those three drugs using chloramphenicol therapy. Review with patients the signs of toxicity of the three drugs as needed, and caution patients to report any of these signs if they appear.

- Patients receiving chloramphenicol succinate may complain of a bitter taste, which lasts for a few minutes after the injection.

Aminoglycosides

Amikacin   Netilmicin
Gentamicin   Streptomycin
Kanamycin   Tobramycin
Neomycin

524 Pocket Nurse Guide to Drugs

Table 46-8 Administration of aminoglycosides

Generic Name	Trade Name	Dosage and Administration
Streptomycin	Streptomycin	INTRAMUSCULAR: *Adults*— 1 to 4 Gm daily in 2 or 3 doses (15 to 25 mg/kg daily). Elderly patients may require less drug. Lower doses are used for long-term treatment of mild tuberculosis. Intravenous route rarely used. *Children*—20 to 40 mg/kg daily in 2 doses.
Neomycin	Mycifradin* Neobiotic Neomycin	ORAL: *Adults*—4 to 8 Gm daily in up to 6 doses. *Children*— 50 to 100 mg/kg daily in 4 doses.
	Myciguent* Neomycin	TOPICAL: *Adults and children*—Commonly used as 0.5% creams and ointments. Also used in numerous combinations with other antibiotics.
Kanamycin	Kantrex*	ORAL: *Adults*—Up to 8 Gm daily in 4 to 6 doses. *Children*—50 mg/kg daily in 4 to 6 doses.

*Available in U.S. and Canada

Actions of Aminoglycosides

The aminoglycosides inhibit early steps in bacterial protein synthesis by binding bacterial ribosomes; aminoglycosides are generally considered more bactericidal than many other antibiotics that inhibit bacterial protein synthesis.

Indications for Aminoglycosides

Streptomycin is used to treat tularemia and bubonic or black plague and in combination with other antibiotics to treat bacterial endocarditis, tuberculosis, brucellosis, and Listeria

Antibiotics 525

Table 46-8 Administration of aminoglycosides—cont'd.

Generic Name	Trade Name	Dosage and Administration
Kanamycin—cont'd.		INTRAMUSCULAR, INTRAVENOUS, INTRAPERITONEAL: *Adults and children*—Not to exceed 15 mg/kg daily, given at 12 hr intervals.
Gentamicin	Garamycin*	INTRAMUSCULAR, INTRAVENOUS: *Adults*—3 to 5 mg/kg daily in 3 doses. *Children*—6 to 7.5 mg/kg daily in 3 doses. *Neonates*—5 mg/kg daily in 3 doses.
Tobramycin	Nebcin*	INTRAMUSCULAR, INTRAVENOUS: *Adults, children, infants*—3 to 5 mg/kg daily in 3 doses.
Amikacin	Amikin*	INTRAMUSCULAR, INTRAVENOUS: *Adults, children, infants*—15 mg/kg daily in 2 or 3 doses. Do not exceed 1.5 Gm daily. Intravenous doses are given by slow infusion.
Netilmicin	Netromycin*	INTRAMUSCULAR, INTRAVENOUS: *Adults*—4 to 6.5 mg/kg daily divided into 3 equal doses.

*Available in U.S. and Canada

infections. *Neomycin* is used orally to reduce bacterial populations in the bowel. *Kanamycin* is used to treat serious infections caused by aerobic gram-negative bacteria other than pseudomonas. *Gentamicin* is used for serious infections caused by aerobic gram-negative bacteria including *Pseudomonas aeruginosa*. *Tobramycin* is used primarily for *Pseudomonas aeruginosa* but sometimes substitutes for gentamicin in other kinds of infections. *Amikacin* is primarily used for *Pseudomonas aeruginosa* infections resistant to other aminoglycosides. *Netilmicin* is used for serious infections caused by aerobic gram-negative bacteria.

Nurse Alert for Aminoglycosides

- Aminoglycosides may damage kidney tubules and glomeruli, leading to rapid clinical deterioration as the drug accumulates.
- Aminoglycosides may impair balance and damage hearing. Patients may need to be tested before and during therapy to assess progressive deterioration in these functions. Tinnitus, hearing loss, feelings of "fullness" in the ear are signs of auditory damage. Diminished balance suggests vestibular damage.

Parenteral Administration of Aminoglycosides

- *Intravenous kanamycin:* Dilute the prescribed dose in Normal Saline, 5% Normal Saline, or 5% Dextrose in Water to a concentration of 500 mg in 100 to 200 ml and administer over 30 to 60 minutes.
- *Intravenous gentamicin:* Dilute a single dose in 50 to 200 ml of Normal Saline or 5% Dextrose in Water. The concentration should not exceed 0.1% (1 mg/ml). Administer each dose over 30 to 60 minutes.
- *Intravenous tobramycin:* Dilute an adult dose in 50 to 100 ml of 5% Dextrose in Water or Normal Saline and administer over 30 to 60 minutes. For pediatric doses, consult the literature.
- *Intravenous amikacin:* Dilute 500 mg in 200 ml of Normal Saline or 5% Dextrose in Water and administer over 30 to 60 minutes. For pediatric doses, consult the literature.
- *Intravenous netilmicin:* Dilute a single dose in 50 to 200 ml of diluent, and administer over a period of 30 minutes to 2 hours.

Side Effects of Aminoglycosides

The aminoglycosides commonly cause ototoxicity, renal toxicity, and neuromuscular blockade, as shown below. Other effects of aminoglycoside therapy include nausea, vomiting,

Table 46-9   Ototoxicity

Drug	Vestibular	Hearing	Renal Toxicity	Neuromuscular Blockade
Streptomycin	May affect 75% of patients receiving 2 Gm daily for 2 to 4 mo and 25% of patients receiving 1 Gm daily.	Loss usually partial but may be complete; affects 4% to 15% of patients receiving drug longer than 1 wk.	Not common unless high drug doses are used and the urine is acid.	May occur following peritoneal lavage; reversed by neostigmine and/or calcium.
Neomycin	Not common.	Irreversible hearing loss progressing to complete deafness is common.	Reversible, progressive kidney toxicity causing an increase in blood urea.	Occurs following peritoneal lavage; usually reversed by neostigmine.
Kanamycin	Vertigo or other symptoms of vestibular damage affect about 7% of patients receiving high doses.	Up to 30% of patients receiving high doses suffer detectable hearing loss; fewer patients develop complete deafness.	Blood urea and creatinine may rise; hematuria and other signs of renal irritation may occur. Most signs of	Occurs following peritoneal lavage; usually not reversed by neostigmine and occasionally not

cont'd. next page

Table 46-9 Ototoxicity—cont'd.

Drug	Vestibular	Hearing	Renal Toxicity	Neuromuscular Blockade
Kanamycin—cont'd.			damage disappear when drug is discontinued.	reversed by calcium.
Gentamicin	About 2% of treated patients suffer permanent mild to severe vestibular damage.	Less frequent than vestibular damage and usually involves high tone hearing loss.	Acute renal failure has occurred. Blood urea and creatinine may rise; proteinuria may occur. Damage is usually but not always reversible.	May occur, but is less common than with above three aminoglycosides.
Tobramycin	One to 11% of treated patients show measurable impairment.	Incidence is the same as for vestibular damage.	Serum creatinine may be elevated, but the incidence may be less than for gentamicin or amikacin.	Expected from animal studies.

Amikacin	Lower incidence than hearing impairment.	Three to 11% of treated patients may show measurable hearing impairment.	More patients show rise in serum creatinine than for gentamicin. Up to 20% of patients may be affected.	Expected from animal studies.
Netilmicin	Possible but less likely than hearing loss.	One to 2% of treated patients show hearing impairment.	Three to 8% of treated patients show some sign of changes in renal function.	May be twice as potent as gentamicin in producing blockade.

530   Pocket Nurse Guide to Drugs

drug fever, paresthesias, hypotension, and elevations of transaminase levels (SGOT, SGPT) and bilirubin.

Nursing Implications for Aminoglycosides

- Signs of ototoxicity include tinnitus, roaring in ears, decreased hearing, feelings of fullness in the ears, nausea, dizziness, ataxia, and vertigo. A baseline audiometric test and periodic tests during the course of therapy should be done if practicable, and aminoglycoside therapy discontinued if there is a loss of high frequency perception. Newborn infants of mothers who received aminoglycosides during pregnancy or labor may suffer ototoxicity. Elderly persons and patients with preexisting tinnitus, vertigo, hearing loss, or who have previously received ototoxic drugs will need especially careful evaluations.

- Signs of renal toxicity include oliguria and increasing urine specific gravity. There may be proteinuria, appearance of casts or cells in the urine, and increased creatinine clearance. Blood work indicative of possible renal toxicity would include increasing blood urea nitrogen (BUN), nonprotein nitrogen (NPN), serum creatinine, and elevated serum concentrations of the specific drug. The potential for renal toxicity is increased if other nephrotoxic drugs are given concomitantly. Monitor the patient's fluid intake and output and keep the patient well hydrated.

- Neuromuscular blockade caused by aminoglycoside therapy is most frequently seen in patients receiving other neuromuscular blocking agents during surgery and patients with myasthenia gravis or Parkinson's disease. Apnea has been reported after too-rapid administration of an intravenous bolus. Monitor the respiratory rate of patients receiving aminoglycosides, especially those with myasthenia gravis or those during the early postoperative period. Administer intravenous aminoglycosides slowly.

- Because of the possibility of vertigo or hypotension, patients should be cautioned not to rise suddenly from a supine position.

- Serum concentrations of a specific drug are frequently used

Antibiotics **531**

to help regulate the dose. To interpret these levels correctly, blood is drawn at specific intervals before (trough level) and after (peak level) a dose of the drug is given. It is important to administer the drug on the prescribed schedule and to be familiar with the institution's procedures for blood sample collections for serum aminoglycoside levels so that errors are not made.

- Oral neomycin impairs absorption of other oral drugs, such as penicillin V, digitalis preparations, and vitamin B_{12}. Patients receiving neomycin who are also receiving any of the three drugs should be regularly evaluated for the continuing effect of these medications.

- Patients receiving oral aminoglycosides may absorb a relatively small amount of the drug from the gastrointestinal tract. In some sensitive patients the amount absorbed may be sufficient to cause renal or ototoxicity, so patients should be regularly evaluated.

- With topical preparations of aminoglycosides, nephrotoxicity and ototoxicity are rare but possible side effects. Factors influencing the likelihood of toxicity would include the frequency of applications, the size of the area to which the preparation is being applied, whether the skin surface was intact, and the amount and kind of other ototoxic and nephrotoxic drugs the patient might be receiving concomitantly. Photosensitivity has been reported in patients using gentamicin topical preparations. Caution patients using gentamicin topical preparations to avoid direct exposure to the sun or ultraviolet light.

- Pain at the injection site can accompany the intramuscular use of any aminoglycoside.

- A separate form of gentamicin, without preservatives, is available for intrathecal administration.

- The aminoglycosides are incompatible with other medications in the same syringe. For other incompatibilities, see the manufacturer's literature or consult the pharmacist.

- *Intramuscular streptomycin:* Dilute the powder with 0.9% Sodium Chloride Injection or Sterile Water for Injection as directed on the vial.

Polymyxins

Colistin sulfate
Colistimethate sodium (colistin methane sulfonate)
Polymyxin B sulfate

Actions of Polymyxins

Polymyxins alter the permeability of bacterial cell membranes, causing the loss of required small molecules and ions from the cell, leading to inevitable cell death.

Indications for Polymyxins

Colistin, polymyxin B, and colistimethate are used as reserve drugs for the treatment of infections caused by *Pseudomonas aeruginosa*.

Nurse Alert for Polymyxins

- Polymyxins usually cause reversible nephrotoxicity, which if not recognized may lead to further drug accumulation and further damage, with rapid clinical deterioration.

Parenteral Administration of Polymyxins

- *Parenteral colistimethate sodium*
    a. For intramuscular use, reconstitute with Sterile Water for Injection as directed on the vial.
    b. For intravenous use, it can be administered as reconstituted for intramuscular use and given as a bolus slowly over 3 to 5 minutes. It can also be further diluted with appropriate fluids (see literature) and administered over 1 to 2 hours.
- *Polymyxin B sulfate*
    a. For intravenous use, dissolve 500,000 units of the drug in 300 to 500 ml of 5% Dextrose in Water. The dose should not be administered in less than 60 to 90 minutes.
    b. For intrathecal use, dissolve 500,000 units in 10 ml Sodium Chloride Injection to produce a concentration of 50,000 units per ml.

Antibiotics 533

Table 46-10 Administration of polymyxins

Generic Name	Trade Name	Dosage and Administration
Colistin sulfate	Coly-Mycin S*	ORAL: *Children and infants*—5 to 15 mg/kg daily in 3 doses. The oral form is not used for adults.
Colistimethate sodium (colistin methane sulfonate)	Coly-Mycin M*	INTRAMUSCULAR, INTRAVENOUS: *Adults and children*—2.5 to 5 mg/kg daily in 2 to 4 doses up to 300 mg daily. Dosage must be reduced if renal impairment exists.
Polymyxin B sulfate	Aerosporin*	INTRAMUSCULAR: *Adults and children*—25,000 to 30,000 units/kg daily in 4 to 6 doses. INTRAVENOUS: *Adults and children*—15,000 to 25,000 units/kg daily by infusion in 300 to 500 ml 5% dextrose. INTRATHECAL: *Adults*—50,000 units daily in single dose. *Children under 2 yr*—20,000 units in single daily dose.

*Available in U.S. and Canada

Side Effects of Polymyxins

Polymyxins may cause significant neurotoxicity, nephrotoxicity, and neuromuscular blockade. The neurotoxicity may produce symptoms of numbness, tingling of the extremities, generalized pruritus, dizziness, paresthesias, confusion, slurring of speech, ataxia, convulsions and coma at higher doses.

534   **Pocket Nurse Guide to Drugs**

Nursing Implications for Polymyxins

- See nursing implications for nephrotoxicity and neuromuscular blockade listed for aminoglycosides on pp. 530-531.
- The likelihood of neurotoxic side effects occurring is increased when the polymyxins are given to patients with myasthenia gravis, those receiving other potentially neurotoxic drugs, those receiving neuromuscular blocking agents, or those receiving magnesium, quinidine, or quinine parenterally. If side effects occur, discontinue the drug and notify the physician.
- There are a variety of products containing polymyxin B in combination with other drugs. Examples include Neosporin and Neo-Polycin, both of which are ointments that contain polymyxin B, bacitracin, and neomycin.

Sulfonamides

Single component formulations
    Sulfacytine
    Sulfadiazine
    Sulfamethizole
    Sulfamethoxazole
    Sulfasalazine
    Sulfisoxazole
Fixed oral combinations
    Sulfamethoxazole and trimethoprim
    Sulfamerazine and sulfadiazine
    Sulfamerazine, sulfadiazine, and sulfamethazine
    Sulfamethoxazole and phenazopyridine
    Sulfamethizole and phenazopyridine
    Sulfisoxazole and phenazopyridine
Topical agents
    Mafenide acetate
    Silver sulfadiazine
    Sulfacetamide
    Sulfisoxazole

Actions of Sulfonamides

Sulfonamides are metabolic inhibitors that block bacterial synthesis of folic acid from paraaminobenzoic acid and other

Antibiotics **535**

precursors, with a bacteriostatic action against affected organisms.

Indications for Sulfonamides

Sulfonamides are active against a wide range of gram-positive and gram-negative bacteria, as well as Nocardia, Chlamydia, and Actinomyces, although resistance by many organisms has become widespread. *Sulfacytine* is used for urinary tract infections. *Sulfadiazine* is used for nocardiosis, rheumatic fever prophylaxis, and meningitis by susceptible organisms. *Sulfamethizole* and *sulfamethoxazole* are used for urinary tract infections. *Sulfasalazine* is used in the treatment of ulcerative colitis. *Sulfisoxazole* is used for urinary tract infections, nocardiosis, and systemic infections caused by sensitive organisms. All the *oral sulfonamide combinations* are used for urinary tract infections; *sulfamethoxazole* is used additionally for otitis media and enteritis due to sensitive Shigella. The combination of *sulfamethoxazole and trimethoprim* is used to treat pneumocystis pneumonia. The *sulfonamides used topically* are effective against a broad spectrum of pathogens, including *Pseudomonas aeruginosa.*

Parenteral Administration of Sulfonamides

- Parenteral sulfisoxazole:
  a. For intramuscular use, dissolve as directed on the ampule with Sterile Water for Injection and administer. There may be pain at the injection site.
  b. For intravenous use, further dilute the dissolved drug to a 5% solution (e.g., combine a 5 ml ampule with 35 ml Sterile Water for Injection; only this diluent should be used). Administer slowly, about 1 ml per minute or through slow infusion. For further information, consult the manufacturer's literature or the pharmacist.

Side Effects of Sulfonamides

Sulfonamides commonly cause allergic reactions, including skin rashes, pruritus, fever, and anaphylaxis. Nausea, vomiting, diarrhea, pancreatitis, hepatitis, and stomatitis may occur. Central nervous system alterations may include headache, ataxia, hallucinations, and convulsions. Aplastic anemia

Text continued on p. 540

536 Pocket Nurse Guide to Drugs

Table 46-11 Administration of sulfonamides

Generic Name	Trade Name	Dosage and Administration
Single Component Formulations		
Sulfacytine	Renoquid	ORAL: *Adults*—500 mg loading dose, then 250 mg 4 times daily. Not for children under 14 yr.
Sulfadiazine		ORAL: *Adults*—single loading dose of 2 to 4 Gm, then 2 to 4 Gm daily in 3 to 6 doses. *Children over 2 mo*—75 mg/kg to load, then 150 mg/kg daily in 4 to 6 doses. INTRAVENOUS: *Adults*—100 mg/kg daily in 4 doses after a 50 mg/kg loading dose. *Children over 2 mo*—50 mg/kg, then 100 mg/kg daily in 4 doses.
Sulfamethizole	Thiosulfil*	ORAL: *Adults*—0.5 to 1 Gm, 3 or 4 times daily. *Children over 2 mo*—30 to 45 mg/kg daily in 4 doses.
Sulfamethoxazole	Gantanol*	ORAL: *Adults*—single 2 Gm loading dose, then 1 Gm 2 or 3 times daily. *Children over 2 mo*—50 to 60 mg/kg loading dose, then 25 to 30 mg/kg twice daily, not to exceed 75 mg/kg daily.
Sulfasalazine	Azulfidine SAS-500*	ORAL: *Adults*—3 to 4 Gm daily in divided doses. *Children*—40 to 60 mg/kg daily in 3 to 6 doses.
Sulfisoxazole	Gantrisin*	ORAL: *Adults*—2 to 4 Gm loading dose, then 4 to 8

Antibiotics 537

	SK-Soxazole		Gm daily in 3 to 6 doses. *Children over 2 mo*—75 mg/kg loading dose, then 150 mg/kg daily in 4 to 6 doses. INTRAMUSCULAR, INTRAVENOUS, SUBCUTANEOUS: *Adults*—50 mg/kg initial dose, then 100 mg/kg daily in 2 to 4 doses. *Children*—smaller volumes per injection site are used.

Fixed Combinations

Sulfamethoxazole 400 mg Trimethoprim 80 mg	Bactrim* Septra*	Tablet / Per 5 ml solution for IV infusion	*Adults*—2 tablets every 12 hr. *Children*—8 mg/kg trimethoprim and 40 mg/kg sulfamethoxazole daily in 2 doses. *Adults, children*—As for oral route.
Sulfamerazine 250 mg Sulfadiazine 250 mg	Sulfonamide Duplex	Per 5 ml suspension for oral use	*Adults*—2 to 4 Gm total sulfonamide loading dose, then 2 to 4 Gm daily in 3 to 6 doses. *Children* 75 mg/kg to load, then 150 mg/kg daily in 4 to 6 doses.

cont'd. next page

†Trade name not available in U.S.
*Available in U.S. and Canada

Table 46-11 Administration of sulfonamides—cont'd.

Generic Name		Trade Name	Dosage and Administration
Fixed Combinations—cont'd.			
Sulfamerazine 167 mg Sulfadiazine 167 mg Sulfamethazine 167 mg	Tablet or per 5 ml suspension	Neotrizine Quadetts Triple Sulfa	As for sulfamerazine, sulfadiazine combination.
Sulfamethoxazole 500 mg Phenazopyridine 100 mg	Tablet	Azo-Gantanol	*Adults*—4 tablets to load, then 2 tablets every 12 hr for 3 days.
Sulfamethizole 250 or 500 mg Phenazopyridine 50 mg	Tablet	Thiosulfil-A Uremide	*Adults*—2 to 4 tablets 2 or 3 times daily. *Children*—30 to 45 mg of sulfamethizole per kg daily in 4 doses.
Sulfisoxazole 500 mg Phenazopyridine 50 mg	Tablet	Azo-Gantrisin Suldiazo	*Adults*—4 to 6 tablets to load, then 2 tablets every 12 hr for 3 days. *Children*—Dose as for sulfisoxazole alone.
Topical Agents			
Mafenide acetate	Cream: 85 mg mafenide acetate/Gm.	Sulfamylon*	To prevent infections in second and third degree burns.
Silver sulfadiazine	Cream: 10 mg/Gm	Silvadene Flamazine†	To prevent infections in second and third degree burns.

Sulfacetamide	Solution: 10%, 15%, or 30% Ointment: 10%	Bleph Liquifilm* Sulamyd* Sulf-10*	Ophthalmic only.
Sulfisoxazole	Solution: 4% Ointment: 4%	Gantrisin* Ophthalmic*	Ophthalmic only.

†Trade name not available in U.S.
*Available in U.S. and Canada

Nursing Implications for Sulfonamides

- The sulfonamides displace oral anticoagulants, oral hypoglycemics, and methotrexate from protein binding sites resulting in higher than desired serum levels of these drugs. Patients receiving oral anticoagulants should be alert to increased bleeding or bruising, whereas patients receiving oral hypoglycemics should be warned that they may have difficulty with hypoglycemia. Patients receiving methotrexate may have more trouble with drug related side effects.
- The sulfonamides bear a chemical similarity to some other classes of drugs (certain goitrogens, diuretics, and oral hypoglycemic agents). Rarely, patients taking sulfonamides may develop or experience goiter production, diuresis, or hypoglycemia.
- Patients receiving sulfonamides should be well hydrated, with an intake of 2000 to 2500 ml per day (for an adult) if possible.
- Phenazopyridine will color urine orange-red. Any patients receiving a sulfonamide in combination with phenazopyridine should be so warned.
- Azulfidine can also cause alopecia and reduced sperm count. It should be given in evenly divided doses throughout the 24 hours, with no period between doses, even at night, exceeding 8 hours. It should be given after meals when possible. It also causes an orange-yellow color to the skin and urine.
- Patients receiving sulfamethizole should be warned that the drug can cause the urine and skin to be yellow-orange in color.
- Sulfonamides may cause photosensitivity. Caution patients to avoid exposure to the sun or ultraviolet light.
- Both mafenide and silver sulfadiazine are used in the treatment of burns, although mafenide can cause pain and can contribute to electrolyte imbalance. Both creams should be applied with sterile gloves to the burned areas. Both

work less effectively in the presence of pus, debris, and blood, so regular cleaning of the wounds is recommended. Dressings are not necessary, although patients may request them. Because the rate of absorption through the skin cannot be easily measured, it is recommended that routine serum sulfonamide levels be determined to monitor for possible toxic levels.

Other Drugs for Urinary Tract Infections

Nitrofurantoin
Nalidixic acid
Cinoxacin
Trimethoprim

Actions of Other Drugs for Urinary Tract Infections

Trimethoprim inhibits tetrahydrofolic acid (THFA) synthesis and prevents THFA formation in bacteria. Nitrofuratoin apparently inhibits certain bacterial enzymes required for proper metabolism of sugar and other compounds. Nalidixic acid and cinoxacin have a bactericidal action involving direct interference with DNA replication in susceptible bacteria.

Indications for Other Drugs for Urinary Tract Infections

Trimethoprim is used similarly to the sulfonamides but is more active against the gram-negative bacteria Proteus, Klebsiella, and Serratia and is not useful alone against Chlamydia or Nocardia. *Nitrofurantoins* are effective against a variety of bacteria, including most common pathogens of the urinary tract except usually Pseudomonas and Proteus. *Nalidixic acid* and *cinoxacin* are effective against a variety of gram-negative bacteria; cinoxacin is used to treat urinary tract infections in adults but is not recommended for children.

Nurse Alert for Other Drugs for Urinary Tract Infections

- Nitrofurantoin should be used only with caution in pregnancy.

542 Pocket Nurse Guide to Drugs

■ The safety of cinoxacin in pregnancy has not yet been established.

Table 46-12 Administration of other drugs for urinary tract infections

Generic Name	Trade Name	Dosage and Administration
Nitrofurantoin	Furadantin Furalan Nitrex	ORAL: *Adults*—50 to 100 mg 4 times daily. *Children*—5 to 7 mg/kg daily in 4 divided doses. The drug should not be given to children under 3 mo.
Nitrofurantoin macrocrystals	Macrodantin*	As for nitrofurantoin.
Nalidixic acid	NegGram*	ORAL: *Adults*—1 Gm 4 times daily for 1 to 2 wk. Prolonged use may require cutting dosage back to 2 Gm or less daily. *Children under 12 yr*—55 mg/kg daily in 4 divided doses, initially. For long-term therapy the dose may be reduced to 33 mg/kg daily. *Children under 3 mo* should not receive this drug.
Cinoxacin	Cinobac	ORAL: *Adults*—1 Gm daily in 2 or 4 divided doses for 7 to 14 days.
Trimethoprim	Proloprim* Trimpex	ORAL: *Adults*—100 mg every 12 hr. *Children*—the drug has not been extensively tested in children and is not recommended.

*Available in U.S. and Canada

Side Effects of Other Drugs for Urinary Tract Infections

Trimethoprim is less toxic than the sulfonamides but may have similar side effects and may affect the bone marrow. *Nitrofurantoin* may cause anorexia, nausea, emesis, rashes, allergies, reversible blood dyscrasias, hemolytic anemia, alopecia, tooth-staining with oral suspensions, pneumonitis or pulmonary fibrosis over extended therapy, and potentially serious neuropathy. *Nalidixic* acid may cause central nervous system toxicity marked by mental instability, convulsions, headache, dizziness, and visual disturbances; other side effects may include rashes, photosensitivity, and hemolytic anemia. *Cinoxacin* may cause central nervous system effects similar to those of nalidixic acid although less commonly.

Nursing Implications for Other Drugs for Urinary Tract Infections

- Occasionally, patients taking nitrofurantoin develop pulmonary complications that manifest as acute pneumonitis: cough, dyspnea, wheezing, fluid infiltration, or pulmonary edema. Caution the patient to report any of these signs immediately. With long-term therapy, the pulmonary sensitivity reaction may develop insidiously, with fatigue, malaise, cough, dyspnea, and changes on x-ray film, including pulmonary fibrosis.
- Warn the patients receiving nitrofurantoin that oral suspensions may stain the teeth. To help prevent this, suspensions can be well diluted in milk or juices before taking.
- Nitrofurantoin will turn the urine brown.
- Patients taking nitrofurantoin should be kept well hydrated, with an intake of 2000 to 2500 ml per day (in the adult) if possible.
- Patients taking oral anticoagulants should be alerted that while taking nalidixic acid they will be more prone to toxic effects of the anticoagulants. Caution them to be alert for bruising and bleeding.
- Nalidixic acid may cause false positive reactions when urine is tested with Benedict's solution, Fehling's solution,

Pocket Nurse Guide to Drugs

or Clinitest tablets. While taking nalidixic acid and nitrofurantoins, patients who must monitor urine sugar concentration should use Clinistix or Tes-Tape.

- Resistance to nalidixic acid, when it occurs, does so within the first couple of days of therapy. Follow-up cultures should be done 2 or 3 days after starting therapy to check for sterility.
- Patients receiving nalidixic acid should be kept well hydrated with a daily intake of 2000 to 2500 ml (in the adult) if possible.
- Patients receiving cinoxacin with normal renal function should be kept well hydrated with a daily intake of 2000 to 2500 ml (adults) if possible.

Antituberculosis Drugs

First-line antituberculosis drugs
    Isoniazid, or isonicotinic acid hydrazide (INH)
    Ethambutol
    Rifampin
    Streptomycin
    Para-aminosalicylic acid (PAS)
    Aminosalicylate acid sodium salt
Second-line antituberculosis drugs
    Capreomycin
    Cycloserine
    Ethionamide
    Pyrazinamide

Actions of Antituberculosis Drugs

Isoniazid alters several metabolic processes in mycobacteria. The exact mechanism of *ethambutol* is unknown, but it alters the formation of several cellular metabolites in mycobacteria. *Rifampin* inhibits DNA-dependent RNA polymerase in sensitive organisms and halts gene transcription and protein synthesis. *Streptomycin* inhibits protein synthesis in sensitive bacteria and mycobacteria. *Para-amino salicylic acid (PAS)* inhibits mycobacterial growth by interfering with folic acid metabolism.

Indications for Antituberculosis Drugs

Of the first line antituberculosis drugs, *isoniazid* is the drug of choice and is most effective against *Mycobacterium tuberculosis,* with *Mycobacterium kansaii* less sensitive. *Ethambutol* is effective only against mycobacteria and is often used as one of the drugs in intermittent therapy programs. *Rifampin* has a broader spectrum of effectiveness against different species of mycobacteria but is limited in use because of its toxicity. *Streptomycin* is often used as part of a combined drug regimen for initial therapy. *PAS* is currently used less often in combined drug initial therapy, since ethambutol and rifampin have been introduced.

The second-line drugs, or reserve drugs, are used with strains of mycobacteria resistant to first-line drugs or when the patient develops an intolerable reaction to the first-line drugs.

Nurse Alert for Antituberculosis Drugs

- With ethambutol and rifampin, pregnant women and nursing mothers should be observed to detect whether the drug may be harming the fetus or infant.
- Patients with malnutrition, alcoholism, diabetes, or liver or renal dysfunction may be at greater risk for isoniazid toxicity.
- Fetuses and nursing infants may be at risk with mothers receiving isoniazid.
- Elderly patients are more sensitive to the ototoxic effects of streptomycin.

Parenteral Administration of Antituberculosis Drugs

- *Parenteral isoniazid:* Reconstitute the drug as directed on the vial. Pain may occur at the injection site following intramuscular administration. If the drug crystallizes in the vial, warm the solution to room temperature to redissolve.

Side Effects of Antituberculosis Drugs

Of the first-line drugs, *isoniazid* may cause peripheral neuropathy, hepatotoxicity and liver failure or hepatitis, and

546 **Pocket Nurse Guide to Drugs**

Table 46-13 Administration of antituberculosis drugs

Generic Name	Trade Name	Dosage and Administration
First-line Drugs		
Isoniazid or isonicotinic acid hydrazide (INH)	Niconyl Nydrazid Rimifon† Teebaconin	ORAL: *Adults*—300 mg daily maximum. *Children*—10 to 20 mg/kg daily. INTRAMUSCULAR, INTRAVENOUS: As for oral.
Ethambutol	Myambutol*	ORAL: *Adults*—15 mg/kg in a single daily dose. *Children under 13 yr* should not receive the drug. ORAL: *Adults*—25 mg/kg in a single daily dose for 2 mo, after which dose may be reduced to 15 mg/kg daily. ORAL: *Adults*—45 to 50 mg/kg twice weekly.
Rifampin	Rifadin* Rimactane*	ORAL: *Adults*—600 mg daily in 1 dose. *Children*—10 to 20 mg/kg up to 600 mg daily.
Streptomycin		INTRAMUSCULAR: *Adults*—1 Gm daily for 2 to 4 mo or longer. After initial therapy dosage may be reduced to 1 Gm 2 or 3 times weekly. *Children and elderly patients*—may require smaller doses.

*Available in U.S. and Canada
†Available in Canada only

Antibiotics **547**

Table 46-13 Administration of antituberculosis drugs—cont'd.

Generic Name	Trade Name	Dosage and Administration
First-line Drugs—cont'd.		
Para-aminosalicylic acid (PAS)	Aminosalicylic Acid Teebacin Acid	ORAL: *Adults*—10 to 12 Gm daily in 3 or 4 doses. *Children*—200 to 300 mg/kg daily in 3 or 4 doses.
Aminosalicylate acid sodium salt (10.9% sodium)	PAS Sodium Parasal Sodium Teebacin	ORAL: *Adults*—12 to 15 Gm daily in 2 or 3 doses. *Children*—200 to 300 mg/kg daily in 3 or 4 doses.
Second-line Drugs		
Capreomycin	Capastat Sulfate*	INTRAMUSCULAR: *Adults*—15 to 20 mg/kg daily in single dose. Not recommended for children.
Cycloserine	Seromycin	ORAL: *Adults*—15 mg/kg daily in 2 doses up to maximum daily dose of 1 Gm. Dosage not established for children.
Ethionamide	Trecator SC	ORAL: *Adults*—0.5 to 1 Gm daily in 1 to 3 doses. Dosage not established for children.
Pyrazinamide		ORAL: *Adults*—20 to 35 mg/kg daily up to 3 Gm. Dosage not established for children.

*Available in U.S. and Canada
†Available in Canada only

Pocket Nurse Guide to Drugs

occasionally allergies, blood dyscrasias, gastric distress, and metabolic acidosis. *Ethambutol* causes visual disturbances, and, rarely, allergic reactions or peripheral neuritis. *Rifampin* may cause gastrointestinal upset, central nervous system disturbances, orange-red coloring of body fluids, liver function alterations or jaundice, and in high doses an immune reaction with a flu-like syndrome of chills, fever, vomiting, diarrhea, and myalgia. The toxicity may progress to renal failure. *Streptomycin* commonly causes ototoxicity and other side effects seen with aminoglycoside antibiotics (see pp. 526, 530). *PAS* commonly causes gastrointestinal irritation, allergic reactions such as rashes but including exfoliative dermatitis and hepatitis.

Of the second-line drugs, *capreomycin* may cause nephrotoxicity, low blood potassium levels, and eighth cranial nerve toxicity. *Cycloserine* may cause central nervous system toxicity, including psychotic reactions. *Ethionamide* may cause nausea and vomiting induced by central nervous system effects and may cause liver toxicity. *Pyrazinamide* may cause hepatotoxicity and hyperuricemia.

Nursing Implications for Antituberculosis Drugs
Isoniazid

- Patients receiving isoniazid should be questioned about numbness, tingling, paresthesias, and feelings of heaviness in the arms and legs as this may indicate the development of peripheral neuropathy. Some physicians will choose to treat all patients who are taking isoniazid with pyridoxine prophylactically to prevent the peripheral neuropathy rather than waiting until symptoms develop.
- Symptoms of hepatitis include fever, jaundice, right upper quadrant abdominal pain, and sometimes changes in the appearance of stools. Encourage the patient to report any unusual symptoms.
- Phenytoin may be potentiated in patients taking isoniazid, so it may be necessary to monitor phenytoin blood concentrations and even to reduce the dosage while patients are taking isoniazid. Caution patients to be alert to signs of phenytoin toxicity (Chapter 37).

Antibiotics **549**

- Patients should be encouraged to avoid the use of alcohol.
- Taking isoniazid with meals may reduce gastric irritation.
- A wide variety of side effects has been attributed to isoniazid therapy, but a causal relationship has not always been found. Encourage patients to return for routine follow-up and to report any symptoms that seem unusual.

Ethambutol

- Encourage patients to report any visual changes they experience. Pretreatment ophthalmological examinations are probably indicated only in patients with cataracts, diabetic retinopathy, and optic neuritis, but careful questioning and assessment of visual ability should be done with all patients during follow-up visits.

Rifampin

- Alert patient to the fact that body fluids (tears, sweat, feces, and urine) may turn orange-red while they are receiving therapy. Soft contact lenses may become permanently stained.
- Liver abnormalities are the most common side effect of this drug. Symptoms that may indicate liver dysfunction include anorexia, malaise, jaundice, or a change in the stools. Instruct the patient to report any unusual feelings or symptoms.
- Abdominal distress, aching joints and muscles, and leg cramps are often reported after initiation of therapy but will usually disappear in a few weeks.
- Encourage patients not to miss rifampin doses. An immunological reaction characterized by dyspnea, wheezing, purpura, thrombocytopenia, and anaphylactic-type reactions have occurred with intermittent therapy or when the drug has been resumed after a lapse of days or weeks.
- Patients taking coumarin anticoagulants, methadone, oral hypoglycemic agents, digitalis, oral contraceptives, or replacement doses of corticosteroids may find the effectiveness of these drugs decreased, resulting in a need for a change in dosage. Persons relying on oral contraceptives for

550   Pocket Nurse Guide to Drugs

birth control may wish to use additional or alternate methods of birth control while receiving rifampin therapy.

- It is recommended that rifampin be taken 1 hour before or 2 hours after a meal if it can be tolerated that way.

Streptomycin

This drug is discussed earlier in this chapter.

Para-aminosalicylic acid

- Gastrointestinal upset is a very common problem with PAS and is often the source of patient noncompliance. Encourage patients to take the drug with meals, antacids, or a snack. It is unpleasant to take; a 12 Gm per day adult dose requires consumption of 24 of the 500 mg tablets.
- Because of the rare but serious side effect of exfoliative dermatitis, the patient should be cautioned to report immediately the appearance of any rash or skin changes.
- Hepatic dysfunction may be manifested by malaise, jaundice, anorexia, change in stools, and fever. Instruct patients to report any unusual sign or symptom.
- Patients receiving oral anticoagulants may require a change in dosage of their anticoagulant.
- Discoloration of the tablets indicates deterioration; the tablets should be discarded and a new supply obtained.
- Because PAS is excreted primarily in the urine, patients should be encouraged to maintain a good intake (2000 to 2500 ml per day in the adult) to prevent crystalluria.

Antileprosy Drugs

Dapsone
Clofazimine
Rifampin
Sulfoxone sodium

Indications for Antileprosy Drugs

Dapsone is the most reliable and least toxic of the antileprosy drugs. Alternative drugs are used with resistant infections or when toxic effects are intolerable.

Antibiotics **551**

Table 46-14 Administration of antileprosy drugs

Generic Name	Trade Name	Dosage and Administration
Dapsone	Avlosulfon*	ORAL: *Adults*—up to 100 mg daily. *Children*—1.4 mg/kg daily.
Clofazimine	Lamprene	ORAL: *Adults*—100 mg daily. (Investigational only.)
Rifampin	Rifadin* Rimactane*	ORAL: *Adults*—600 mg daily.
Sulfoxone sodium	Diasone Sodium	ORAL: *Adults*—330 mg daily.

*Available in U.S. and Canada

Side Effects of Antileprosy Drugs

Dapsone and *sulfoxone sodium* cause gastrointestinal distress, including nausea, vomiting and abdominal pain, and headache, vertigo, tinnitus, and hemolytic reactions that are more common in patients with glucose-6-phosphate dehydrogenase deficiency. *Clofazimine* causes gastrointestinal distress, and imparts a dark red color to skin and other tissues. *Rifampin* causes liver toxicity and abdominal distress.

Nursing Implications for Dapsone

- Complete blood counts should be done before initiating therapy with dapsone and at regular intervals during therapy. Drug-related blood dyscrasias can include agranulocytosis and aplastic anemia. Instruct the patient to report symptoms of malaise, fever, sore throat, jaundice, or purpura.
- Dermatitis is a rare side effect but may be serious, as exfoliative dermatitis can ensue. The patient should be cautioned to report the appearance of any skin changes.
- Peripheral neuropathy is a rare but definite complication that can occur. Patients should be instructed to report any tingling, heaviness, numbness, unusual sensations, or paresthesias that occur in the arms and legs.

Antifungal Agents

47

Drugs for systemic fungal infections
- Amphotericin B
- Flucytosine
- Hydroxystilbamidine isethionate
- Ketoconazole
- Miconazole nitrate

Drugs for topical fungal infections
- Acrisorcin
- Amphotericin B
- Clioquinol or iodochlorhydroxyquin
- Clotrimazole
- Ciclopirox olamine
- Econazole nitrate
- Griseofulvin
- Haloprogin
- Miconazole
- Nystatin
- Tolnaftate
- Undecylenic acid
- Calcium undecylenate

Drugs for Systemic Fungal Infections

Actions of Drugs for Systemic Fungal Infections

Amphotericin B selectively damages membranes containing ergosterol (fungal membranes); the action is not entirely selective and may damage some cholesterol-containing mammalian cell membranes. *Flucytosine* is apparently converted to a cytotoxic agent in sensitive fungi. *Ketoconazole* inhibits the synthesis of ergosterol, thereby impairing fungal cell membrane function, and limits the development of invasive hyphae by fungal cells, thereby enhancing the ability of the host immune system to eliminate the fungi.

Indications for Drugs for Systemic Fungal Infections

Amphotericin B is used to treat a broad spectrum of fungal diseases including those caused by Histoplasma, Blastomyces, Cryptococcus, Aspergillus, and others and may also be used to treat systemic Candida and Coccidioides infections. *Flucytosine* is used to treat Cryptococcus and Candida infections. *Ketoconazole* is used for Histoplasma and Paracoccidioides infections and may be effective for patients with disseminated Candidiasis, Blastomycosis, Coccidioidomycosis, and Cryptococcosis. *Hydroxystilbamidine* is used only to treat patients with Blastomycosis. *Miconazole* is used systemically as well as topically for Candida, Cryptococcus, and Aspergillus infections.

Nurse Alert for Drugs for Systemic Fungal Infections

- Because of toxic effects, amphotericin therapy often has to be discontinued early.
- Ketoconazole is generally contraindicated in pregnancy and should be used with caution during lactation.

Side Effects of Drugs for Systemic Fungal Infections

Amphotericin B may cause headache, chills, fever, nausea, vomiting, renal damage with prolonged therapy, and anemia and electrolyte disturbance over time. *Flucytosine* may cause nausea and diarrhea in one-fourth of patients, and reportedly blood dyscrasias and transient liver abnormalities. *Ketoconazole* causes nausea and pruritis in less than 5% of patients, and less frequently dizziness, nervousness, headache, and liver damage; gynecomastia is noted in 10% of males. *Hydroxystilbamidine* commonly causes nausea, vomiting, malaise, and headache and less commonly dizziness, paresthesias, blood dyscrasias, incontinence, and facial edema; hypotension and tachycardia may result from too rapid infusion. *Miconazole* may cause thrombophlebitis, gastrointestinal distress, blood dyscrasias, and allergic reactions.

554   Pocket Nurse Guide to Drugs

Table 47-1   Administration of drugs for systemic fungal infections

Generic Name	Trade Name	Dosage and Administration
Amphotericin B	Fungizone*	INTRAVENOUS: *Adults and children*—0.25 to 1 mg/kg per day infused at 0.1 mg/ml in 5% dextrose over 6 hr. Total drug course usually less than 4 Gm.
Flucytosine	Ancobon Ancotil†	ORAL: *Adults and children*—50 to 150 mg/kg daily in 4 doses. Lower drug doses are required when renal function is impaired.
Hydroxystilbamidine isethionate		INTRAVENOUS: *Adults*—225 mg in 200 ml of 5% dextrose or saline daily. Total drug course usually less than 8 Gm.
Ketoconazole	Nizoral	ORAL: *Adults*—200 to 400 mg daily in a single dose. Higher doses have been suggested to improve response. *Children weighing less than 20 kg*—50 mg once daily. *Children 20 to 40 kg*—100 mg once daily. *Children over 40 kg*—200 mg once daily.

*Available in U.S. and Canada
†Available in Canada only

Antifungal Agents

Table 47-1 Administration of drugs for systemic fungal infections—cont'd.

Generic Name	Trade Name	Dosage and Administration
Miconazole nitrate	Monistat-IV*	*Adults*—Highly variable, depending upon the causative organism. Daily doses as low as 200 mg or as high as 3.6 Gm, divided into 3 equal doses, may be indicated. *Children*—Total daily dose 20 to 40 mg/kg with no single infusion exceeding 15 mg/kg.

*Available in U.S. and Canada
†Available in Canada only

Nursing Implications for Drugs for Systemic Fungal Infections

Amphotericin B

- Patients receiving amphotericin B via intravenous infusion may be hospitalized for 6 weeks or longer for the course of therapy.
- Most patients will suffer some side effects while receiving amphotericin B. Monitor the temperature and vital signs at regular intervals (every two to four hours) while the drug is infusing. Common complaints include headache, fever, chills, nausea, anorexia, vomiting, and diarrhea. Infrequently seen side effects include hypertension or hypotension, coagulation defects, tinnitus, rash, and vertigo; anaphylactic reactions are rare. Treatment of side effects is symptomatic, and as it becomes clear what an individual patient's response will be, the anticipatory use of supportive therapy should proceed. Thus the patient may receive, in

556   Pocket Nurse Guide to Drugs

addition to amphotericin B, antiemetics, antipyretics, antihistamines, or steroids.

- Most patients will show some degree of renal damage; therefore appropriate studies (BUN, NPN, serum creatinine, creatinine clearance) should be done prior to therapy and at weekly intervals during therapy. In addition, serum electrolytes should be monitored twice a week, since hypokalemia is frequently observed.
- Parenteral administration:
  a. See the manufacturer's literature for complete instructions about dilution. The final concentration should be less than 0.1 mg/ml.
  b. If an in-line intravenous filter is being used, the mean pore diameter should not be less than 1.0 μm.
  c. Thrombophlebitis often occurs; the addition of a small amount of heparin to the infusion may help. No other drugs should be added to the infusion. Avoid extravasation.
  d. The drug is light-sensitive so the medication must be protected from direct sunlight during infusion.
  e. Administer over 2 to 6 hours or longer. The use of an electronic infusion monitor may be appropriate.
  f. During infusions, monitor the temperature and vital signs. Fluid intake and output should be monitored during the course of therapy.
  g. The intravenous preparation is a suspension. Gently agitate or rotate the IV bottle several times while the drug is infusing.
- When amphotericin is used topically, there are virtually no side effects.

Flucytosine

- Blood work should be done at regular intervals to monitor for hematopoietic, renal, and hepatic changes that can occur. Most commonly, the drug produces neutropenia, eosinophilia, thrombocytopenia, and elevations of hepatic enzymes, BUN, and creatinine.
- If nausea occurs, it may be reduced by giving the capsules a few at a time over a 15- to 20-minute period.

Ketoconazole

- Administer this drug on an empty stomach, 1 hour before or two hours after eating, for best absorption. Do not administer within two hours of antacids or H_2 histamine-receptor blocking drugs such as cimetidine.
- Instruct the patient to report the development of any side effects, especially signs of hepatitis or liver dysfunction: jaundice, right-upper-quadrant abdominal pain, change in the color or consistency of stools, nausea. Monitor liver function tests at regular intervals.

Miconazole

- Nausea and vomiting may be reduced by giving an antiemetic or antihistamine before administering the drug, by not giving miconazole at mealtimes, and by reducing the rate of infusion.
- Interaction with the coumarin anticoagulants results in enhancement of the anticoagulant effect; reduction in the dose of anticoagulant may be needed. Caution the patient to be alert for signs of bleeding and bruising.
- For dilution, see the manufacturer's literature. The rate of infusion should be 30 to 60 minutes per dose.

Griseofulvin

- Griseofulvin interferes with the activity of warfarin-type anticoagulants. It may be necessary to increase the dose of anticoagulants.

Nystatin

- When nystatin is used to treat oral *Candida* infections, a drug suspension is used. The patient's mouth should be free of food particles when the suspension form is administered. Instruct the patient to place one half of the dose in each side of the mouth and to hold it as long as possible before swallowing.
- The vaginal suppositories can also be used orally. Instruct the patient to suck on the tablet-like suppository to allow for prolonged contact in the mouth. The dose should not be chewed and swallowed.

Drugs for Topical Fungal Infections

Acrisorcin
Amphotericin B
Clioquinol or iodochlorhydroxyquin
Clotrimazole
Ciclopirox olamine
Econazole nitrate
Griseofulvin
Haloprogin
Miconazole
Nystatin
Tolnaftate
Undecylenic acid
Calcium undecylenate

Indications for Drugs for Local Fungal Infections

Acrisorcin is used only for tinea versicolor. *Amphotericin B* is used for Candida infections of skin or mucous membranes. *Cloquinol* is used for localized dermatophytoses. *Clotrimazole* is used for a broad spectrum of antifungal activity. *Griseofulvin* is used for tinea infections except for tinea versicolor. *Ciclopirox* and *econazole* are used for tinea infections including tinea versicolor. *Haloprogin* is used for tinea and other superficial fungal infections. *Miconazole* is used for dermatophytosis of Candida infections. *Nystatin* is used in different forms for Candida infections of the intestinal tract, skin, and vagina. *Tolnaftate* is used for tinea infections only. *Undecylenic acid* is used for athlete's foot and ringworm in areas other than around nails or hairy areas. *Calcium undecylenate* is used for tinea cruris, diaper rash, and other skin irritations of groin area.

Nurse Alert for Drugs for Topical Fungal Infections

- With female patients with vaginal Candida infections, male sexual partners should also be treated to avoid reinfection.
- Do not use clotrimazole, ciclopirox, econazole, haloprogin, miconazole, or tolnaftate around the eyes.

Antifungal Agents 559

- Do not use ciclopirox with occlusive dressings.
- Diabetics and others with impaired circulation should use undecylenic acid and calcium undecylenate only with the physician's advice.
- Intravaginal medications should be used during pregnancy only when the physician considers it absolutely necessary.

Side Effects of Drugs for Local Fungal Infections

Acrisorcin may cause blisters and skin irritation. *Amphotericin B* may cause local tissue irritation. *Cloquinol* may cause mild skin irritation. *Clotrimazole* may cause skin irritation, pruritus, and urticaria. *Griseofulvin* may cause blood dyscrasias, headache, gastrointestinal disturbances, neuritis, allergic reactions, and hepatotoxicity. *Ciclopirox* and *econazole* may cause redness, itching, burning, and stinging of the skin. *Haloprogin* and *miconazole* may cause local tissue irritation or maceration. *Nystatin* in oral forms may cause nausea, vomiting, and diarrhea, and in topical applications may cause skin irritation.

Nursing Implications for Drugs for Local Fungal Infections

- Instruct patients to report any local irritation (rash, burning, pruritus) or any systemic symptoms that occur.
- Ascertain that women can accurately and correctly use the applicator supplied with intravaginal preparations. Use of the agent should continue during the menstrual period. Some women may find better treatment results if sanitary napkins are worn, not tampons. The routine use of douches is not recommended; consult the physician.

Table 47-2 Administration of drugs for local fungal infections

Generic Name	Trade Name	Dosage and Administration
Acrisorcin	Akrinol	TOPICAL: *Adults and children*—cream (2 mg/Gm) applied twice daily.
Amphotericin B	Fungizone*	TOPICAL: *Adults and children*—3% cream, lotion, or ointment applied 2 to 4 times daily.
Clioquinol or iodochlorhydroxyquin	Vioform*	TOPICAL: *Adults and children*—3% cream, ointment, or powder applied several times daily.
Clotrimazole	Gyne-Lotrimin Lotrimin	TOPICAL: *Adults and children*—1% cream or solution applied twice daily.
	Mycelex Myclo†	INTRAVAGINAL: *Adults*—Tablets or creams containing 100 mg inserted once daily.
Ciclopirox olamine	Loprox	TOPICAL: *Adults*—1% cream applied twice daily.
Econazole nitrate	Ecostatin*	TOPICAL: *Adults*—1% cream applied twice daily.
Griseofulvin	Fulvicin* Grifulvin Grisactin	ORAL: *Adults*—500 mg microcrystalline form in single or divided daily dose. *Children*—10 mg/kg daily.
Haloprogin	Halotex*	TOPICAL: *Adults and children*—1% cream or solution applied twice daily.
Miconazole	Monistat*	TOPICAL: *Adults and children*—2% cream or lotion applied twice daily.
		INTRAVAGINAL: *Adults*—2% cream once daily.

Antifungal Agents

Nystatin	Candex Mycostatin* Nilstat* O-V Statin	ORAL: *Adults and children*—0.5 to 1 million units 3 times daily. *Infants*—0.1 to 0.2 million units 4 times daily. TOPICAL: *Adults and children*—ointments, creams, lotions, (0.1 million units/Gm) applied twice daily. INTRAVAGINAL: *Adults*—tablets, 0.1 to 0.2 million units daily.
Tolnaftate	Aftate Tinactin*	TOPICAL: *Adults and children*—1% cream, gel, solution, powder, or aerosol applied twice daily.
Undecylenic acid	Desenex* Ting Undecylenic compound Unde-Jen	TOPICAL: *Adults and children*—ointment (5%, with 20% zinc undecylenate), powder (2%, with 20% zinc undecylenate), 10% solution, 2% soap applied twice daily.
Calcium undecylenate	Caldesene Cruex	TOPICAL: *Adults and children*—10% powder applied as needed.

*Available in U.S. and Canada
†Available in Canada only

Antiviral Agents

48

Vaccines
  Hepatitis B
  Influenza
  Mumps
  Poliomyelitis
  Rabies
  Rubella
  Rubeola
  Smallpox
  Yellow fever

Antiviral drugs
  Acyclovir
  Amantadine
  Idoxuridine
  Methisazone
  Trifluridine
  Vidarabine

Actions of Antiviral Agents

Vaccines induce the formation of antibodies in healthy individuals prior to exposure to the viral disease. *Amantadine* acts by blocking the process by which virus particles enter the cell and release their genetic material. *Acyclovir* is activated by viral thymidine kinase and inhibits the viral DNA polymerase present in the infected cell, effectively halting the virus production. *Idoxuridine* and *trifluridine* are incorporated into DNA in place of the normal thymidine, preventing normal DNA replication and halting virus formation, but will also harm rapidly growing normal host cells. *Methisazone* blocks replication of vaccinia virus and various pox viruses. *Vidarabine* is activated by host cell enzymes to selectively inhibit viral DNA polymerase.

Indications for Antiviral Agents

Vaccines for poliomyelitis, rubella, rubeola, and mumps are administered prophylactically to children. Influenza vaccine is used in flu season for patients at high risk. Smallpox vaccine, now that smallpox has been eliminated from world populations, is given to persons working in laboratories with variola virus. Yellow fever vaccine is given to persons travelling to areas of high exposure. Rabies vaccine is used to treat persons bitten by a rabid animal, or one suspected of being rabid. Hepatis B vaccine is given to those at high risk of acquiring hepatitis B (eg., patients with frequent blood transfusions, operating room personnel). Amantadine has limited capability to treat influenza type A after symptoms have appeared, and normally is used prophylactically with high-risk patients, particularly the elderly or others for whom influenza may lead to life-threatening complications. Amantadine is also used to treat Parkinson's disease (see Ch. 8). Acyclovir is used intravenously, orally, and topically for lesions of genital herpes and for mucocutaneous herpes simplex in immunocompromised patients; it is being studied for herpes zoster infections. Idoxuridine is used topically for herpes simplex infections of the cornea, conjunctiva, and eyelids. Methisazone, once used prophylactically for smallpox exposures, is used to treat vaccinia infections such as vaccinia eczema and vaccinia gangrenosa. Trifluridine is used topically for herpes infections of the eye. Vidarabine is used topically for herpes eye infections and intravenously for herpetic encephalitis and other herpes infections.

Nurse Alert for Antiviral Agents

- Rubella vaccine should be given to females before puberty because the disease is most dangerous for fetuses in the first trimester.
- Amantadine should be used cautiously if at all in elderly patients with cerebral arteriosclerosis or patients with a history of epilepsy.

Side Effects of Antiviral Agents

Amantadine may cause amphetamine-like stimulation of the central nervous system, lethargy, ataxia, slurred speech, and other CNS symptoms; toxic reactions are more common if kidney failure is present and the drug accumulates in the bloodstream. *Acyclovir* may crystallize in the renal tubule and

Pocket Nurse Guide to Drugs

Table 48-1 Administration of antiviral agents

A. Administration of Vaccines

Disease	Characteristics of Vaccine	When Administered
Poliomyelitis	Oral vaccine (trivalent) containing attenuated live polio virus mimics natural form of disease without risk of central nervous system involvement.	At 2, 4, 6 and 18 mo of age or at 2, 4, and 18 mo; boosters at 6 yr.
Rubella (German measles)	Attenuated live rubella vaccine confers long-term resistance.	After 15 mo of age; especially important that females be immunized before puberty, since disease is most dangerous for fetuses in first trimester.
Measles (rubeola)	Attenuated live virus vaccine stimulates protective antibodies in 95% of children receiving it.	After 15 mo of age.
Mumps	Attenuated live virus vaccine stimulates protective antibodies in 95% of those receiving it.	After 15 mo of age.

Influenza	Inactivated viruses of types causing recent outbreaks. Differs from year to year.	During flu season to patients at high risk.
Smallpox	Success of vaccination is judged by response at vaccination site.	Given to persons working in laboratories with variola virus.
Yellow fever	Live attenuated virus confers resistance on most persons receiving injection.	After 6 mo of age to persons traveling to areas of high exposure.
Rabies	Killed, fixed virus confers resistance to most patients exposed to infection.	Used after being bitten by rapid animal or animal suspected of being rabid, or prophylactically to high risk individuals.

Table 48-1   Administration of antiviral agents—cont'd.

B. Administration of Antiviral Drugs

Generic Name	Trade Name	Dosage and Administration
Acyclovir	Zovirax*	ORAL: 200 mg 4 times daily. INTRAVENOUS: *Adults*—5 mg/kg infused at a constant rate over 1 hr, repeated every 8 hr. *Children under 12*—250 mg/M^2 infused at a constant rate over 1 hr, repeated every 8 hr. TOPICAL: 5% ointment applied directly to initial lesions of genital herpes.
Amantadine	Symmetrel*	ORAL: *Adults*—100 mg twice daily. *Children*—4.4 to 8.8 mg/kg, up to 150 mg daily.
Idoxuridine	Dendrid Herplex Liquifilm* Stoxil	OPHTHALMIC: *Adults and children*—0.1% solution, 0.5% ointment used 5 times daily.
Trifluridine	Viroptic	OPHTHALMIC: *Adults and children*—1% solution applied up to 9 times daily.
Vidarabine	Vira-A*	OPHTHALMIC: *Adults and children*—3% ointment used 5 times daily. INTRAVENOUS: *Adults and children*—15 mg/kg daily by slow continuous infusion for 12 to 24 hr.

*Available in U.S. and Canada

Antiviral Agents **567**

cause nephrotoxicity if administered as a rapid bolus; phlebitis may occur at the injection site with intravenous administration. *Idoxuridine* used topically in the eye may cause corneal pitting defects and may interfere with corneal epithelial regeneration and healing; systemic reactions may include anorexia, nausea, stomatitis, vomiting, alopecia, blood dyscrasias, and cholestatic jaundice. *Idoxuridine* is also potentially mutagenic and carcinogenic. *Methisazone* affects liver function and may interfere with the metabolism of a number of drugs including barbituates and alcohol. *Trifluridine* administered topically in the eye may cause burning of the conjunctiva and cornea and swelling of the eyelids; it is potentially mutagenic and carcinogenic. *Vidarabine* may cause transient gastrointestinal distress including anorexia, nausea, vomiting and diarrhea, and malaise, superficial punctate keratitis, allergic reactions, rash, and more rarely central nervous system disturbances such as tremors, dizziness, ataxia, confusion, and hallucinations; high doses are cytotoxic and cause blood dyscrasias; the drug is teratogenic and potentially carcinogenic.

Nursing Implications for Antiviral Agents

- See Ch. 8 for nursing implications for amantadine.
- Vidarabine must be given via slow infusion. Rapid or bolus injections are to be avoided. See the manufacturer's literature for dilution instructions.

Acyclovir

- The sterile powder for intravenous infusion should be used only for that purpose; it should not be administered topically, intramuscularly, orally, subcutaneously, or in the eye.
- Dilute the sterile powder for infusion as directed by the manufacturer. This solution should be further diluted to a concentration of approximately 7 mg/ml or lower. More concentrated solutions may cause venous irritation and phlebitis. The dose should then be administered over at least one hour.
- Inspect the intravenous insertion site frequently for signs of irritation or phlebitis.

568   **Pocket Nurse Guide to Drugs**

- Monitor the fluid intake and urine output of patients receiving the intravenous preparation. Nephrotoxicity can be minimized when the patient is well hydrated. Force fluids to 2500 to 3000 ml per day, unless otherwise indicated.
- Topical acyclovir: Sufficient ointment should be used to cover the lesions. For best results, the patient should not omit applications or stop therapy before the prescribed course has been completed. A finger cot or rubber glove should be worn on the hand of the individual applying the ointment to reduce the possibility of spreading the infection.

Antiparasitic Agents*

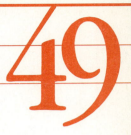

Chloroquine
Diloxanide furoate
Emetine
Furazolidone
Hydroxychloroquine
Iodoquinol (diiodohydroxyquin)
Mebendazole
Metronidazole
Niclosamide
Piperazine
Povidone-iodine
Primaquine
Pyrantel pamoate
Pyrimethamine
Pyrvinium pamoate
Quinacrine
Quinine
Sulfadiazine
Sulfadoxine and pyrimethamine
Sulfamethoxazole and trimethoprim
Tetracycline
Thiabendazole

Actions of Antiparasitic Agents

Chloroquine and *hydroxychloroquine* bind tightly to DNA of infected cells and alter the physical properties of the DNA; they seem to inhibit the ability of the DNA to be replicated or transcribed. The biochemical basis for the amoeba-destroying action of *diloxanide* is not known. *Emetine* may block protein synthesis in eukaryotes, and therefore mammalian cells as well as the amoeba may be sensitive. *Furazolidone* is a nitrofuran similar in action to the nitrofurans used to treat urinary infections (Ch. 46). The amebicidal action of *iodoquinol* is thought to be related to the iodine content of the drug. *Mebendazole* is a broad spectrum antihelminthic agent that

Text continued on p. 576

---

*Because many different drugs are used to treat protozoal and helminthic infestations, and some of the same drugs are used to treat different kinds of infestations, this chapter is organized somewhat differently from others. The drug indications are tabularized along with dosage and administration information, organized according to grouped classes of protozoal and helminthic infestations. Drug trade names are given along with generic names in a special table on toxic and side effects.

Table 49-1   Indications for and administration of antiparasitic agents

Drugs Used to Treat Amebic Infestations (Amebiasis)

Disease Form	Drug Used	Dosage and Administration
Asymptomatic	Iodoquinol	ORAL: *Adults*—650 mg 3 times daily for 3 wks. *Children*—30 to 40 mg/kg divided in 3 doses daily for 3 wks. Maximal daily dosage 2 Gm.
	Diloxanide furoate (investigational)	ORAL: *Adults*—500 mg 3 times daily for 10 days. *Children over 2 yr*—20 mg/kg daily in 3 divided doses for 10 days.
Intestinal symptoms only	Metronidazole	ORAL: *Adults*—750 mg 3 times daily for 10 days. *Children*—35 to 50 mg/kg divided into 3 doses daily for 10 days.
	plus	
	Iodoquinol	As above.
	Emetine	INTRAMUSCULAR (deep), SUBCUTANEOUS: *Adults*—1 mg/kg up to 60 mg daily in a single dose for 5 days. *Children*—same dosage but divided into 2 doses.
	plus	
	Iodoquinol	As above
Abscesses in liver or other organs	Metronidazole	As above
	plus	
	Iodoquinol	As above

	Emetine plus	As above
	Iodoquinol and	As above
	Chloroquine phosphate	ORAL: *Adults*—1 Gm daily for 2 days, then 500 mg daily for 2 or 3 wks. *Children*—10 mg/kg up to 600 mg daily for 3 wks.

Drugs Used to Treat Malaria

Blood forms causing clinical symptoms.	Chloroquine phosphate	ORAL: *Adults*—600 mg initially; 300 mg at 6, 24, and 48 hr. *Children*—10 mg/kg initially; 5 mg/kg at 6, 24, and 48 hr.
	Chloroquine hydrochloride	INTRAMUSCULAR, INTRAVENOUS: *Adults*—3 mg/kg (maximum 900 mg) every 6 hr. *Children*—2 to 3 mg/kg repeated in 6 hr. Not for intravenous use in children under 7 yr.
	Hydroxychloroquine sulfate	ORAL: *Adults*—620 mg initially; 310 mg at 6, 24, and 48 hr. *Children*—10 mg/kg initially; 5 mg/kg at 6, 24, and 48 hr.
	Quinine sulfate	ORAL: *Adults*—650 mg 3 times daily for 10 to 14 days. *Children*—25 mg/kg per day in 3 doses for 10 to 14 days.

cont'd. next page

Table 49-1 Indications for and administration of antiparasitic agents—cont'd.

Disease Form	Drug Used	Dosage and Administration
Blood forms causing clinical symptoms—cont'd.	Quinine dihydrochloride	INTRAVENOUS: *Adults*—600 mg every 8 hr. *Children*—25 mg/kg divided into 2 one hr infusions.
Persistent tissue forms of *Plasmodia (P. ovale, P. vivax)* or gametocytes	Primaquine phosphate	ORAL: *Adults*—15 mg for 14 days following therapy with one of the drugs listed above. *Children*—0.3 mg/kg for 14 days following therapy with one of the drugs listed above.
Chloroquine-resistant *P. falciparum*	Quinine sulfate or hydrochloride plus	As above.
	Pyrimethamine/sulfadoxine	ORAL: *Adults and children over 4 yr*—Tablets contain 25 mg pyrimethamine and 500 mg sulfadoxine. One to 3 tablets as a single dose may be followed with quinine or primaquine.

Drugs Used to Treat Trichomoniasis, Giardiasis, Toxoplasmosis, and Pneumocystosis

Trichomoniasis	Povidone-iodine	VAGINAL: *Adults*—10% gel applied nightly; 10% douche applied every morning. Therapy continues for 2 wk or longer.
	Metronidazole	ORAL: *Adults*—250 mg 3 times daily for 7 to 10 days.

Antiparasitic Agents

Disease	Drug	Dosage
Giardiasis	Quinacrine	ORAL: *Adults*—100 mg 3 times daily for 5 to 7 days. *Children*—7 mg/kg daily in 3 divided doses for 5 days. Daily dose should not exceed 300 mg in children.
	Furazolidone	ORAL: *Adults*—100 mg 4 times daily for 1 wk. *Children*—6 mg/kg daily divided into 4 doses. Not for infants less than one month old.
Toxoplasmosis	Metronidazole	ORAL: *Adults*—250 mg 3 times daily for 7 days.
	Pyrimethamine	ORAL: *Adults*—50 to 100 mg daily for 1 to 2 wk, then 25 mg daily for up to 5 wk. *Children*—1 mg/kg daily in 2 doses for 2 to 4 days. Continue 0.5 mg/kg for 30 days.
	plus Sulfadiazine	ORAL: *Adults*—2 to 4 Gm for 1 or 2 wk, then 1 Gm every 4 to 6 hr for up to 5 wk. *Children*—150 mg/kg total divided in 4 to 6 daily doses after an initial dose equivalent to one-half the daily total.
Pneumocystosis	Trimethoprim with sulfamethoxazole	ORAL: *Adults*—20 mg/kg trimethoprim and 100 mg/kg sulfamethoxazole daily in 4 doses for 2 wk. *Children*—reduced doses are required.

cont'd. next page

Table 49-1   Indications for and administration of antiparasitic agents—cont'd.

Disease Form	Drug Used	Dosage and Administration
Drugs Used to Treat Infestations by Helminths		
Roundworms (ascariasis)	Pyrantel pamoate	ORAL: *Adults and children*—single dose of 11 mg/kg up to 1 Gm.
	Mebendazole	ORAL: *Adults and children*—100 mg twice daily for 3 days.
	Piperazine	ORAL: *Adults*—3.5 Gm in single dose for 2 days. *Children*—75 mg/kg up to 3.5 Gm once daily for 2 days.
Pinworms (enterobiasis)	Mebendazole	ORAL: *Adults and children*—100 mg single dose.
	Pyrantel pamoate	ORAL: *Adults and children*—single dose of 11 mg/kg up to 1 Gm.
	Pyrvinium pamoate	ORAL: *Adults and children*—single dose of 5 mg/kg.
	Piperazine	ORAL: *Adults and children*—65 mg/kg up to 2.5 Gm once daily for 1 wk.
Whipworms (trichuriasis)	Mebendazole	ORAL: *Adults and children*—100 mg daily for 3 days.
	Thiabendazole	ORAL: *Adults and children*—25 mg/kg up to 3 Gm twice daily for 1 or 2 days.

Threadworms (strongyloidiasis)	Thiabendazole	ORAL: *Adults and children*—25 mg/kg up to 3 Gm twice daily for 1 or 2 days.
Hookworms (necatoriasis)	Mebendazole	ORAL: *Adults and children*—100 mg twice daily for 3 days.
	Pyrantel pamoate	ORAL: *Adults and children*—11 mg/kg up to 1 Gm as single dose for 3 days.
	Thiabendazole	ORAL: *Adults and children*—25 mg/kg up to 3 Gm twice daily for 1 or 2 days.
Cutaneous larva migrans	Thiabendazole	ORAL: *Adults and children*—as for hookworms plus topical application of suspension (500 mg/ 5 ml) 4 times daily for 5 days.
Pork roundworms (trichinosis)	Thiabendazole	ORAL: *Adults and children*—25 mg/kg up to 3 Gm twice daily for 2 to 4 days.
Tapeworms (cestodiasis)	Niclosamide	ORAL: *Adults*—2 Gm as a single dose. *Children weighing more than 34 kg*—1.5 Gm as a single dose. *Children 11 to 34 kg*—1 Gm as a single dose. For all patients, tablets should be thoroughly chewed and taken on an empty stomach. For treatment of dwarf tapeworm infestations, doses must be continued for 5 days and repeated two weeks after initial therapy.

blocks glucose uptake in sensitive helminths, thus ultimately destroying the worms. *Metronidazole* acts by attacking amoeba at intestinal and other tissue sites. *Niclosamide* kills cestodes by blocking respiration and glucose uptake in the worms. *Piperazine* is effective against ascarids and pinworms apparently by blocking the action of acetylcholine on the muscles of these parasites, thus paralyzing the worms which are then eliminated by normal peristaltic flow. *Povidone-iodine* has a general antiseptic action produced by the release of free iodine. The exact mechanism of action of *primaquine* is not known. *Pyrantel* is a depolarizing neuromuscular blocking agent that causes spastic paralysis and gradual contraction of the muscle in worms, which are then eliminated by normal peristalsis. *Pyrimethamine* blocks the enzyme dihydrofolate reductase in plasmodia, thus inhibiting certain metabolic transformations. *Pyrvinium* inhibits energy metabolism in facultative anaerobic organisms such as intestinal parasitic worms. *Quinacrine* acts on tapeworms by acting on the attachment organ and causing the worm to release from the intestinal wall and be eliminated. *Quinine's* exact antimalarial action is unknown. The exact mechanism of action of *thiabendazole* is unknown, but it is believed to attack a metabolic process essential in helminths but not found in humans.

Nurse Alert for Antiparasitic Agents

- Children are more sensitive to the side effects of chloroquine and hydroxychloroquine than adults, and patients with liver disease or retinal damage are at greater risk for severe toxic reactions.
- If patients receiving emetine experience tachycardia or ECG changes, the drug should be discontinued.
- Mebendazole may be teratogenic in humans.
- Metronidazole causes an alarming reaction when ethyl alcohol is ingested: intense flushing, nausea, headaches, and abdominal cramps.
- Metronidazole may be teratogenic.

Antiparasitic Agents 577

- The side effects of piperazine may be more severe in patients with renal dysfunction.
- In patients with G-6-PD deficiency, primaquine may cause cyanosis and severe hemolysis, requiring discontinuation of the drug.
- Quinacrine is contraindicated in pregnant women.
- Thiabendazole may alter liver function; patients with preexisting liver disease should be carefully observed for progressive liver damage.

Nursing Implications for Antiparasitic Agents

- Most of these drugs are not recommended for use during pregnancy.
- Individuals contemplating international travel should be referred to the local health department for information regarding diseases that are endemic in areas which are to be visited.
- Giardiasis is endemic in Russia, Mexico, Africa, and other countries and is usually transmitted from contaminated food, fruits, vegetables, and water.
- Amebiasis is found in the United States where unsanitary conditions exist or where living conditions are crowded, as in institutions.
- Trichinosis can be prevented by cooking pork thoroughly. Smoking, drying, and salting are not reliable methods for killing trichinae.
- Hookworms are easily transmitted in endemic areas because the larvae penetrate the skin. It is not possible to completely eradicate this infection, but instructing children and adults to avoid going barefoot outside will decrease the incidence.
- Pinworms are difficult to eliminate because they are so easily transmitted. Adults and children should be instructed to wash their hands before eating and after using the toilet. It is often necessary to treat the entire family for pinworms.
- Roundworms are not so easily transmitted as pinworms, but hygiene, especially handwashing, should be stressed.
- In the case of worms, it is occasionally appropriate to make a public health referral.

Table 49-2   Side effects of antiparasitic agents

Generic Name	Trade Name	Toxicity
Chloroquine	Aralen*	Gastrointestinal distress is most common. Vision changes, central nervous system irritability, hemolysis can occur.
Diloxanide furoate	Furamide	Flatulence is common. Other gastrointestinal symptoms are rare.
Emetine		Gastrointestinal irritation and cardiac toxicity are common.
Furazolidone	Furoxone	Gastrointestinal distress, allergic reactions, and a disulfiram-like reaction may occur. Hemolysis is possible, especially in patients with G-6-PD deficiency.
Hydroxychloroquine	Plaquenil sulfate*	As for chloroquine.
Iodoquinol (Diiodohydroxyquin)	Yodoxin	Gastrointestinal upset and skin eruptions are most common. Blood levels of iodine may rise; optic neuritis may occur rarely.
Mebendazole	Vermox*	Abdominal discomfort may occur. Mebendazole is teratogenic in rats.
Metronidazole	Flagyl* Metryl	Gastrointestinal distress and pelvic discomfort may occur. Bone marrow suppression is possible.
Niclosamide	Niclocide	Mild gastrointestinal upset on day of therapy.
Piperazine	Antepar Vermizine	Gastrointestinal upset may occur. Skin rashes and transient neurological signs may be seen.
Povidone-iodine	Betadine*	Tissue irritation may occur with topically applied drug.

Antiparasitic Agents 579

Primaquine		Gastrointestinal distress can occur. Hemolysis may occur, especially when G-6-PD deficiency exists.
Pyrantel pamoate	Antiminth	Mild gastrointestinal upset and transient changes in liver function occur. Headaches and dizziness are more rare.
Pyrimethamine	Daraprim*	Nausea and vomiting as well as blood dyscrasias occur, especially with higher doses.
Pyrvinium pamoate	Povan	Intestinal distress occurs in some patients. Bright red drug stains teeth, intestinal contents.
Quinine	Generic*	Cinchonism is a dose-related sign of toxicity. Blood dyscrasias and pain on injection occur.
Sulfadiazine	Generic*	Gastrointestinal, allergic, and blood reactions are possible (see Chapter 46).
Sulfadoxine and pyrimethamine	Fansidar	Blood dyscrasias and allergic reactions as expected for sulfonamides (Chapter 46) or for pyrimethamine.
Sulfamethoxazole and trimethoprim	Bactrim* Septra*	Folic acid deficiency or sulfonamide toxicity may occur (see Chapter 46).
Tetracycline		Gastrointestinal distress is common (see Chapter 46).
Thiabendazole	Mintezol*	Gastrointestinal upset is common. Central nervous system effects and reduced liver function may be observed.

*Available in U.S. and Canada

Pocket Nurse Guide to Drugs

- To prevent toxoplasmosis, individuals should be instructed to avoid contact with cat feces. Pregnant women, in particular, should not empty the litter box. In addition, this disease is sometimes transmitted through food.
- For malaria prevention, medication is often prescribed on a weekly basis, starting several weeks to a month before the individual is to go to the malaria infested area. Therapy is continued for 6 weeks to 3 months after leaving the infested area. Reinforce with patients the need to continue the drug for as long as prescribed and to find a way to remember to take the drug on a weekly basis.

Chloroquine and Hydroxychloroquine

- Side effects are mild and usually reversible in antimalarial doses. In the high doses used to treat rheumatoid arthritis or lupus erythematosus, side effects are more common and may result in permanent damage. Of specific concern are retinopathy and other eye changes; patients receiving long-term therapy or high doses of these drugs should have regular ophthalmic examinations. Caution patients to report any visual changes.
- Muscular weakness may develop with long-term therapy. Assess muscle strength and ankle and knee reflexes regularly.
- Patients with a history of psoriasis may experience an exacerbation of their condition while taking these drugs.
- Taking these medications with meals may reduce gastrointestinal irritation.
- For suppression of malaria, patients should choose one day a week on which to take their medication.

Emetine

- Toxicity with emetine is cumulative and may result in degenerative changes in the heart, kidneys, liver, and other organs. Because of these changes and possible cardiac toxicity, patients should remain in bed during therapy and for several days afterward.
- Monitor the pulse and blood pressure regularly during the course of therapy. If possible, the patient could be attached to a cardiac monitor for the course of therapy, or an

Antiparasitic Agents 581

electrocardiogram should be done at least every 2 days. Assess the patient's cardiovascular functioning at regular intervals during therapy, watching for precordial chest pain, dyspnea, tachycardia, arrhythmias, gallop rhythm, palpitations, and hypotension.
- Emetine should be administered by deep subcutaneous or intramuscular injection; the intravenous route should be avoided.

Iodoquinol

- This drug may interfere with thyroid function test, and this action may persist for up to 6 months after the drug is discontinued.
- The relatively high concentration of iodine in this drug may cause certain side effects, including anal irritation and itching, skin changes, and discoloration of skin and nails.

Mebendazole

- The tablet may be chewed, swallowed, or crushed and mixed with food.
- Depending on the form of worm being treated, a single dose may be all that is necessary.

Metronidazole

- Instruct patients to avoid the use of alcohol while taking this drug.
- Caution patients that their urine may turn reddish brown during therapy.
- Patients receiving oral anticoagulants may need a reduction in dose of anticoagulant while taking metronidazole. Caution patients to report any bleeding or excessive bruising.
- If indicated, discuss with female patients the need to treat sexual partners concomitantly if *Trichomonas* in the female seems resistant to treatment or if reinfection occurs.

Intravenous Metronidazole

- Review the manufacturer's literature before preparing the dose. Preparation involves three steps: reconstitution, dilu-

582 Pocket Nurse Guide to Drugs

tion and neutralization, the last step necessary because of the low pH of the solution.

- The intravenous form is to be administered via slow infusion only; do not give via direct infusion (IV push).
- Do not use equipment containing aluminum (e.g., needles or cannulae) which could come in direct contact with the drug.

Piperazine

- It may be necessary to treat all members of a family.
- Because the worms are excreted alive, parents should be cautioned to supervise bowel elimination of children carefully for several days after therapy. The worms may be safely flushed down the toilet.

Povidone-iodine

- Patients should be questioned about possible allergy to iodine prior to use of this drug.
- Review instructions for use carefully before sending the patient home. The gel comes with an applicator, and the usual dose is one applicator full at night followed by a povidone-iodine douche in the morning. It is important that therapy continues even during the menstrual period.
- Povidone-iodine preparations will not stain the skin and are not supposed to stain clothing or bed linens.

Primaquine

- This drug should not be administered to patients who have recently received quinacrine.
- An acute intravascular hemolysis can occur in susceptible patients, especially dark-skinned individuals or blacks. Instruct patients to report any darkening or change in color in urine, which may represent hemoglobinuria.

Pyrimethamine

- Check the dosage carefully. The dose for treatment of toxoplasmosis may be 10 to 20 times as high as the recommended antimalarial dose, and thus side effects are more common.

Antiparasitic Agents 583

- Taking the drug with meals may decrease gastrointestinal irritation and vomiting.
- In usual antimalarial doses, side effects are rare, but with chronic use, folic acid deficiency may result. Symptoms of folic acid deficiency are macrocytic anemia, glossitis, diarrhea, and malabsorption.

Pyrvinium Pamoate

- This drug colors stools and vomitus red and will stain most materials.
- Tablets should be swallowed without chewing to avoid staining the teeth. For patients who cannot swallow tablets, a suspension is available.

Quinacrine

- Inform patients that the drug may cause urine and skin to turn yellow temporarily.
- Patients with a history of psoriasis may experience an exacerbation of their disease while taking this drug.
- For tapeworms, this procedure is often followed:
  a. Before receiving this drug, a cathartic and/or a cleansing enema will be ordered for patients. Some physicians will also request that patients receive a special diet for 24 to 48 hours prior to treatment.
  b. A saline cathartic should be given 1 to 2 hours after treatment. The worms passed will be stained yellow. The stool should be examined for the tapeworm scolex or head.
  c. When given through a nasogastric tube directly into the duodenum, the dose should be diluted in 100 ml of warm water and administered via the tube. The dose should be followed by additional water to flush the tube. The cathartic can be given 30 minutes later via the tube; then the tube can be removed.
  d. When given orally, the dose can be divided into 100 to 200 mg amounts and given at 10-minute intervals until the ordered dose is given. Sodium bicarbonate can be administered with each dose to help prevent nausea and vomiting.

584   Pocket Nurse Guide to Drugs

- For treatment of malaria or giardiasis, the dose should be taken after meals with a full glass of water, tea, or fruit juice.

Quinine

- Observe the patient for signs of cinchonism (see text). Instruct the patient that the physician should be notified if any of these symptoms occur.
- Intravenous dose of quinine dihydrochloride should be dissolved to a concentration of 600 mg in 300 ml, or 200 mg in 100 ml (for adults), and infused over at least a one hour period. Marked hypotension often accompanies this route of administration. Monitor the blood pressure. Administer only with the patient in a supine position. As soon as possible, the patient should be switched to oral medication.

Thiabendazole

- Central nervous system effects occur frequently. Caution patients to avoid driving, operating machinery, or engaging in other hazardous activities requiring mental alertness until the effect of the drug can be evaluated.
- Oral tablets should be chewed before swallowing and should be taken after meals. An oral suspension is also available.

ANTI-NEOPLASTICS

PART XI

Anticancer Drugs: Drugs that Directly Attack DNA

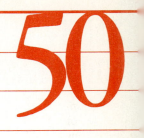

Bleomycin
Busulfan
Carmustine
Chlorambucil
Cisplatin
Cyclophosphamide
Dacarbazine
Lomustine
Mechlorethamine or nitrogen mustard
Melphalan
Mitomycin
Triethylenethiophosphoramide

Actions of Drugs that Directly Attack DNA

Alkylating agents may attack DNA by attaching various compounds to one strand or the other or by forming chemical bonds or cross links between the strands, thereby blocking replication. These actions are lethal only when cells attempt division, but the drugs do not have great specificity and thus have toxic effects on normal tissues with high growth fractions.

Indications for Drugs that Directly Attack DNA

Mechlorethamine is used to treat Hodgkin's disease and other lymphomas and selected leukemias and may be palliative for certain solid tumors and their pleural effusions. *Melphalan* is used to treat multiple myeloma, certain tumors of the reproductive tract, and malignant melanoma. *Chlorambucil* is used to treat lymphocytic leukemias, Hodgkin's disease, lymphomas, and multiple myelomas. *Cyclophosphamide* is used to treat lymphomas, lymphocytic leukemias, and myelomas. *Busulfan* may prolong life in chronic myelocytic leukemia. *Triethylenethiophosphoramide* is used in palliative therapy for certain carcinomas and rarely for lymphomas. *Carmustine* and *lomustine* are used in palliative therapy for tumors of the central nervous system, certain myelomas, and lymphomas. *Dacarbazine* is used to treat malignant melanoma and certain other solid tumors. *Cisplatin* is used for metastatic testicular cancer, genital and urinary tract tumors, and carcinomas in many tissues. *Bleomycin* is used in palliative therapy for lymphomas, squamous cell carcinomas, and testicular and ovarian cancers. *Mitomycin* is used in the treatment of tumors of the stomach, intestine, rectum, pancreas, and other tumors.

Nurse Alert for Drugs that Directly Attack DNA

- Mechlorethamine is a potent vesicant; patients and medical personnel must be carefully protected from contact by using protective clothing and gloves.
- Cancer patients often require many additional drugs to relieve disease symptoms or the side effects of therapeutic drugs; such drugs many include allopurinol to inhibit the formation of uric acid, analgesics, antiemetics, radioactive isotopes for palliative therapy or to control ascites or pleural effusions.
- Vital signs, body weight, fluid input and output records, and the progression of side effects should be monitored throughout therapy.
- Antineoplastic drugs may be mutagenic or teratogenic; they are contraindicated in pregnancy, and women receiving chemotherapy should consider birth control measures.

Side Effects of Drugs that Directly Attack DNA

Mechlorethamine causes bone marrow suppression, nausea and vomiting, arrest of spermatogenesis, menstrual irregularities, fetal toxicity, immunosuppression, and pain and severe

Table 50-1 Administration of drugs that directly attack DNA

Generic Name	Trade Name	Dosage and Administration
Mechlorethamine or nitrogen mustard	Mustargen*	INTRAVENOUS: *Adults*—0.4 mg/kg total dose in 1 or several doses. Doses range from 6 to 10 mg/M^2, depending on the disease. INTRACAVITARY: *Adults*—0.2 to 0.4 mg/kg.
Melphalan	Alkeran*	ORAL: *Adults*—0.15 mg/kg daily for 2 to 3 wk or 0.25 mg/kg daily for 4 days. After recovery of the bone marrow for 1 mo, 2 to 4 mg may be taken daily.
Chlorambucil	Leukeran*	ORAL: *Adults and children*—0.1 to 0.2 mg/kg daily for 3 to 6 wk. Smaller doses may be used for maintenance therapy.
Cyclophosphamide	Cytoxan* Neosar	ORAL: *Adults and children*—1 to 5 mg/kg daily for maintenance. INTRAVENOUS: *Adults and children*—40 to 50 mg/kg total dose over 2 to 5 days for induction of remission. 3 to 5 mg/kg twice weekly for maintenance.
Busulfan	Myleran*	ORAL: *Adults and children*—60 µg/kg daily or 1.8 mg/M^2 body surface area daily.
Triethylenethiophosphoramide	Thiotepa	INTRAVENOUS: *Adults*—0.2 mg/kg for 5 days every 4 wk. TOPICAL: *Adults*—60 mg in solution (sterile water) for application at tumor site.

Carmustine	BiCNU*	INTRAVENOUS: *Adults*—200 mg/M^2 as a single dose or divided into equal doses administered on successive days. Dose may be repeated no more frequently than every 6 wk.
Lomustine	CeeNU*	ORAL: *Adults*—130 mg/M^2 as a single dose. Repeated no more frequently than every 6 wk.
Dacarbazine	DTIC-Dome*	INTRAVENOUS: *Adults*—2 to 4.5 mg/kg for 10 days every mo or 250 mg/M^2 for 5 days every mo.
Cisplatin	Platinol*	INTRAVENOUS: *Adults*—100 mg/M^2 once every 4 wk, after heavy hydration to protect the kidneys. Doses of 20 mg/M^2 daily for 5 days, repeated at 3 wk intervals, are used when vinblastine and bleomycin are also being employed.
Bleomycin	Blenoxane*	INTRAMUSCULAR, INTRAVENOUS, SUBCUTANEOUS: *Adults*—0.25 to 0.50 units/kg weekly or twice weekly initially; decreasing to 1 unit daily or 5 units weekly for maintenance.
Mitomycin	Mutamycin*	INTRAVENOUS: *Adults*—20 mg/M^2 as a single dose or 2 mg/M^2 daily for 5 days separated by a 2-day interval. Neither schedule should be repeated more frequently than every 6 to 8 wk.

*Available in U.S. and Canada

590 **Pocket Nurse Guide to Drugs**

tissue damage if the drug leaks into surrounding tissue. *Melphalan* causes bone marrow suppression, nausea, and vomiting. *Chlorambucil* causes bone marrow suppression, and at high doses central nervous system stimulation, gastrointestinal irritation, liver toxicity, and skin reactions. *Cyclophosphamide* may cause hemorrhagic cystitis, nausea and vomiting, bone marrow suppression, alopecia, immunosuppression, suppression of the menstrual cycle and spermatogenesis, and bladder fibrosis. *Busulfan* may cause bone marrow toxic effects, hemorrhage, and fetal toxicity. *Triethylenethiophosphoramide* causes bone marrow suppression, nausea, and anorexia. *Carmustine* and *lomustine* cause delayed bone marrow suppression (onset 5-6 weeks), nausea and vomiting, and pain at injection sites, which may be severe if infusion is too rapid. *Dacarbazine* causes bone marrow suppression, nausea and vomiting, and pain and tissue damage if the drug leaks into surrounding tissue. *Cisplatin* may cause severe renal damage, nausea and vomiting, ototoxicity, neurotoxicity, and anaphylactic reactions. *Bleomycin* may cause severe, potentially fatal pulmonary toxicity, and commonly causes mucous membrane changes, fever, chills, anorexia, vomiting, anaphylaxis, and skin reactions. *Mitomycin* causes gradual and progressive bone marrow suppression, gastrointestinal irritation, alopecia, renal toxicity, liver toxicity, lung damage, and local necrosis if it contacts skin or soft tissues.

Nursing Implications for Drugs that Directly Attack DNA

General Nursing Implications

- Possible side effects should be fully discussed with the patient and family.
- The patient should understand that the appearance or severity of side effects is a gauge for determining whether the dose of the drug is adequate.
- Every patient's response to the diagnosis and treatment of cancer is unique. Employ nursing interventions as needed for the patient's emotional well-being.
- Menstrual irregularities are common with chemotherapy;

Anticancer Drugs: Drugs that Directly Attack DNA

the patient should keep a record of menstruation and report any unusual symptoms.

- General nursing implications for problems related to the chemotherapy: decreased white blood count, decreased platelet count, anemia, diarrhea, constipation, stomatitis, alopecia, nausea and vomiting, anorexia, and the extravasation of chemotherapeutic agents.

Mechlorethamine

- If the drug comes in contact with the skin, flush with copious amounts of water for 15 minutes, followed by a flush with a 2% sodium thiosulfate solution. If the solution comes in contact with the eye, irrigate with copious amounts of normal saline, then see an ophthalmologist.
- If extravasation of the drug occurs, the manufacturer recommends prompt infiltration of the area with sterile isotonic sodium thiosulfate (1/6 molar), followed by ice compresses for 6 to 12 hours. For a 1/6 molar solution of sodium thiosulfate, dilute 4 ml of Sodium Thiosulfate Injection (10%) with 6 ml of sterile water for injection. For other ways to obtain the sodium thiosulfate solution, consult the manufacturer's literature.
- The drug must be administered immediately after reconstitution. Length of administration should not exceed 5 minutes.
- This drug is one of the most powerful emetics of the chemotherapy agents. Vomiting should be anticipated.

Melphalan

- Administering the dose at night before sleep may make the nausea more tolerable.

Chlorambucil

- The drug has remarkably few side effects. Bone marrow suppression may continue for up to 10 days after the last dose.
- Monitor the uric acid level. Force fluids to 2500 to 3000 ml per day.

Cyclophosphamide

- For hemorrhagic cystitis, encourage the patient to increase the fluid intake, up to several liters per day. This will result in increased need for urination but will help dilute the drug as it passes through. In addition to drinking during the day, instruct the patient to drink a full glass of water at bedtime and, if the patients gets up to void during the night, to drink another full glass at that time. If given orally, it should be given in the morning so adequate hydration can continue all day. If given intravenously, increased hydration should continue for several days.
- Cytoxan 25 and 50 mg tablets contain FD&C yellow number 5 (tartrazine), a coloring that may cause allergic-type responses in some individuals. Whereas overall incidence is rare, persons with aspirin hypersensitivity seem to be more susceptible.
- The patient should be warned that skin and fingernails may darken during the course of therapy; this is temporary.

Busulfan

- Pulmonary reactions, including pulmonary fibrosis, can occur. This first symptom may be shortness of breath or persistent cough.
- Monitor the uric acid level. Force fluids to 2500 to 3000 ml per day.

Carmustine and Lomustine

- Carmustine often causes pain during infusion. Dilute well and administer slowly, over a one to two hour period. Too rapid infusion may produce intensive flushing of the skin and suffusion of the conjunctiva; this side effect last about 4 hours. In addition, extravasation may cause tissue necrosis.
- Accidental contact with reconstituted carmustine may cause transient hyperpigmentation of the skin.
- Administering lomustine at night may decrease the incidence of nausea and vomiting. Administer lomustine on an empty stomach.

Dacarbazine

- Anaphylaxis can occur following administration of this drug. Epinephrine, corticosteroids, antihistamines, and oxygen should be readily available, as well as necessary equipment for possible resuscitation.
- Rarely, photosensitivity has been reported. Caution patients to report any skin changes and to avoid exposure to the sun.
- Extravasation of this drug during therapy may cause pain and tissue necrosis.

Cisplatin

- Anaphylaxis can occur following administration of this drug. Epinephrine, corticosteroids, antihistamines, and oxygen should be readily available, as well as necessary equipment for possible resuscitation.
- To prevent renal toxicity, this drug is usually given concomitantly with a high volume infusion of intravenous fluids, for example, 250 to 500 ml per hour for 4 hours. Some physicians also infuse mannitol during this time. It is important that the fluid infusion not be discontinued until completed, unless the patient's condition warrants it. Monitor fluid intake and output. Monitor the effects of the large fluid volume by assessing blood pressure and pulse, auscultating breath sounds, and monitoring cardiopulmonary status. Monitor the BUN and creatinine levels to assess renal function.
- Assess the patient's hearing before each dose. Instruct the patient to report any ringing or noises in the ear or hearing loss. Hearing loss may be more severe in children. Ideally, audiometric testing should be done before the first dose is given, then on an annual or semiannual basis after that.
- Needles or intravenous infusion sets having aluminum parts that might come in contact with the medications should not be used. If in doubt about the equipment being used, contact the manufacturer.
- This drug causes severe nausea, which is often very difficult to control, even with high doses of antiemetics.

594 **Pocket Nurse Guide to Drugs**

Metoclopramide may be effective in decreasing the nausea which usually accompanies this drug.

- Peripheral neuropathy can occur. Symptoms of this would be numbness, tingling, or other unusual sensations in the extremities. Instruct the patient to report these symptoms if they occur.

Bleomycin

- The pulmonary toxicity of bleomycin is difficult to detect. The first signs and symptoms may be fine rales and dyspnea; there may be changes on the chest x-ray film. This toxicity is usually dose related (in patients receiving more than 400 units total dose) and is more common in elderly persons.
- An anaphylactic-type reaction can occur following administration of this drug. Epinephrine, corticosteroids, antihistamines, and oxygen should be readily available, as well as necessary equipment for possible resuscitation. This reaction seems to be more common in lymphoma patients, so it is suggested that these patients receive a test dose of 1 to 2 units, with the ordered dose withheld until the next day so the patient's response can be monitored.
- Fever may occur as a side effect of this drug. It may appear within a day of receiving the dose, then disappear within 24 hours. In some patients the fever occurs or recurs, accompanied by flulike symptoms, 7 to 10 days after treatment. If the fever occurs, instruct the patient to take and record the temperature every 4 hours, maintain fluid intake (at least 2500 ml per day), and to take antipyretics as ordered. If the fever persists longer than 2 days or exceeds 100° F or 38.3° C, the physician should be notified. Often, the physician will elect to treat the patient with antibiotics, since it is difficult to tell initially if the fever is drug related or due to an infection in the patient.
- Skin problems can occur with this drug, including rash, tenderness, swelling of the fingers, and vesicle formation over pressure points and the palms of the hands. Instruct the patient to report any skin changes.

Mitomycin

- To monitor renal effects, assess serum creatinine and BUN levels regularly. Monitor the fluid intake and output.
- Fever may occur as a side effect of this drug. Instruct the patient to take the temperature at regular intervals; if fever occurs, to maintain fluid intake (at least 2500 ml per day), and to take antipyretics as directed. If the fever persists longer than 2 days, or exceeds 100° F or 38.3° C, the physician should be notified. Because it is often difficult to differentiate a fever due to drug therapy from one due to infection, the physician may elect to treat the patient with antibiotics.

Anticancer Drugs: Drugs that Block DNA Synthesis

51

Cytarabine, or Ara-C
Floxuridine
Fluorouracil, or 5-FU
Hydroxyurea
Mercaptopurine
Methotrexate
Procarbazine hydrochloride
Thioguanine

Actions of Drugs that Block DNA Synthesis

Some of these drugs are enzyme inhibitors that prevent the action of an enzyme necessary for DNA synthesis; others are chemically similar to the natural purines and pyrimidines used to form DNA and may be incorporated into DNA, making it unstable and nonfunctional.

Indications for Drugs that Block DNA Synthesis

Cytarabine is used to induce and maintain remission in leukemia patients. *Fluorouracil* is used as palliative therapy for solid tumors that are incurable; topical fluorouracil is used to treat multiple actinic (solar) keratoses. *Floxuridine* is used in palliative therapy for solid tumors that are incurable. *Mercaptopurine* and *thioguanine* are used to produce remissions in leukemia, especially those of childhood. *Methotrexate* is used to treat choriocarcinoma, to maintain remission in childhood lymphoblastic leukemia, and for palliative therapy or treatment of certain lymphomas and solid tumors. *Procar-*

bazine is used for palliative therapy for Hodgkin's disease, lymphomas, and certain brain tumors and bronchogenic carcinoma. *Hydroxyurea* is used to treat melanoma, myelocytic leukemia, carcinoma of the ovary, and carcinomas of the head and neck.

Nurse Alert for Drugs that Block DNA Synthesis

- Cancer patients often require many additional drugs to relieve disease symptoms or the side effects of therapeutic drugs; such additional drugs many include allopurinol to inhibit the formation of uric acid, analgesics, antiemetics, radioactive isotopes for palliative therapy or to control ascites for pleural effusions.
- Because most antineoplastic drugs may be mutagenic or teratogenic, they are contraindicated in pregnancy; women receiving chemotherapy should consider birth control measures.
- Vital signs, body weight, and the progression of side effects should be monitored throughout therapy.

Side Effects of Drugs that Block DNA Synthesis

Cytarabine may cause nausea and vomiting, bone marrow suppression, immunosuppression, and liver toxicity. *Fluorouracil* and *floxuridine* may cause gastrointestinal and hematologic toxicity, including inflammation of the membranes of the mouth and pharynx, nausea, vomiting, diarrhea, duodenal ulcers, bowel perforation, blood dyscrasias, and alopecia; topical applications may cause pain, dermatitis, swelling, and scarring. *Mercaptopurine* and *thioguanine* commonly cause immunosuppression, bone marrow suppression, and delayed hematological toxicity. *Methotrexate* commonly causes gastrointestinal toxicity, severe damage of gastrointestinal mucosal lining, stomatitis, bowel perforation, bone marrow depression, and immunosuppression. *Procarbazine* causes bone marrow depression, gastrointestinal disturbances, and neurological reactions. *Hydroxyurea* causes bone marrow suppression, and less commonly gastrointestinal disturbances, renal impairment, and skin reactions.

Table 51-1 Administration of drugs that block DNA synthesis

Generic Name	Trade Name	Dosage and Administration
Cytarabine, or Ara-C	Cytosar*	INTRAVENOUS BOLUS: *Adults and children*—100 mg/M² daily for 10 days or until toxicity intervenes or remission occurs. INTRAVENOUS INFUSION: *Adults and children*—100 to 200 mg/M² daily for 10 days or until toxicity intervenes or remission occurs. SUBCUTANEOUS: *Adults and children*—1 mg/kg once or twice per wk.
Fluorouracil, or 5-FU	Adrucil* Efudex* Fluoroplex*	INTRAVENOUS: *Adults*—12 mg/kg for 4 days as initial therapy. Less frequent administration of the same dose is used for maintenance therapy when toxicity permits. TOPICAL: *Adults*—used as 1%, 2%, or 5% solution or cream.
Floxuridine	FUDR	INTRAARTERIAL: *Adults*—0.1 to 0.6 mg/kg over 24 hr.
Mercaptopurine	Purinethol*	ORAL: *Adults and children over 5 yr*—2.5 mg/kg/day initially. May continue for weeks if toxicity does not supervene.
Thioguanine		ORAL: *Adults*—2 mg/kg daily initially. May continue for weeks if toxicity does not supervene.
Methotrexate	Mexate	ORAL: *Adults and children*—2.5 to 25 mg daily for various lengths of time, depending on the disease.

		INTRAMUSCULAR: *Adults and children*—15 to 30 mg daily for 5 days.
		INTRAVENOUS: *Adults and children*—0.4 mg/kg daily for 4 days of therapy or twice weekly to maintain remissions.
		INTRATHECAL: *Adults and children*—0.2 to 0.5 mg/kg up to 12 mg total. Administered every 2 to 5 days until response is noted.
Procarbazine hydrochloride	Matulane	ORAL: *Adults*—100 to 200 mg daily for the first wk; then 300 mg daily until bone marrow toxicity intervenes. On recovery of marrow, drug may be continued at 50 to 100 mg daily. *Children*—doses between 50 and 100 mg daily.
Hydroxyurea	Hydrea*	ORAL: *Adults*—doses range from 20 to 30 mg/kg daily up to 80 mg/kg every 3 days. *Children*—doses not established.

*Available in U.S. and Canada

Nursing Implications for Drugs that Block DNA Synthesis

General Nursing Implications

- Possible side effects should be fully discussed with the patient and family.
- The appearance or severity of side effects is a gauge for determining whether the dosage of the drug is adequate.
- Every patient's response to the diagnosis and treatment of cancer is unique. Employ nursing interventions as needed for the patient's emotional well-being.
- Menstrual irregularities are common with chemotherapy; the patient should keep a record of menstruation.
- Other nursing implications important for problems related to chemotherapy: decreased white blood count, decreased platelet count, anemia, diarrhea, constipation, stomatitis, alopecia, nausea and vomiting, anorexia, and the extravasation of chemotherapeutic agents.

Cytarabine

- Fever may occur as a side effect of this drug. Instruct the patient to take the temperature at regular intervals: if fever occurs, maintain fluid intake (at least 2500 ml per day), and take antipyretics as directed. If the fever persists longer than 2 days, or exceeds 100° F or 38.3° C, the physician should be notified. Because it is often difficult to differentiate a fever due to drug therapy from one due to infection, the physician may elect to treat the patient with antibiotics.

Fluorouracil and Floxuridine

- Fluorouracil may be diluted and given as an infusion or as a bolus.
- Some unusual side effects that can occur include darkening of the veins where infused, tearing (increased lacrimation), and cerebellar dysfunction manifested as gait abnormalities. Skin changes have also been reported, including photosensitivity. Instruct the patient to report any skin changes and to avoid prolonged direct exposure to the sun.

Methotrexate

- There are a variety of medications that should not be taken with methotrexate, at least in the usual doses. Remind the patient to keep all health care personnel informed of all medications being taken.
- This drug is sometimes prescribed for treatment for psoriasis. The epithelium of the patient with psoriasis is dividing more rapidly than normal skin and thus may respond to the drug therapy.
- Patients taking vitamin preparations that contain folic acid may have an altered response to methotrexate.
- To monitor for renal toxicity, measure the fluid intake and output. Monitor the BUN and creatinine levels.
- Prolonged use can result in liver toxicity. Monitor liver function tests. Assess the patient for development of jaundice.
- Leucovorin rescue may be used with high dose methotrexate. The patient is kept well hydrated. The urine may be alkalinized to increase the solubility of the methotrexate; usually sodium bicarbonate is used.
- Skin rash may appear as a side effect. Some physicians feel this is a sign of toxicity and that it warrants discontinuing the drug. Instruct the patient to report any skin changes.

Procarbazine

- The patient should be cautioned to avoid the use of alcohol while receiving procarbazine. Review with the patient the disulfiram (Antabuse) type reaction that may occur if alcohol is consumed (flushing, headache, nausea, hypertension).
- Foods with a known high tyramine content should be avoided by the patient receiving procarbazine.

Hydroxyurea

- If the patient is unable to swallow capsules, the contents of the capsules may be emptied into a glass of water and taken immediately.

Anticancer Drugs: Drugs that Block RNA and Protein Synthesis

52

Asparaginase
Dactinomycin
Doxorubicin
Daunorubicin
Mithramycin

Actions of Drugs that Block RNA and Protein Synthesis

These drugs inhibit the rapid proliferation of cancer cells by blocking the formation of RNA or interfering with the use of RNA as a template for protein synthesis. Except for asparaginase, which has some selectivity, these drugs are not highly specific for cancer cells and interfere with RNA and protein synthesis in any rapidly dividing normal tissue.

Indications for Drugs that Block RNA and Protein Synthesis

Asparaginase is used to induce remission in acute lymphocytic leukemia in children. *Dactinomycin* is used to treat choriocarcinoma, Wilms' tumor, and the various sarcomas. *Doxorubicin* is used to treat leukemias, lymphomas, sarcomas, and squamous cell carcinomas of the head and neck, genitourinary carcinomas, and lung cancer. *Daunorubicin* is used for leukemias and neuroblastomas. *Mithramycin* is used

Anticancer Drugs: Drugs that Block RNA and Protein Synthesis   603

to treat embryonal cell carcinoma and certain metastatic bone tumors associated with hypercalcemia.

Nurse Alert for Drugs that Block RNA and Protein Synthesis

- Dactinomycin is a very toxic and highly corrosive drug and must be handled and administered with great care.
- Vital signs, body weight, and the progression of side effects should be monitored throughout therapy.
- Cancer patients often require many additional drugs to relieve disease symptoms or the side effects of therapeutic drugs; such additional drugs may include allopurinol to inhibit the formation of uric acid, analgesics, antiemetics, radioactive isotopes for palliative therapy or to control ascites or pleural effusions.
- Because most antineoplastic drugs may be mutagenic or teratogenic, they are contraindicated in pregnancy; women receiving chemotherapy should consider birth control measures.

Side Effects of Drugs that Block RNA and Protein Synthesis

Asparaginase may cause allergic or anaphylactic reactions, central nervous system depression, impaired renal and liver function, bleeding, and hyperglycemia. *Dactinomycin* commonly causes bone marrow depression, gastrointestinal irritation, nausea and vomiting, cheilitis, ulcerative stomatitis, dysphagia, pharyngitis, abdominal pain, proctitis, skin reactions, alopecia, hematological changes such as aplastic anemia, and erythema. *Doxorubicin* and *daunorubicin* cause bone marrow depression, gastrointestinal irritation, alopecia, heart toxicity such as ECG changes and congestive heart failure, and local necrosis if the drugs contact skin or soft tissues. *Mithramycin* causes gastrointestinal irritation, nausea and vomiting, anorexia, lowered blood concentrations of calcium, potassium, and phosphorus, skin reactions, liver and kidney toxicity, potentially life-threatening bleeding episodes, and local necrosis if it contacts skin or soft tissues.

604   Pocket Nurse Guide to Drugs

Table 52-1   Administration of drugs that block RNA and protein synthesis

Generic Name	Trade Name	Dosage and Administration
Asparaginase	Elspar	INTRAMUSCULAR: *Children*—6000 i.u./M^2 with doses administered every 3 days for one mo. INTRAVENOUS: *Adults and children*—200 i.u. (international units)/kg daily for 28 days, or 1000 i.u./kg daily for 10 days when used after prednisone and vincristine.
Dactinomycin	Cosmegen*	INTRAVENOUS: *Adults*—0.5 mg daily for no more than 5 days in succession. Recovery period must be allowed between courses of drug. *Children*—0.015 mg/kg for 5 days.
Doxorubicin	Adriamycin*	INTRAVENOUS: *Adults*—60 to 75 mg/M^2 as a single injection repeated no more often than every 4 wk.
Daunorubicin	Cerubidine*	INTRAVENOUS: 30 to 60 mg/M^2 through a running line daily for 3 days. Treatment may be repeated every 3 to 6 weeks.
Mithramycin	Mithracin	INTRAVENOUS: *Adults*—0.025 to 0.050 mg/kg every other day for 8 doses.

*Available in U.S. and Canada

Nursing Implications for Drugs that Block RNA and Protein Synthesis

General Nursing Implications

- Side effects should be fully discussed with the patient and the family.

Anticancer Drugs: Drugs that Block RNA and Protein Synthesis

- The appearance or severity of side effects is a gauge for determining whether the dose of the drug is adequate.
- Every patient's response to the diagnosis and treatment of cancer is unique. Employ nursing interventions as needed for the patient's emotional well-being.
- Menstrual irregularities are common with chemotherapy; the patient should keep a record of menstruation.
- Other patient problems requiring nursing interventions include: decreased white blood count, decreased platelet count, anemia, diarrhea, constipation, stomatitis, alopecia, nausea and vomiting, anorexia, and the extravasation of chemotherapeutic agents.

Asparaginase

- Monitor the urine and blood sugar concentrations regularly. Diabetics may find it necessary to increase insulin or oral hypoglycemic doses during therapy.
- Because of the frequency of allergic responses, it is recommended that the patient be monitored closely during asparaginase administration. Epinephrine, corticosteroids, antihistamines, and oxygen should be readily available, as well as personnel, drugs, and equipment for resuscitation. The possibility of an allergic response should be anticipated with each dose.
- Check the temperature every 4 hours during treatment as fatal hyperthermia has been reported.
- Bleeding tendencies may occur as a side effect and may be due to decreased platelets and/or decreased clotting factors. Regardless of the cause, patients should be cautioned to report any bruising or bleeding, or development of petechiae.
- Because of the high incidence of allergic reactions, it is recommended that each patient be tested prior to receiving the first dose of asparaginase. Note that a negative skin test does not completely rule out the possibility of an allergic response to the larger chemotherapy dose.
- Pancreatitis can occur as a result of therapy. Signs and symptoms might include abdominal pain, enlarged pancreas (felt as an abdominal mass), tachycardia, jaundice, and elevation of serum amylase values.

Pocket Nurse Guide to Drugs

Dactinomycin

- Extravasation should be avoided. See the patient care implications for extravasation.
- Administer over 5 minutes for intravenous push. When given as intravenous drip, administer over 1 hour.

Doxorubicin and Daunorubicin

- There is no agreement as to the best way to monitor for cardiac toxicity. Some physicians recommend monitoring the ECG for changes, and some feel the most predictive sign is persistent reductions in the QRS voltage. Other practitioners feel that echocardiography is the best tool. The toxicity is dose related. At a total dose of less than 400 mg per M^2, cardiac toxicity is rare; many physicians use 550 mg per M^2, total dose, as the highest possible dose that can be given safely. If there has been radiation to the heart, toxicity can occur at a lower dose than the values listed.

Mithramycin

- Because of the effect of this drug on calcium, potassium, and phosphorus, serum electrolyte levels should be monitored regularly.
- In addition to monitoring platelets, the prothrombin time or bleeding time should be checked. Instruct the patient to report any bleeding or bruising. Often the first sign of bleeding difficulties with this drug is a severe nosebleed or hematemesis (vomiting of blood).
- Observe the patient for possible renal failure. Monitor the fluid intake and output and regularly check the BUN and creatinine levels. The patient with a history of renal failure should receive only one half the usual dose.
- This drug can also cause liver damage. Monitor the lactic dehydrogenase (LDH) level.

Anticancer Drugs: Drugs that Block Mitosis

53

Vincristine sulfate, or VCR
Vinblastine sulfate, or VLB
Etoposide

Actions of Drugs that Block Mitosis

Vincristine and vinblastine arrest mitosis and cell division by disrupting the structure of the microtubules that compose the mitotic spindle of a dividing cell, ultimately causing the death of these cells. Etoposide prevents cells from entering mitosis.

Indications for Drugs that Block Mitosis

Vincristine is used to treat acute leukemia, lymphomas, various sarcomas, and Wilms' tumor. *Vinblastine* is used in palliative treatment of various lymphomas and selected carcinomas of other tissues. *Etoposide* is used for refractory testicular tumors, leukemias, and small-cell lung carcinoma.

Nurse Alert for Drugs that Block Mitosis

- Vital signs, body weight, and the progression of side effects should be monitored throughout therapy.
- Additional drugs that relieve disease symptoms or the side effects of therapeutic drugs; may include: allopurinol to inhibit the formation of uric acid, analgesics, antiemetics, radioactive isotopes for palliative therapy or to control ascites or pleural effusions.

608 Pocket Nurse Guide to Drugs

- Antineoplastic drugs are contraindicated in pregnancy; women receiving chemotherapy should consider birth control measures.

Side Effects of Drugs that Block Mitosis

Vincristine causes alopecia, abdominal pain, constipation, peripheral neuropathy, and local necrosis if it comes in contact with skin or other soft tissue. *Vinblastine* causes bone marrow suppression, peripheral neuropathy, mental depression, headache, nausea and vomiting, stomatitis, diarrhea, constipation, alopecia, and local necrosis in contact with skin or soft tissue. *Etoposide* causes bone marrow suppression.

Nursing Implications for Drugs that Block Mitosis
General Nursing Implications

- Side effects should be fully discussed with the patient and family.

Table 53-1   Administration of drugs that block mitosis

Generic Name	Trade Name	Dosage and Administration
Vincristine, or VCR	Oncovin*	INTRAVENOUS: *Adults*—1.4 mg/M^2 as a single dose. *Children*— 2 mg/M^2 as a single dose.
Vinblastine, or VLB	Velban Velbe†	INTRAVENOUS: *Adults*—0.15 to 0.2 mg/kg once weekly. Doses must start at 0.1 mg/kg and increase gradually. Final dose is limited by bone marrow toxicity.
Etoposide VP-16	VePesid*	ORAL: *Adults*—100 mg/M^2 daily for 5 days. *Children*—dose has not been established. INTRAVENOUS: *Adults*—50 to 75 mg/M^2 daily for 5 days. *Children*—dose has not been established.

*Available in U.S. and Canada
†Available in Canada only

Anticancer Drugs: Drugs that Block Mitosis **609**

- The appearance or severity of side effects is a gauge for determining whether the dose of the drug is adequate.
- Every patient's response to the diagnosis and treatment of cancer is unique. Employ nursing interventions as needed for the patient's emotional well-being.
- Menstrual irregularities are common with chemotherapy; the patient should keep a record of menstruation and report any unusual symptoms.
- Other patient problems requiring nursing interventions include: decreased white blood count, decreased platelet count, anemia, diarrhea, constipation, stomatitis, alopecia, nausea and vomiting, anorexia, and the extravasation of chemotherapeutic agents.

Vincristine

- To monitor for peripheral neuropathy, check deep tendon reflexes, sensory loss, gait abnormalities. Instruct the patient to report any unusual sensations, tingling, or numbness of the feet or hands.
- In addition to constipation, this drug can cause paralytic ileus, especially in children. Keep a record of the frequency of bowel movements. Auscultate for the presence of bowel sounds before each meal.
- The routine use of a stool softener, starting before the vincristine is administered, is usually necessary.
- An unusual side effect that can occur with this drug is jaw pain.
- Orthostatic hypotension can occur after long-term use. Caution patients to move slowly from lying to sitting or standing positions. If, on changing position quickly, the patient feels dizzy or lightheaded, the patient should sit or lie down.

Vinblastine

- Orthostatic hypotension can occur after long-term use. Caution patients to move slowly from lying to sitting or standing positions. If, on changing positions quickly, the patient feels dizzy or lightheaded, the patient should sit or lie down.
- Jaw pain can occur as an unusual side effect of this drug.

610   Pocket Nurse Guide to Drugs

Etoposide

- Peripheral neuropathy has been reported. Instruct the patient to report any numbness, tingling, or other unusual sensations of the fingers, hands, or feet.
- Orthostatic hypotension has been reported. Instruct the patient to move slowly from a lying to sitting or standing position. If the patient feels dizzy or lightheaded on arising, the patient should sit or lie down. In the hospital, it might be appropriate to monitor the blood pressure.
- Blood pressure should be taken every 15 minutes during the administration of this drug.
- Anaphylaxis can occur with VP-16. Epinephrine, corticosteroids, antihistamines, and oxygen should be readily available, as well as personnel, drugs, and equipment for resuscitation.
- Administer the prescribed dose over at least one hour to decrease the side effect of hypotension.
- Contact with the skin should be avoided. Personnel preparing this drug should wear gloves.

Drugs to Control Cancer of Specific Tissues

54

Androgens
    Dromostanolone propionate
    Testolactone
Estrogens
    Polyestradiol phosphate
    Diethylstilbestrol diphosphate
    Estramustine phosphate
    sodium
Antiestrogens
    Tamoxifen

Progestins
    Megestrol acetate
    Medroxyprogesterone acetate
Glucocorticoids
    Prednisone
Adrenal antagonist
    Mitotane
    Streptozocin

Actions of Drugs to Control Cancer of Specific Tissues

These drugs are effective anticancer agents because they interact with specific receptors on or in certain cells. The drugs derived from hormones interact with cells bearing specific receptors for the hormone. The sex steroids enter sensitive cells and are transported to the cell nucleus, where they alter RNA and protein synthesis and thus change the cell function. The glucocorticoids suppress lymphoid tissue by acting on the specific receptors in that tissue for glucocorticoids.

Indications for Drugs to Control Cancer of Specific Tissues

Dromostanolone and *testolactone* are used in palliative therapy for selected carcinomas of the breast in postmeno-

611

pausal women. *Polyestradiol* and *diethylstilbestrol* are used in palliative therapy for prostatic carcinoma. *Estramustine* is used for palliative treatment for selective carcinomas of the breast. *Tamoxifen* is used in palliative treatment for advanced carcinoma of the breast. *Megestrol* is used in palliative therapy for advanced carcinoma of the breast or endometrium. *Medroxyprogesterone* is used in palliative therapy for advanced carcinoma of the endometrium or kidney. *Prednisone* is used to treat lymphoblastic leukemias and lymphomas, especially in children. *Mitotane* is used to control adrenal cortical carcinoma. *Streptozocin* is used in treatment of insulin-secreting islet cell tumors of the pancreas.

Nurse Alert for Drugs to Control Cancer of Specific Tissues

- Vital signs, body weight, and the progression of side effects should be monitored throughout therapy.
- Additional drugs used to relieve disease symptoms or the side effects of therapeutic drugs may include: allopurinol to inhibit the formation of uric acid, analgesics, antiemetics, radioactive isotopes for palliative therapy or to control ascites or pleural effusions.
- Antineoplastic drugs are contraindicated in pregnancy; women receiving chemotherapy should consider birth control measures.

Side Effects of Drugs to Control Cancers of Specific Tissues

Both *dromostanolone* and *testolactone* may cause virilism, increased libido, nausea, edema, hypercalcemia, and pain and irritation at the injection site. *Polyestradiol* and *diethylstilbestrol* may cause edema, hypercalcemia, mood changes, breast tenderness, abdominal cramps, increased pigmentation of breast areola, nausea and vomiting, and increased risk of thromboembolic disease. *Estramustine* may produce the same toxicity as other estrogens (see also Ch. 39), and may include adverse reactions to the nitrogen mustard component. *Tamox-*

ifen may cause hot flashes, nausea and vomiting, vaginal discharge or bleeding, menstrual disturbances, and skin rashes. *Megestrol* increases the risk of breast cancer and thromboembolic disease. *Medroxyprogesterone* causes menstrual irregularities, breast tenderness, rashes, and increased risk of thrombolytic disease. Both of these progestins may also cause vision changes, fluid retention, and pain and tissue changes at the injection site. *Prednisone* causes the symptoms of glucocorticoid excess (see Ch. 36) and in long-term use may produce Cushing's syndrome. *Mitotane* commonly causes gastrointestinal disturbances, central nervous system toxicity, lethargy or dizziness, changes in blood pressure, abnormalities of the eye, hemorrhagic cystitis, and skin reactions. *Streptozocin* causes renal toxicity.

Nursing Implications for Drugs to Control Cancers of Specific Tissues

General Nursing Implications

- Side effects should be fully discussed with the patient and family.
- The appearance or severity of side effects is a gauge for determining whether the dose of the drug is adequate.
- Every patient's response to the diagnosis and treatment of cancer is unique. Employ nursing interventions as needed for the patient's emotional well-being.
- Menstrual irregularities are common with chemotherapy; the patient should keep a record of menstruation and report any unusual symptoms.
- Other nursing implications important for problems related to the chemotherapy: decreased white blood count, decreased platelet count, anemia, diarrhea, constipation, stomatitis, alopecia, nausea and vomiting, anorexia, and the extravasation of chemotherapeutic agents.

Androgens and Estrogens

- Patient care implications for these categories of drugs are discussed in Chapters 44 and 39.

Table 54-1   Administration of drugs to control cancer of specific tissues

Generic Name	Trade Name	Dosage and Administration
Androgens		
Dromostanolone propionate	Drolban	INTRAMUSCULAR: *Adults*—100 mg 3 times weekly for 8 to 12 wk.
Testolactone	Teslac	ORAL: *Adults*—250 mg 4 times daily for 12 wk. INTRAMUSCULAR: *Adults*—100 mg 3 times weekly for 12 wk.
Estrogens		
Polyestradiol phosphate	Estradurin	INTRAMUSCULAR (DEEP): *Adults*—40 to 80 mg every 2 to 4 wk for at least 3 mo.
Diethylstilbestrol diphosphate	Stilphostrol	INTRAVENOUS: *Adults*—500 mg in 300 ml of saline or 5% dextrose on the first day; 1 Gm/300 ml diluent for subsequent 5 days or longer. Maintain with 250 to 500 mg IV once or twice weekly thereafter, or with oral dosage. ORAL: *Adults*—50 to 200 mg 3 times daily.
Estramustine phosphate sodium	EMCYT*	ORAL: One 140 mg capsule for each 10 kg body weight daily in 3 or 4 doses. Therapy continues for 30 to 90 days or longer.
Antiestrogens		
Tamoxifen	Nolvadex*	ORAL: *Adults*—10 or 20 mg twice daily.

Drugs to Control Cancer of Specific Tissues

Progestins		
Megestrol acetate	Megace*	ORAL: *Adults*—40 to 320 mg daily in divided doses for at least 2 mo for endometrial carcinoma; 160 mg daily, divided into 4 doses, for breast cancer.
Medroxyprogesterone acetate	Depo-Provera*	INTRAMUSCULAR: *Adults*—400 to 1000 mg in weekly injections.
Glucocorticoids		
Prednisone	Deltasone* Meticorten	ORAL: *Adults and children*—10 to 100 mg daily.
Adrenal Antagonist		
Mitotane	Lysodren*	ORAL: *Adults*—6 to 15 mg/kg initially, daily in 3 or 4 doses. Daily dose may be increased gradually to 2 to 16 Gm.
Pancreatic Antagonist		
Streptozocin	Zanosar	INTRAVENOUS: 1 to 1.5 Gm/M² weekly or 500 mg/M² daily for 5 days at 6 week intervals.

*Available in U.S. and Canada

616 **Pocket Nurse Guide to Drugs**

Tamoxifen

- Decreases in the platelet count of 50,000 to 100,000 have been reported, but this is rarely associated with bleeding problems.
- Hypercalcemia may occur, usually in patients with bone metastases.
- Other side effects include hot flashes and abnormal uterine bleeding. Instruct the patient to report any vaginal bleeding or discharge.
- Fluid retention may be a problem. Have the patient check weight at regular intervals. Monitor the blood pressure.
- At high doses, there may be retinal changes, eventually leading to areas of blindness. Before beginning therapy, the patient should have a visual field examination, and an ophthalmological examination on a yearly basis.

Progestins

- See Ch. 40 for nursing implications.

Glucocorticoids

- See Ch. 36 for nursing implications.

Mitotane

- Treatment with mitotane may cause drowsiness and decreased mental alertness. Caution patients to avoid hazardous activities requiring mental alertness (e.g., driving, operating machinery) until the effects of the drug can be evaluated.
- Monitor the blood pressure every 4 hours for hypertension. Orthostatic hypotension can also occur. Instruct the patient to move slowly from lying to sitting or standing positions. Symptoms of hypotension include dizziness, lightheadedness, and syncope. If the patient feels dizzy, the patient should sit or lie down.
- Visual side effects include blurring of vision, diplopia, and lens opacities. Caution the patient to report any visual changes. Test for visual acuity on a regular basis.

Streptozocin

- Monitor blood and urine sugar levels, as hyperglycemia has been reported. Diabetics may find it necessary to increase the dose of insulin or oral hypoglycemic agents while receiving therapy.
- Renal damage may be a problem. Monitor the fluid intake and output. Monitor the BUN, serum creatinine, and urinary protein levels.

APPENDIX A

Representative Common Drug Interactions

Pocket Nurse Guide to Drugs

Drug or Drug Classes Interacting	Mechanism and Result of Interaction	Comment
Acetaminophen and alcohol (ethanol)	Chronic alcohol abuse and high doses of acetaminophen both damage the liver. Additive effects of these agents may be fatal.	This interaction is most important for alcoholics with liver damage from chronic alcohol ingestion.
Acetaminophen and chloramphenicol	Acetaminophen may increase the elimination half-life of chloramphenicol. As a result, chloramphenicol may accumulate, increasing the risk of dose-dependent bone marrow suppression.	This interaction can usually be avoided by selecting an alternative agent for one of the drugs.
Alcohol (ethanol) and barbiturates or chloral hydrate (sedative-hypnotics)	Central nervous system depression caused by alcohol may greatly enhance the action of other depressant drugs leading to severely impaired motor activity, unconsciousness, respiratory depression, and death, as the dose increases.	In addition to sedative-hypnotics, many other classes of drugs may produce this interaction: Antihistamines producing marked sedation alone, e.g. diphenhydramine or chlorpheniramine; Benzodiazepines, especially diazepam; Meprobamate;

		Opioids, such as morphine and codeine; Phenothiazines, especially chlorpromazine; Phenylbutazone; Propoxyphene; Tricyclic antidepressants, especially amitriptyline.
Alcohol (ethanol) and disulfiram	Disulfiram blocks metabolism of ethanol, leading to accumulation of toxic metabolites. Symptoms are flushing, hypotension, headache, nausea, and difficulty in breathing. Some sensitive persons experience more serious cardiovascular reactions.	This very striking interaction with ethanol is observed with several drugs in addition to disulfiram: Cefamandole, cefoperazone, and moxalactam; Chlorpropamide, a sulfonylurea; Procarbazine; Metronidazole.
Allopurinol and dicumarol or warfarin (anticoagulants)	Allopurinol may interfere with the metabolism of the anticoagulants by enzyme systems in the liver. As a result, the anticoagulants accumulate and may cause dangerous bleeding episodes.	Only a few patients may show this serious interaction but all patients receiving both drugs should be carefully watched for excessive action of the anticoagulant.

cont'd. next page

Pocket Nurse Guide to Drugs

Drug or Drug Classes Interacting	Mechanism and Result of Interaction	Comment
Allopurinol and cyclophosphamide or mercaptopurine (cytotoxic anticancer drugs)	Allopurinol is chemically related to cytotoxic nucleotide analogs and may have additive effects with other cytotoxic agents. The result is excessive toxicity as if from an overdose of the anticancer drug.	Allopurinol is often administered to cancer patients to prevent excess uric acid formation. Doses of the anticancer agents listed may need to be reduced when allopurinol is added.
Aspirin (salicylates) and antacids	Antacids may promote excretion of salicylates by alkalinizing the urine. Antacids such as sodium bicarbonate or magnesium aluminum hydroxide can reduce salicylate concentrations in blood to subtherapeutic levels.	This interaction is most important for those patients receiving high doses of salicylates for extended periods.
Aspirin (salicylates) and dicumarol or warfarin (anticoagulants)	Aspirin interferes with platelet aggregation and thus has anticoagulant activity even at low doses. The additive effects of aspirin with other potent anticoagulants may cause serious bleeding, a reaction intensified by the tendency of aspirin to cause gastrointestinal bleeding.	This interaction is most important for patients regularly receiving anticoagulants who begin regular dosing with aspirin.
Aspirin (salicylates) and	Salicylates induce gastrointestinal	Several drugs may irritate the

gastrointestinal irritants	bleeding which may worsen the effects of other irritant drugs. Glucocorticoids may mask the symptoms of ulceration and may allow perforation or hemorrhage to occur before the condition is noticed.	gastrointestinal mucosa enough to cause bleeding or even ulceration: Alcohol; Glucocorticoids; Phenylbutazone.
Aspirin (salicylates) and probenecid or sulfinpyrazone (uricosuric agents)	The ability of both drugs to promote uric acid excretion is diminished when the drugs are combined.	Patients should not receive aspirin and probenecid or sulfinpyrazone concurrently.
Chloramphenicol and phenytoin	Chloramphenicol inhibits enzymes in the liver that metabolize phenytoin. As a result, phenytoin elimination may be impaired and the drug may accumulate to toxic levels.	During acute therapy with chloramphenicol, patients on phenytoin should be carefully monitored to prevent toxicity. Some physicians prefer to choose an alternative antibiotic, if possible.
Chlordiazepoxide, diazepam, flurazepam, lorazepam (benzodiazepines) and central nervous system depressants	Central nervous system depression produced by benzodiazepines is additive with that of other drugs. The result may be dangerous and potentially fatal central nervous system depression.	Benzodiazepines may cause this interaction with: Alcohol; Antihistamines; Antipsychotic drugs; Barbiturates; Opiate analgesics; Tricyclic antidepressants.

cont'd. next page

Drug or Drug Classes Interacting	Mechanism and Result of Interaction	Comment
Chlorthalidone, ethacrynic acid, furosemide, or thiazides (potassium-depleting diuretics) and corticosteroids	Both corticosteroids and the diuretics listed can cause loss of potassium from the body over a period of time.	Potassium supplements may be required to prevent severe depletion.
Cimetidine and chlordiazepoxide or diazepam (benzodiazepines)	Cimetidine seems to inhibit the liver enzymes that degrade diazepam and chlordiazepoxide. Patients on cimetidine who then receive one of these benzodiazepines might be expected to accumulate the benzodiazepine and show excessive drowsiness, ataxia, and other signs of benzodiazepine overdose.	This interaction does not occur with oxazepam or lorazepam because these benzodiazepines are not metabolized by the liver in the same way as diazepam and chlordiazepoxide. Patients should be warned about driving or carrying out other hazardous tasks when receiving cimetidine and diazepam or chlordiazepoxide.
Cimetidine and dicumarol or warfarin (anticoagulants)	Cimetidine is an inhibitor of liver enzymes that metabolize many of the anticoagulants. Therefore, cimetidine causes accumulation of the anticoagulants, increasing the risk of overdose and bleeding.	This interaction makes careful monitoring of prothrombin times necessary when a person who has been stabilized on an anticoagulant has cimetidine added.

Representative Common Drug Interactions 625

Cimetidine and phenytoin	Cimetidine may inhibit the liver enzymes that metabolize phenytoin, leading to phenytoin accumulation and intoxication.	Symptoms of phenytoin intoxication are often mild but additive; bone marrow depression with cimetidine is also possible. Phenytoin blood levels may need monitoring.
Cimetidine and propranolol (beta-adrenergic receptor blocker)	Cimetidine is an inhibitor of liver enzymes that may metabolize many beta-adrenergic blocking agents. Propranolol concentrations are elevated when cimetidine is also administered; dangerous bradycardia has resulted.	In addition to propranolol, other similarly metabolized beta-adrenergic blocking agents may cause similar interactions.
Cimetidine and theophylline	Cimetidine inhibits the enzymes in the liver that metabolize theophylline, causing accumulation and theophylline toxicity.	This interaction may require that theophylline levels be monitored during cimetidine therapy to prevent theophylline toxicity.
Clofibrate and dicumarol or warfarin (anticoagulants)	Clofibrate greatly enhances the anticoagulant activity of warfarin and dicumarol by displacing the anticoagulants from plasma-binding proteins and possibly by other mechanisms.	Doses of the anticoagulants may need to be reduced significantly to avoid dangerous overdosage and bleeding.

cont'd. next page

Pocket Nurse Guide to Drugs

Drug or Drug Classes Interacting	Mechanism and Result of Interaction	Comment
Dicumarol and chlorpropamide or tolbutamide (sulfonylureas)	Metabolism of the sulfonylureas may be reduced. The drugs may also compete for plasma protein-binding sites. Both actions tend to increase blood concentrations of active sulfonylurea. The most commonly reported result is an acute hypoglycemic reaction.	This interaction may be controlled by using a different anticoagulant or by carefully monitoring blood concentrations of the drugs.
Digoxin (digitalis glycoside) and chlorthalidone, ethacrynic acid, furosemide, or thiazides (potassium-depleting diuretics)	Since hypokalemia (low blood potassium) increases the likelihood of digitalis toxicity, concurrent use of digitalis preparations and one of the potassium-depleting diuretics may lead to dangerous cardiac arrhythmias.	This interaction may be prevented by using a potassium supplement.
Digoxin (digitalis glycoside) and quinidine or quinine	Quinidine and its chemical relative quinine slow renal excretion of digoxin, which may double serum concentrations of digoxin and lead to digoxin toxicity.	These drugs should be used together only if serum concentrations of digoxin can be carefully monitored.
Doxycycline and phenobarbital	Barbiturates can induce enzymes in the	Other tetracyclines are eliminated to a

	liver that may aid in eliminating doxycycline from the body. As a result, doxycycline metabolism may increase and inadequate concentrations of the antibiotic may appear in blood.	greater degree by renal mechanisms and are therefore less likely to suffer from this interaction.
Erythromycin and theophylline	Patients receiving high doses of theophylline may accumulate toxic concentrations of theophylline when erythromycin is also added. The mechanism is unknown.	This interaction seems most important for patients receiving high doses, but all patients receiving both drugs should be watched closely for theophylline toxicity.
Furosemide and phenytoin	The diuretic activity of a fixed dose of furosemide may be drastically reduced in a patient receiving phenytoin. The mechanism is not understood.	Increased doses of furosemide may be required to maintain control of symptoms.
Gentamicin and ethacrynic acid or furosemide (loop diuretics)	The loop diuretics and the aminoglycoside antibiotics are both capable of impairing balance and causing hearing loss. When given together, especially in high doses, the risk of ototoxicity seems to be greater.	Although this interaction is best documented with gentamicin, it is also a possibility with other aminoglycosides (amikacin, kanamycin, neomycin, netilmicin, streptomycin, tobramycin).

cont'd. next page

Drug or Drug Classes Interacting	Mechanism and Result of Interaction	Comment
Indomethacin and propranolol or thiazides (antihypertensives)	Indomethacin elevates blood pressure and interferes with the adequate control of hypertension by a variety of drugs.	Blood pressure control needs to be carefully monitored in hypertensive patients who are given indomethacin.
Levodopa and chlordiazepoxide or diazepam (benzodiazepines)	Some patients receiving both drugs lose the antiparkinsonian action of levodopa. The mechanism of this interaction is not known.	Patients receiving both drugs should be closely observed to assure that parkinsonian symptoms are being adequately controlled.
Methyldopa and lithium carbonate	Lithium tends to accumulate in the blood of patients receiving methyldopa. The brain may also be sensitized to the effects of lithium.	Serum concentrations of lithium may need monitoring in patients receiving methyldopa.
Methyldopa and levodopa	Each of these drugs may enhance the effects of the other by unknown mechanisms. Side effects of levodopa may also worsen.	Doses of either or both drugs may need to be reduced.
Methyltestosterone or methandrostenolone (anabolic steroids) and dicumarol or warfarin (anticoagulants)	Anabolic steroids may enhance the anticoagulant effects of warfarin or dicumarol, possibly by effects on metabolism. The result is an increased risk of bleeding episodes.	This interaction should be expected and the dose of anticoagulant reduced accordingly.

Oral contraceptives and barbiturates, phenytoin, or primidone (anticonvulsants)	The anticonvulsants may induce liver enzymes that degrade the steroid components of oral contraceptives. The result may be unexpected pregnancy.	Break-through bleeding may signal contraceptive failure. Mechanical contraception may be required, although some women may be protected with different doses of oral contraceptives.
Oral contraceptives and rifampin	Rifampin may induce enzymes in the liver that metabolize the steroid components of progestin-only or combined estrogen-progestin oral contraceptives. The result may be unexpected pregnancy.	Other antibiotics may also increase the failure rate of oral contraceptives: Penicillins, especially ampicillin; Tetracyclines, e.g. oxytetracycline.
Phenobarbital and dicumarol or warfarin (anticoagulants)	Barbiturates can induce enzymes in the liver that metabolize the anticoagulants. As a result, the effect of the anticoagulant is reduced or lost.	Many physicians would prefer to avoid the interaction by substituting another drug for the barbiturate.
Phenobarbital and sodium valproate	Sodium valproate increases the serum concentrations of phenobarbital by an unknown mechanism. As a result, excessive sedation can occur.	When these drugs are combined to treat epilepsy, doses of phenobarbital may need to be reduced.

cont'd. next page

Drug or Drug Classes Interacting	Mechanism and Result of Interaction	Comment
Phenylbutazone and acetohexamide, chlorpropamide, glyburide, or tolbutamide (hypoglycemic agents)	Phenylbutazone may lower excretion, metabolism, and protein binding of the hypoglycemic agents. These actions may result in accumulation of the hypoglycemic agents and may trigger an acute hypoglycemic reaction.	The same effect may be produced by oxyphenbutazone, a metabolite of phenylbutazone.
Phenylbutazone and dicumarol or warfarin (anticoagulants)	Phenylbutazone and its metabolite oxyphenbutazone can displace the anticoagulants from plasma protein binding sites and may also interfere with metabolism of the anticoagulants. These actions greatly enhance the anticoagulant activity of fixed doses of dicumarol or warfarin and may cause dangerous bleeding.	This interaction is so well documented and potentially so serious that many physicians choose not to use these drugs together.
Phenytoin and dicumarol or warfarin (anticoagulants)	Phenytoin toxicity may be enhanced and anticoagulant drug effect may be either diminished or enhanced as a result of multiple interacting effects on metabolism.	The possibility of this interaction requires that the clinical effects of both drugs be carefully monitored during therapy.

Phenytoin and disulfiram	Disulfiram may inhibit enzymes in the liver that metabolize phenytoin. As a result, phenytoin may accumulate to toxic levels.	This interaction would normally be avoided by withholding disulfiram, or possibly by substituting a different anticonvulsant.
Phenytoin and folic acid	Folic acid deficiency can occur in patients chronically receiving anticonvulsants. Attempts to supplement with folic acid may hasten the metabolic clearance of the anticonvulsants. The result is lower blood concentrations of the anticonvulsant with the danger of loss of seizure control.	This interaction may also occur between folic acid and primidone.
Phenytoin and isoniazid	Isoniazid inhibits the enzymes in the liver that metabolize phenytoin. As a result, serum concentrations of phenytoin can rise to dangerous levels.	Patients receiving both drugs should be carefully monitored for accumulation of phenytoin. Slow acetylators of isoniazid are more at risk of this interaction than are fast acetylators.

cont'd. next page

632 Pocket Nurse Guide to Drugs

Drug or Drug Classes Interacting	Mechanism and Result of Interaction	Comment
Phenytoin and phenylbutazone	Phenylbutazone displaces phenytoin from plasma protein-binding sites and inhibits the metabolism of phenytoin by enzymes in the liver. Both actions tend to increase the serum concentration of active phenytoin. Serious accumulation and toxicity can result.	Phenytoin dosage may need to be reduced to avoid toxicity when both drugs are administered. Oxyphenbutazone, a metabolite of phenylbutazone, is presumed to behave similarly to the parent drug.
Phenytoin and sulfamethoxazole (sulfonamides)	Sulfonamides can interfere with enzyme systems in the liver that metabolize phenytoin. As a result, phenytoin may accumulate to dangerous levels.	This interaction is best documented with sulfamethoxazole and the preparation of sulfamethoxazole combined with trimethoprim. The interaction is best avoided by selecting an alternate antibiotic. If a sulfonamide must be used, care should be taken to monitor phenytoin blood levels.
Propoxyphene and carbamazepine	Propoxyphene raises serum levels of carbamazepine by unknown mechanisms. The result may be excessive carbamazepine toxicity.	This interaction is often avoided by substituting a different analgesic for propoxyphene.

Interacting drugs	Mechanism	Comments
Propranolol and epinephrine	Beta-adrenergic block drugs like propranolol which block both beta-1 and beta-2 receptors prevent beta-adrenergic stimulation of the heart by direct-acting sympathomimetics. With epinephrine the remaining unopposed alpha-adrenergic effects may drastically slow the heart.	This interaction is more likely with the non-selective beta-adrenergic blocking drugs.
Propranolol and insulin or sulfonylureas (hypoglycemic agents)	Propranolol may increase the frequency of serious hypoglycemic reactions, and may mask the tachycardia that often warns of impending hypoglycemia.	Diabetic patients receiving any non-selective beta-adrenergic blocking drug should be warned of the increased risk of insidious onset of hypoglycemia.
Propranolol and verapamil	These drugs depress contractility of the heart by independent mechanisms. Given together, depression of cardiac function may be severe.	Propranolol is a relative contraindication for the use of verapamil. Other beta-adrenergic blockers may show the same interaction.

cont'd. next page

Drug or Drug Classes Interacting	Mechanism and Result of Interaction	Comment
Quinidine and barbiturates, phenytoin, or primidone (anticonvulsants)	The anticonvulsants may increase enzymes in the liver that metabolize quinidine. Therefore, quinidine is rapidly removed from the body and the antiarrhythmic effect may be lost.	This interaction is especially dangerous during the periods when the anticonvulsant is started or withdrawn from a patient who has been stabilized on a set dose of quinidine.
Rifampin and digitoxin (digitalis glycoside)	Rifampin induces drug-metabolizing enzymes in the liver, thereby increasing elimination of digitoxin. As a result, the serum concentration of digitoxin falls, with concurrent loss of digitalis action.	This interaction requires the patients receiving both drugs be carefully watched for signs that the digitalis effect is being lost.
Theophylline and ephedrine	When used together to treat asthma, these drugs are no more effective than theophylline alone, but seem to produce additive toxicity. The mechanism is unknown.	This combination offers no advantage and the potential for disadvantages. Therefore, the direct combination should be avoided.
Thiazide diuretics or chlorthalidone and insulin or sulfonylureas (hypoglycemic agents)	Thiazide and related diuretics raise blood glucose concentrations, which may impair diabetic control.	These drugs can be used together so long as the dose of the hypoglycemic agent is adjusted to maintain diabetic control.

Representative Common Drug Interactions 635

Drug combination	Mechanism	Management
Thiazide diuretics or chlorthalidone and lithium carbonate	Lithium concentrations in the blood are raised by the concurrent use of thiazide or related diuretics. Dangerous accumulation of lithium may result over a long period of time.	Lithium levels in the blood must be carefully monitored if thiazides or related diuretics are also administered.
Thyroid hormones and dicumarol or warfarin (anticoagulants)	Thyroid hormones seem to increase the rate of breakdown of blood factors. The anticoagulants inhibit synthesis of the factors. Combining the drugs results in a marked anticoagulant effect that may lead to dangerous bleeding episodes.	Patients must be closely monitored when adjusting the dose of anticoagulant in a patient receiving thyroid hormones, or when adding thyroid hormones, in a patient previously stabilized on a dose of anticoagulant.
Tolbutamide and chloramphenicol or rifampin	Chloramphenicol and rifampin inhibit enzymes in the liver that metabolize tolbutamide. As a result, tolbutamide accumulates and acute hypoglycemia may occur.	Many physicians prefer to avoid the interaction when possible by substituting another antibiotic. Chlorpropamide and possibly other sulfonylureas may behave similarly to tolbutamide.

cont'd. next page

Drug or Drug Classes Interacting	Mechanism and Result of Interaction	Comment
Warfarin and barbiturates, griseofulvin, or rifampin	Barbiturates, rifampin, and possibly griseofulvin may induce enzymes in the liver that metabolize warfarin. As a result, warfarin is eliminated more rapidly and adequate anticoagulation may be lost.	Warfarin doses may be increased to offset the effects of increased metabolism but there is risk of bleeding if the inducing drugs are suddenly withdrawn.
Warfarin and metronidazole or sulfamethoxazole/trimethoprim	Metronidazole inhibits the enzymes in the liver that metabolize warfarin whereas sulfamethoxazole/trimethoprim may have other effects. Both antimicrobial preparations markedly enhance the anticoagulant activity of warfarin.	This interaction should be expected when warfarin is combined with either antimicrobial agent. Doses of warfarin should be reduced to prevent dangerous bleeding episodes.
Warfarin and sulindac	Sulindac in some way enhances the anticoagulant activity of warfarin and possibly other anticoagulants. Bleeding may result.	For some patients reducing the dosage of warfarin may control the interaction. Others may require discontinuation of the sulindac.

APPENDIX B

Vaccines Useful in Preventing Bacterial or Rickettsial Diseases

Disease	Characteristics of Vaccine	When Administered
Bubonic plague	Inactivated *Yersinia pestis* confers immunity.	Administered during outbreaks, or to persons heavily exposed. Injections are normally spaced over 4 to 12 mo, with a booster as needed to protect against continued exposure.
Cholera	Killed strains of *Vibrio cholerae* confer resistance.	Used for persons entering a country where cholera is known to exist.
Diphtheria, Tetanus, and Pertussis (whopping cough)	This combination known as DTP contains adsorbed toxoids and a vaccine to protect against all three illnesses.	Given routinely in four doses to children between the ages of 2 mo and 7 yr, at fixed intervals. Additional protection may be needed against tetanus in the event of injury.
Meningitis	Meningococcal polysaccharide mixtures give protection against Group A, Group C, or both serogroups.	Only for outbreaks or for exposed persons who also receive antibiotics to protect against infections by the more common serogroup B.
Pneumococcal pneumonia	Mixed capsular material from cultured pneumococci confers resistance to lobar pneumonia and bacteremia caused by one of the strains used as a source of capsular material.	Given only to high-risk patients such as those with chronic organ dysfunction, weak convalescents, or those older than 50 years of age.

Tetanus and Diphtheria	Mixed adsorbed toxoids, called Td, are used for immunization of patients over 6 yr old.	Used for routine prophylaxis in those patients who have not received DPT.
Tetanus toxoid	Adsorbed tetanus toxoid confers immunity; boosters required every 10 yr.	May be used for routine immunization, although DTP is preferred. Most common use is following an injury with risk of tetanus infection.
Tuberculosis	Attenuated strain of *Mycobacterium bovis* confers variable temporary immunity.	Given to exposed but uninfected patients who cannot receive drug therapy. May be repeated in 2 to 3 mo.
Typhoid	Killed *Salmonella typhosa* gives prolonged protection; boosters needed after 3 yr if exposure is repeated.	Used for persons known to have been exposed, or for persons traveling where typhoid is endemic.
Typhus	Killed *Rickettsia prowazekii* confers resistance; boosters are required in 6 to 12 mo if exposure is repeated.	Used for persons entering areas where exposure to the louse-borne disease is likely.

cont'd. next page

APPENDIX C

Physical Symptoms Produced by Common Poisons

Symptoms	Poisoning Agent
Mental/Motor	
Drowsiness, coma	Acetaminophen
	Alcohols
	Antihistamines
	Carbon monoxide
	Insulin
	Opioids (codeine, etc.)
	Salicylates
	Scopolamine
	Sedative-hypnotic drugs
	Tranquilizers
	Tricyclic Antidepressants
Excitation, twitching, convulsions	Aminophylline
	Atropine
	CNS stimulants
	Carbon monoxide
	Cyanide
	Local anesthetics
	Organophosphate insecticides
	Phenothiazines
Agitation, delirium	Alcohols
	Aminophylline
	Atropine
	LSD (lysergic acid diethylamide)
	Lead
	Marijuana
	PCP (phencyclidine)
	Physostigmine

Physical Symptoms Produced by Common Poisons 641

Symptoms	Poisoning Agent
Paralysis	Botulism
	Heavy metals
Ataxia (motor incoordination)	Alcohols
	Anticonvulsants
	Carbon monoxide
	Hallucinogens
	Heavy metals
	Hydrocarbons
	Sedative-hypnotics
	Tranquilizers

Cardiovascular/Renal

Pulse rate increased	Alcohols
	Amphetamine
	Aspirin
	Atropine
	Cocaine
	Parasympatholytics
	Sympathomimetics
Pulse rate decreased	Digitalis
	Opioids
	Parasympathomimetics
Hypertension	Amphetamine
	Sympathomimetics
Hypotension	Alcohols
	Aminophylline
	Aspirin
	Muscarine
	Nitrates, nitrites
	Opioids
	Sedative-hypnotics
	Tranquilizers
Oliguria, anuria	Carbon tetrachloride
	Ethylene glycol
	Heavy metals
	Methanol
	Mushrooms
	Petroleum distillates

cont'd. next page

642 Pocket Nurse Guide to Drugs

Symptoms	Poisoning Agent
Oral Gastrointestinal	
Acetone odor	Acetone
	Alcohol
	Salicylates
Almond odor	Cyanide
Garlic odor	Arsenic
	Dimethyl sulfoxide
	Phosphorus
	Organophosphate insecticides
Dry mouth	Amphetamine
	Antihistamines
	Atropine
	Opioids
	Phenothiazines
Excessive salivation	Arsenic
	Corrosives
	Mercury
	Mushrooms
	Organophosphate insecticides
Prolonged vomiting	Aminophylline
	Corrosives
	Food poisoning
	Heavy metals
	Salicylates
Pupillary	
Dilated pupils	Alcohol
	Anticholinergics
	Antihistamines
	CNS stimulants
	CNS depressants
Constricted pupils	Mushrooms
	Organophosphate insecticides
	Opioids
Nystagmus	Sedative-hypnotics

Physical Symptoms Produced by Common Poisons

Symptoms	Poisoning Agent
Dermatological	
Jaundiced skin	Arsenic
	Carbon tetrachloride
	Mushrooms
	Naphthalene
Flushed skin	Alcohol
	Antihistamines
	Anticholinergics
Cherry red skin	Carbon monoxide
	Cyanide
	Nitrites
Pulmonary	
Rapid breathing	Amphetamine
	Carbon monoxide
	Methanol
	Petroleum distillates
	Salicylates
Depressed respiration	Alcohol
	Opioids
	Sedative-hypnotics
	Tranquilizers
Wheezing	Mushrooms
	Opioids
	Organophosphate insecticides
	Petroleum distillates

APPENDIX D

Common Conversions

Table D-1   Conversion of units between systems

Apothecaries		Metric
15 gr	=	1 Gm*
1 dr	=	4 Gm
1 oz	=	32 Gm
15 m	=	1 ml
1 f dr	=	4 ml
1 f oz	=	30 ml†

Household		Metric
1 t	=	5 ml
1 T	=	14 ml
1 pt	=	480 ml (or 500 ml)
1 qt	=	960 ml (or 1000 ml)
1 gal	=	3.84 L (or 4 L)
1 lb (avoirdupois)	=	0.46 kg or 1 kg = 2.2 lb

*Two factors have been used for converting grains to milligrams. The older conversion factor is 65 mg = 1 gr. This factor is the basis for aspirin and acetaminophen formulations (i.e., a 5 gr aspirin tablet contains 325 mg of aspirin). The newer conversion factor agreed on is 60 mg = 1 gr. This new conversion factor is easier to use for drugs, such as morphine, that are frequently administered in small doses (fractions of grains). For example, ¼ gr of morphine equals 15 mg, using the new conversion factor. One needs to remember that these factors are simply agreed on for ease of calculation.
†30 ml has been agreed on as the equivalent for 1 f oz. rather than the more exact approximation of 32 ml, since 30 ml is more conveniently and accurately estimated in most clinical glassware.

Table D-2   Systems of units in common use in the United States

System	Unit of Mass	Unit of Volume
Metric	Gram (Gm)	Liter (L)
Apothecaries	Grain (gr)	Minims (m)
Household	Pound (lb)	Pint (pt)

Common Conversions 645

Table D-3 Equivalents within systems

System	Equivalents
Metric	1.0 Gm = 0.001 kg
	1.0 Gm = 1000 mg
	1.0 L = 1000 ml
Apothecaries	1.0 gr = ⅟₆₀ dram (dr or L) = ⅟₄₈₀ oz
	60 gr = 1 dr
	8 dr = 1 oz (or K)
	1.0 minim (m) = ⅟₆₀ f dr = ⅟₄₈₀ f oz
	60 m = 1 f dr (or f L)
	8 f dr = 1 f oz (or f K)
Household	1.0 lb = 16 oz
	1.0 pt = ½ quart (qt) = ⅛ gallon (gal)
	1.0 pt = 16 f oz = 32 tablespoonsful (T)
	1.0 T = 3 teaspoonsful (t)

APPENDIX E

Abbreviations

Table E-1 Abbreviations encountered in physicians' orders and prescriptions

Abbreviation	Latin Phrase	Translation
ad lib.	ad libitum	freely; as much or as often as wanted
aa. (or $\overline{aa}$)	ana	of each
a.c.	ante cibum	before meals
b.i.d.	bis in die	twice daily
$\bar{c}$	cum	with
gtt.	guttae	drops
h.s.	hora somni	at bedtime
non rep.	non repetatur	do not repeat
o.d.	oculus dexter	right eye
o.s.	oculus sinister	left eye
o.u.	oculus uterque	both eyes
p.c.	post cibum	after meals
p.o.	per os	by mouth
p.r.	per rectum	by rectal route
p.r.n.	pro re nata	according to circumstances
q.s.	quantum sufficit	as much as is necessary
q.d.	quaque die	every day
q.h.	quaque hora	every hour
q. 4 h.		every 4 hours
q.i.d.	quarter in die	four times daily
ss. (or $\overline{ss}$)	semis	one half
stat.	statim	immediately
t.i.d.	ter in die	three times daily

Abbreviations 647

Table E-2 Abbreviations for various units

Unit	Abbreviation Used in this Text	Other Acceptable Abbreviations
Gram	Gm	gm, g
Milligram	mg	mgm
Microgram	μg	mcg
Liter	L	l
Milliliter	ml	cc*

*Used for gases only.

Generic Drug Index

A

absorbable gelatin film 270, 279, 281, 282
absorbable gelatin sponge 270, 279, 281
acebutolol 176, 177, 181
acetaminophen 78, 370, 371, 373, 374, 399
acetazolamide 91, 92, 98, 103, 136, 143, 203, 218-220
acetazolamide sodium, sterile 136, 144
acetohexamide 426, 434, 436
acetophenazine 24, 36
acetophenazine maleate 25, 39
acetylcysteine 362, 366, 367
acetylsalicylic acid 370, 372
acrisorcin 552, 558, 560
acyclovir 562, 563, 565, 567, 568
adrenocorticotropic hormone (ACTH) 92, 98, 211, 402, 408-411, 412, 416, 422
albuterol 342, 343, 348, 349
alcohol 80, 165, 166, 191, 266, 301, 317, 371, 376, 430, 549, 576, 581, 601
allopurinol 395-397, 399, 597, 603
alphaprodine 73
alphaprodine hydrochloride 71, 74
alprazolam 3, 11, 12
alseroxylon 176, 184
aluminum carbonate 310, 312, 451
aluminum hydroxide gel 310, 312, 451
amantadine 108, 109, 112, 113, 114, 562, 563, 565, 567
ambenonium 122, 125
ambenonium chloride 122, 124
amcinonide 412, 417

amikacin 496, 523, 525, 526, 528
amiloride 203, 216-218
aminocaproic acid 270, 278, 279, 280, 281-283
aminophylline 194, 342, 350-352, 354
aminosalicylate acid sodium salt 497, 544, 547
amitriptyline 44
amitriptyline hydrochloride 43, 46
ammonium chloride 365, 366
ammonium chloride solution 246
amobarbital 3, 5, 6
amobarbital sodium 93
amoxapine 43, 48, 49
amoxicillin 496, 498, 499, 502, 504, 505
amoxicillin and K clavulanate 496, 498, 502
amphetamine 246
amphetamine sulfate 54, 56, 58, 67
dl-amphetamine sulfate 58
amphotericin B 234, 552-556, 558, 560
ampicillin 461, 496, 498, 499, 502
amyl nitrate 156, 164, 169, 201
anisindione 270, 273
anisotropine methylbromide 300, 304
antidiuretic hormone (ADH) 402, 403, 406, 407, 411
ara-c 596, 598
ascorbic acid 294
aspirin 78, 245, 275, 370-372, 374, 382-384, 387, 390, 399, 416
aspirin, buffered 372

650 Pocket Nurse Guide to Drugs

aspirin, aluminum 372
atenolol 176, 177, 181
atracurium 122, 129, 130
atropine 125, 127, 128, 129, 137,
    194, 252, 253, 254, 258, 262,
    264, 266, 300, 307, 327, 328
atropine sulfate 136, 137, 138,
    302, 307
auranofin 390-392
aurothioglucose 390, 392
azatadine maleate 375, 378
azathioprine 399
azlocillin sodium 496, 498, 502,
    504
azulfidine 540

B

bacitracin 132, 497, 511, 513,
    516, 517, 534
baclofen 108, 116, 117, 118, 120,
    121
beclomethasone 350, 354, 356,
    412, 417
beclomethasone dipropionate 342,
    354, 355
belladonna extract, leaf, tincture
    300, 302, 303, 309
bendroflumethiazide 203, 211, 213
benzathine penicillin G 496, 498,
    500
benzocaine 148, 150
benzonatate 362, 366, 367
benzoxinate hydrochloride 148,
    150
benzphetamine 63, 67
benzphetamine hydrochloride 54,
    63, 64
benzquinamide 316
benzquinamide hydrochloride 316,
    322, 325
benzthiazide 203, 211, 212
benztropine 109
benztropine mesylate 108, 110
beta-adrenergic receptor
    antagonists 156, 164
betamethasone 412, 417

bethanechol 300, 301, 307
bethanechol chloride 300, 302
bile salts 338-340
biperiden 110
bisacodyl 329, 330, 332
bishydroxycoumarin 270, 272
bismuth subsalicylate 326, 327
bleomycin 586-588, 590, 594
bretylium 253, 254, 257, 262,
    264, 266
bretylium tosylate 252, 257, 264
bromocriptine 465, 468
bromocriptine mesylate 465, 466,
    468
brompheniramine maleate 375,
    378
buclizine hydrochloride 316, 318
bumetanide 203, 206, 209, 210
bupivacaine 149, 151, 152
bupivacaine hydrochloride 148
buprenorphine 72, 73
buprenorphine hydrochloride 71,
    74
busulfan 586-588, 590, 592
butabarbital 3, 5, 6
butamben picrate 148, 150
butorphanol 72, 73, 77
butorphanol tartrate 71, 74
butyrophenone 301

C

caffeine 68, 69, 311, 314
caffeine sodium benzoate 54, 66,
    69
calcifediol 438, 448-450
calcitonin 438, 448-450
calcitriol 438, 448-450
calcium 241, 247
calcium carbaspirin 370, 372
calcium carbonate 310, 312
calcium channel blockers 165, 164
calcium gluconate 244, 246, 448
calcium iodide 365, 366
calcium undecylenate 552, 558,
    560
candicidin 552
capreomycin 497, 544, 547, 548

Generic Drug Index 651

carbachol 136, 142
carbamazepine 91, 92, 93, 99, 103, 106, 311, 314, 402-404, 407
carbenicillin disodium 496, 498, 503
carbenicillin indanyl sodium 496, 498, 503, 504
carbidopa 92
carbidopa-levodopa 108, 109, 112, 113
carbinoxamine 377
carbinoxamine maleate 375, 377, 378
carboprost tromethane 478, 480, 481
carboxymethylcellulose 332
carboxymethylcellulose sodium 329
carisoprodol 108, 116, 118
carmustine 586-588, 590, 592
carphenazine 24, 36
carphenazine maleate 25, 29
cascara 330
cascara sagrada 329, 332
castor oil 329, 333
castor oil emulsified 329, 333
catopril 176, 179, 180, 186, 189, 200
cefaclor 497, 505, 506
cefadroxil monohydrate 496, 505, 506
cefamandole 510
cefamandole nafate 497, 506, 509
cefazolin 510
cefazolin sodium 496, 505, 506
cefonicid sodium 497, 506, 509
cefoperazone 510
cefoperazone sodium 497, 507, 509
ceforanide 497, 506
cefotaxime 510
cefotaxime sodium 497, 508, 509
cefotixin 510
cefotixin sodium 497, 507, 509
ceftizoxime 510
ceftizoxime sodium 497, 508, 509

cefuroxime 510
cefuroxime sodium 497, 507, 509
cephalexin 496, 505, 506
cephalothin 510
cephalothin sodium 496, 505, 506
cephapirin 510
cephapirin sodium 496, 505, 506
cephradine 496, 505, 506, 510
chlophedianol 362, 366, 367
chloral hydrate 3, 17, 18, 19, 20
chlorambucil 586, 588, 590, 591
chloramphenicol 266, 496, 521, 522, 523
chloramphenicol sodium succinate 496, 521-523
chloramphenicol palmitate 496, 521, 522
chlorazepate 3, 11, 12, 91, 93, 103, 314
chlorazepate dipotassium 99
chlordiazepoxide 3, 11, 12, 17, 311, 314, 458
chloroprocaine 149
chloroprocaine hydrochloride 148, 151
chloroquine 569, 576, 578
chloroquine hydrochloride 571
chloroquine phosphate 571
chlorotheophylline 376
chlorphenesin 108, 116, 118
chlorpheniramine 377
chlorpheniramine maleate 375, 377, 378
chlorpromazine 24, 25, 36, 41, 317
chlorpromazine hydrochloride 24, 26, 316, 320
chlorpropamide 426, 434, 436
chlorprothixene 24, 31, 37
chlorthalidone 203, 211, 214
chlorthiazide 203, 211, 212, 215, 402-404, 406
chlorthiazide sodium 203, 211, 212
chlortrianisene 454, 456
chlorzoxazone 108, 116, 119, 120
cholestyramine 233, 285, 288, 289

652 Pocket Nurse Guide to Drugs

cholestyramine resin 285, 286, 287
choline salicylate 382, 384
choline theophyllinate 342, 350, 353
ciclopirox olamine 552, 558, 560
cimetidine 16, 193, 267, 310, 311, 313, 314, 315, 340, 423, 557
cimetidine hydrochloride 310, 313
cinoxacin 497, 541, 542, 543
cisplatin 586-588, 590
citrated caffeine 54, 66, 69
citrate phosphate dextrose (CPD) 239
citrate phosphate dextrose adenine (CPDA-1) 239
citric acid 365, 366
clavulanate 502
clemastine 375, 377, 378
clinadamycin 132, 497, 511, 513, 516, 517
clindamycin palmitate 497, 511, 514
clindamycin phosphate 497, 511, 514
clinidium bromide 300, 304
clioquinol 552, 558, 560
clocortolone 412, 417
clofazimine 497, 550, 551
clofibrate 285-287, 289, 402-404, 407, 408
clomiphene 467
clomiphene citrate 465, 466
clonazepam 91, 92, 98, 101, 103, 105
clonidine 178, 180, 187, 188, 189, 197
clonidine hydrochloride 176, 185
clortermine 63, 67
clortermine hydrochloride 54, 63, 64
clotrimazole 552, 558, 560
cloxacillin 499
cloxacillin sodium 496, 498, 501
cocaine 149
cocaine hydrochloride 148, 150
codeine 362-364, 370
codeine phosphate 71, 73, 74, 326, 327, 364

codeine sulfate 71, 74, 326, 327, 364
colchicine 395-398
colestipol 285, 287-289
colestipol hydrochloride 285, 286
colistimethate sodium 496, 532, 533
colistin methate sulfonate 496, 532, 533
colistin sulfate 496, 532, 533
cortisol 412, 419, 420
cortisone 98, 412, 417
cosyntropin 412, 416, 422
coumarin 258, 289, 399, 523, 557
cromolyn 354, 356, 357
cromolyn sodium 342, 354, 355
crystalline amino acids 236, 237, 240, 242, 249, 251
curare 122, 128, 129, 131, 132
cyanocobalamin 296, 297
cyclandelate 156, 171, 173
cyclizing hydrochloride 316, 318
cyclizing lactate 316, 318
cyclobenzaprine 108, 116, 119, 120
cyclomethycaine sulfate 148, 150
cyclopentolate 137
cyclopentolate hydrochloride 136, 137, 138
cyclophosphamide 586-588, 590, 592
cyclopropane 68
cycloserine 497, 544, 547, 548
cyclothiazide 203, 211, 214
cycrimine hydrochloride 108, 110
cyproheptadine hydrochloride 375, 378
cytarabine 596-598, 600

D

dacarbazine 586-588, 590, 592
dactinomycin 602-604, 606
danthron 329
dantrolene 108, 116, 117, 118, 120
dantrolene sodium 120, 121
dapsone 497, 550, 551
daunorubicin 602-604, 606

Generic Drug Index 653

deanol 54, 56, 60
deferoxamine 291, 294, 295
deferoxamine mesylate 291, 293
dehydrocholic acid 338-340
demecarium 141
demecarium bromide 136, 142
demeclocycline hydrochloride 497, 518, 519
deserpidine 184
deserpine 176
desipramine 44
desipramine hydrochloride 43, 46
deslanoside 228, 231, 232, 252, 253, 357
desmopressin acetate 402-404, 406
desonide 412, 417
desoximetasone 412, 417
desoxycorticosterone 412, 417
dexamethasone 355, 412, 416, 418
dexamethasone sodium 342, 354
dexchlorpheniramine maleate 375, 379
dextran 236, 237, 239, 242, 249, 278
dextroamphetamine sulfate 54, 56, 68
dextromethorphan 362, 363
dextromethorphan hydrobromide 362, 365
dextrose in saline 237, 241, 250
dextrose in water 236, 238
dextrothyroxine 285-287, 290
diazepam 3, 11, 13, 17, 83, 86-88, 91-93, 97, 98, 102, 103, 105, 108, 116-121, 266, 311, 314
diazoxide 176, 177, 179, 180, 187, 189, 200, 266
dibucaine 148, 149, 152
dibucaine hydrochloride 148, 150
dichlorphenamide 136, 144
diclonine148
diclonine hydrochloride 148, 150
dicloxacillin sodium 496, 498, 501
dicoumarol 270, 272
dicyclomine hydrochloride 300, 306
dienestrol 454, 456
diethylpropion 63, 67

diethylpropion hydrochloride 54, 63, 64
diethylstilbestrol (DES) 454, 456, 458, 612
diethylstilbestrol diphosphate 611, 614
diflorasone 412, 418
diflunisol 382-384
digitalis 196, 208, 211, 233-235, 245, 247, 253, 254, 264, 265, 286, 287, 289, 290, 448, 531, 549
digitalis leaf 228, 231
digitoxin 10, 228, 230-232, 252, 253, 256, 268
digoxin 228, 230-232, 252, 253, 256, 268, 269, 311, 315
dihydroergotamine (DHE) 272
dihydrogenated ergot alkaloids 156, 171, 173
dihydrotachysterol 438, 448-450
dihydroxyaluminum aminoacetate 310, 312
dihydroxyaluminum sodium carbonate 310, 312
diiiodohydroxyquin 569, 578
diloxanide 569
diltiazem 176, 179, 180, 186, 189, 200
dimenhydrinate 316, 317, 381
dimercaprol (BAL) 226
dinoprostone 478, 480, 481
dinoprost tromethamine 478, 480, 481
diphemanil methylsulfate 300, 301, 304
diphenhydramine 108, 317, 362, 367, 375, 376
diphenhydramine hydrochloride 111, 308, 316, 318, 362, 365, 375, 377, 379, 381
diphenhydrinate 376
diphenidol 316, 317, 324, 325
diphenidol hydrochloride 316, 322
diphenoxylate 326-328
diphenylpyraline hydrochloride 375, 379
dipivefrin 136, 143

654 **Pocket Nurse Guide to Drugs**

disopyramide 253, 255, 260, 262, 265, 268, 269
disopyramide phosphate 252
disulfiram 3, 19, 21, 22, 23, 266, 601
dobutamine 157, 160, 162, 228, 229
dobutamine hydrochloride 156, 158
docusate calcium 329, 335
docusate sodium 329, 335
domperidone 316, 317, 322
dopamine 157, 160, 162, 163, 228, 229, 265, 300
dopamine hydrochloride 156
doxapram 54, 66, 68, 69, 70
doxepin 43, 44
doxepin hydrochloride 43, 46
doxorubicin 602-604, 606
doxycycline 10, 497, 518-521
doxylamine 376
doxylamine succinate 375, 379
dromostanolone 611, 612
dromostanolone propionate 611, 614
droperidol 83, 86, 87, 89, 316, 317, 320
dyphylline 342, 350, 352

E

econazole nitrate 552, 558, 560
echothiophate 141
echothiophate iodide 136, 142
edrophonium 123, 125, 126, 129
edrophonium chloride 122, 124
elanapril 176, 179, 186, 189, 200
electolytes 250
emetine 569, 570, 578, 580, 581
enflurane 68, 83, 84
ephedrine 161, 228, 229, 342, 349
ephedrine sulfate 342, 343, 358, 360
epinephrine 141, 145, 146, 149, 151, 152, 153, 156, 157, 160-163, 376, 392, 449, 593, 594, 605
epinephrine (base) 342, 349

epinephrine bitartrate 136, 143, 344
epinephrine borate 136
epinephrine hydrochloride 136, 143, 156, 158, 344, 358, 360
epinephrine (racemic) 344
epinephryl borate 143
ergocalciferol 438, 448-450
ergonovine maleate 478, 480
erythrityl tetranite 156, 164, 166
erythromycin 219, 497, 511, 512, 515-517
erythromycin base 497, 511, 512
erythromycin estolate 497, 511, 512, 517
erythromycin ethylsuccinate 511, 512
erythromycin gluceptate 497, 511, 512
erythromycin lactobionate 497, 511, 512, 515, 517
erythromycin stearate 497, 511, 512
estradiol 454, 456
estradiol cypionate 454, 458
estradiol valerate 454, 458
estramustine 612
estramustine phosphate sodium 611, 614
estrogen 454, 455, 456, 460, 461, 464, 467, 469-471, 475
estrogen, conjugated 454, 456, 458
estrogen, esterified 454, 457, 458
estrogenic substance 454, 457
estrone 454, 457, 459
estropipate 454, 457
ethacrynic acid 203, 206-208, 210
ethambutol 497, 544, 547, 548
ethchlorvinyl 3, 17, 18, 20, 45
ethinamate 3, 18, 20
ethinyl estradiol 454, 457, 459, 472, 473
ethionamide 497, 544, 547, 548
ethopropazine 108, 111
ethosuximide 91, 92, 96
ethotoin 91, 96

Generic Drug Index 655

ethylestrenol 489, 490
ethynodiol diacetate 469, 472
etidocaine 149, 152
etidocaine hydrochloride 148
etomidate 83, 86, 87, 89
etoposide 607, 608
eucatropine hydrochloride 136, 137, 139

F

fat emulsions 237, 240, 242, 249, 251
fenfluramine 63, 66, 67
fenfluramine hydrochloride 54, 63, 64
fenoprofen 382, 383, 386, 387, 389
fentanyl 71, 73, 74, 83
fentanyl citrate 83, 86, 89
ferrocholinate 291, 292
ferroglycine sulfate 291, 292
ferrous fumarate 291, 292
ferrous gluconate 291, 292
ferrous sulfate 291, 292
floxuridine 596-598, 600
flucytosine 552-554, 556
fludrocortisone 418
flumethasone 412, 419
flunisolide 342, 354, 355, 412, 418
flunitrazepam 83, 86, 87, 89
fluocinolone 412, 419
fluocinonide 412, 419
fluoperazine 25
fluorometholone 412, 419
fluorouracil 596-598, 600
fluoxymesterone 459, 484, 485, 487
fluphenazine 24, 25, 36
fluphenazine decanoate 29
fluphenazine ethanoate 29
fluphenazine hydrochloride 25, 29, 316, 321
fluprednisolone 412, 419
flurandrenolide 412, 419
flurazepam 3, 11, 14
folic acid 266, 291, 296-298

follicle stimulating hormone (FSH) 402, 408-411, 465
5-FU 596, 598
furazolidine 569, 573, 578
furosemide 203, 206, 207, 208, 210, 229

G

gallamine 128, 129
gallamine triethiodide 122, 130
gemfibrozil 285-287, 289
gentamicin 496, 523, 524, 526, 528, 531
gitalin 228, 231
glipizide 426, 434, 436
gluceptate 515
glucopyrrolate 300, 304
glutamic acid hydrochloride 338, 339
glutethimide 3, 18, 19, 20
glyburide 426, 434, 436
glycerin 136, 144, 145, 147, 329
glycerin suppositories 329, 333, 335
glycerol guaiacolate 362, 364
gold salts 390
gold sodium thiomalate 390, 392
griseofulvin 552, 557, 558, 560
growth hormone (GH) 402, 408-411
guaifenesin 362-364
guanabenz 178, 180, 188, 189
guanabenz acetate 176, 185, 197
guanadrel 176, 177, 178, 180, 184, 195
guanethidine 41, 177, 178, 180, 187, 188, 195
guanethidine sulfate 176, 184, 195

H

halazepam 3, 11, 14
halcinonide 412, 419
haloperidol 24, 25, 32, 37, 52, 316
haloprogin 552, 558, 560
halothane 68, 83, 84
heparin 250, 270-272, 274-276, 279

656 Pocket Nurse Guide to Drugs

hepatitis B 562, 563
hetastarch 236, 237, 239, 242, 249
hexafluorenium 122, 128, 131
hexocyclium methylsulfate 300, 304
hexylcaine hydrochloride 148, 150
homatropine 137
homatropine hydrobromide 136, 137, 138
homatropine methylbromide 300, 306
human albumin 236, 237, 239, 241
human chorionic gonadotropin (HCG) 465-468
hydralazine 177, 179, 180, 188, 189, 197, 198
hydralazine hydrochloride 176, 185
hydrochloric acid 338-340
hydrochlorothiazide 203, 211, 212
hydrochlorothiazine 191
hydrocodone 363
hydrocodone bitartrate 362, 365
hydrocortisone 412, 419, 420
hydroflumethiazide 203, 211, 213
hydromorphone hydrochloride 71, 73, 74
hydroxocobalomin 291, 296
hydroxyamphetamine hydrobromide 136, 137, 140
hydroxychloroquine 390, 391, 569, 576, 578
hydroxychloroquine sulfate 390, 392, 571, 580
hydroxymagnesium aluminate 310
hydroxyprogesterone 462, 463
hydroxystilbamidine 553
hydroxystilbamidine isethionate 552, 554
1, 5-hydroxytryptophan 92
hydroxyurea 596, 597, 599, 601
hydroxyzine hydrochloride 3, 18, 20, 21, 316, 319, 375, 379
hydroxyzine pamoate 3, 18, 20, 21, 316, 319, 375, 379

hyoscyamine hydrobromide 300, 303
hyoscyamine sulfate 300, 303
hypertonic dextrose solution 236, 237, 239, 241, 249
hypertonic saline solution 237
hypotonic saline solution 236

I

ibuprofen 382, 383, 386, 389
idoxuridine 562, 563, 566, 567
imipramine 43, 44
imipramine hydrochloride 43, 47
imipramine pamoate 43, 47
indapamide 203, 211, 214
indomethacin 193, 382, 383, 385, 388
influenza 562, 564
iodine 444, 445, 448
iodoquinol 569, 570, 571, 578, 581
insulin 105, 147, 163, 211, 250, 290, 398, 409, 411, 423, 426, 430-435, 437, 475, 605, 617
insulin, extended zinc suspension 426, 428
insulin, injection 426, 427
insulin, isophane suspension 426, 428
insulin, prompt zinc suspension 426, 427
insulin, protamine zinc suspension 426, 428
insulin, zinc suspension 426, 428
interstitial cell stimulating hormone (ICSH) 402, 408, 410
intralipid 236
iodinated glycerol 362, 364
iodochlorhydroxyquin 552, 558, 560
ipecac 365, 366
iron-dextran 291, 292, 295
isocarboxazid 43, 49, 50
isoethane 348, 349
isoethane hydrochloride 342, 345
isoethane mesylate 342, 345

Generic Drug Index 657

isoflurane 83, 84
isoflurophate 136, 141, 143, 145
isoniazid 258, 266, 497, 544-546, 548, 549
isonicotinic acid hydrazide (INH) 497, 544, 546
isopropamide iodide 300, 304
isoproterenol 157, 160, 162, 194, 349
isoproterenol hydrochloride 156, 158, 342, 345
isoproterenol sulfate 342, 345
isosorbide 136, 144, 145
isosorbide dinitrate 156, 164, 166, 228, 229
isotonic dextrose in water 237
isotonic saline solution 236, 237, 247, 248
isoxsuprine 156, 172, 173

K

kanamycin 224, 496, 523, 524, 526, 527
karaya gum 329, 332
ketamine 83, 86, 87, 89
ketoconazole 552-554, 557

L

labetalol 178, 188, 195
labetalol hydrochloride 176, 183
lactated Ringer's solution 236-238, 241, 246
lactulose 329-331, 335, 337
leucovorin 296, 298, 601
leucovorin calcium 291, 296, 297
levallorphan 82
levallorphan tartrate 71, 74
levarterenol 42, 156, 157, 160, 162, 194, 196, 263
levarterenol bitartrate 156, 158, 163
levodopa 108, 109, 112, 113, 115, 116
levonorgestrel 469, 472
levopropoxyphene 362, 367

levopropoxyphene napsylate 362, 365
levorphanol tartrate 71, 73, 80
levothyroxine 439
levothyroxine sodium (TU) 438-440
lidocaine 93, 103, 148, 149, 150, 152, 153, 246, 252, 253, 254, 258, 262, 263, 264, 266, 267
lidocaine hydrochloride 91, 99, 148, 150
lincomycin 132, 497, 511, 514, 515, 517
liothyronine sodium (TU) 438, 439, 441
liotrix 438, 439, 441, 442
liposyn 236
lithium 206, 211, 222, 224, 247
lithium carbonate 43, 51, 52, 204, 443
lithium citrate 43, 51, 52
lomustine 586-588, 590, 592
loperamide 326-328
lorazepam 3, 11, 14
loxapine 24, 37, 266
loxapine succinate 25, 34
luteinizing hormone (LH) 402, 408-411, 465
luteotropic hormone (LTH) 402

M

mafenide acetate 497
magaldrate 310, 312
magnesium 534
magnesium carbonate 310, 312
magnesium citrate 329, 334, 337
magnesium hydroxide 310, 312, 329, 334
magnesium oxide 310, 312
magnesium phosphate 329, 334
magnesium salicylate 382-384
magnesium sulfate 132, 329, 334
magnesium sulfate solution 236-238, 241, 246
magnesium trisilicate 310, 312

658   Pocket Nurse Guide to Drugs

mannitol 136, 144, 145, 203, 222, 223, 224, 593
mannitol hexanitrate 224
maprotiline 43, 48
mazindol 54, 63, 64, 67
mebendazole 569, 570, 573, 576, 578, 581
mecamylamine 178, 246
mechlorethamine 586-588, 591
meclizing hydrochloride 316, 319
meclofenamate 383, 386
meclofenamate sodium monohydrate 382
medroxyprogesterone 462, 463, 612, 613
medroxyprogesterone acetate 611, 615
medrysone 412, 420
mefenamic acid 370, 371, 373, 374
megestrol 462, 463, 612, 613
megestrol acetate 611, 615
melphalan 586, 588, 590, 591
menadiol phosphate sodium 283
menadiol sodium diphosphate 270, 279, 280, 281, 283
menadione 270, 279, 280, 282, 284
menadione sodium bisulfate 270, 279, 280, 281, 283
menotropins 465-468
mepenzolate bromide 300, 304
meperidine 72, 73, 77, 80
meperidine hydrochloride 71, 75
mephentermine 157, 160, 161, 202
mephentermine sulfate 156, 159
mephenytoin 91, 95
mephobarbital 5, 91, 92, 94
mepivacaine 148, 149, 152
meprednisone 412, 420
meprobamate 3, 18, 19, 21, 458
mercaptomerin sodium 203, 224, 225
mercaptopurine 399, 596-598
mersalyl 203, 224, 225, 226
mesoridazine 24, 36, 42
mesoridazine besylate 25, 28

mestranol 472, 473, 475
mesylate 176
metaproterenol 348, 349
metaproternol sulfate 342, 346
metaraminol 157, 160-163, 196
metaraminol bitartrate 156, 159
methacycline hydrochloride 497, 518, 519
methadone 72, 73, 82, 549
methadone hydrochloride 71, 75
methamphetamine hydrochloride 54, 56, 59, 458
methandriol 489, 490
methandrostenolone 489
methantheline bromide 300, 305
methazolamide 136, 144, 203, 218, 220
methdilazine 376
methdilazine hydrochloride 375, 379
methicillin 499, 504
methicillin sodium 496, 498, 501
methimazole 438, 443, 446
methisazone 562, 563, 567
methixene hydrochloride 300, 306
methocarbamol 108, 116, 117, 119
methohexital 87
methohexital sodium 83, 86, 88
methotrexate 296, 540, 586-598, 601
methoxamine 157, 160, 162
methoxamine hydrochloride 156, 159
methoxyflurane 83, 84
methscopolomine bromide 300, 303
methsuximide 91, 92, 96
methyclothiazide 203, 211, 214
methylcellulose 329, 332
methyldopa 176, 177, 178, 180, 185, 187, 189, 191, 197
methylergonovine maleate 478, 480
methylphenidate 56, 57, 62
methylphenidate hydrochloride 54, 56, 59
methylprednisolone 412, 420

Generic Drug Index 659

methyltestosterone 458, 484, 485, 487
methyprylon 3, 17, 18, 20
metoclopramide 300-302, 307, 308, 315, 316, 317, 323, 594
metocurine 122, 128, 129
metocurine iodide 130
metolazone 203, 211, 214
metoprolol 176, 177, 181, 193
metyrapone 412, 416, 422
metyrosine 179
mezlocillin 504
mezlocillin sodium 496, 498, 503
microfibrillar collagen hemastat 270, 279, 281
micronazole 552, 553, 557, 558, 560
micronazole nitrate 552, 555
mineral oil 329, 334
mineral supplements 237, 249, 250
minicycline hydrochloride 497, 518-521
minoxidil 176, 177, 179, 180, 186, 189, 198
mithramycin 602-604, 606
mitomycin 586-588, 590, 594
mitotane 611-613, 615
molindone 24, 37
molindone hydrochloride 25, 34
morphine 72, 73, 79
morphine sulfate 71, 75
moxalactam 510
moxalactam disodium 497, 508, 509
mumps 562, 564

N

nadolol 176, 177, 181
nafcillin 499, 504
nafcillin sodium 496, 498, 501
nalbuphine 73, 77
nalbuphine hydrochloride 71, 75
nalidixic acid 497, 541-544
naloxone 82
naloxone hydrochloride 71, 80
naltrexone 71, 80, 82

nandrolone decanoate 489, 490
nandrolone phenpropionate 489, 490
naphazoline 359
naphazoline hydrochloride 358, 360
naproxen 382, 383, 386, 389
naproxen sodium 382, 386
neomycin 496, 523, 524, 526-528, 531, 534
neostigmine 122, 123, 126, 127, 128, 129, 300, 301, 307, 308
neostigmine bromide 122, 124, 125
neostigmine methylsulfate 122, 125, 300, 302, 309
netilmicin 496, 523, 525, 526, 529
niacin 285-287, 289, 290
niacinamide 290
niclosamide 569, 575, 576, 578
nicotinamide 290
nicotinic acid 285, 286, 290
nicotinyl alcohol 156, 172, 173
nifedipine 176, 179, 180, 189, 199
nitrofurantoin 497, 541-544
nitrogen mustard 586, 588
nitroglycerin 156, 164, 166, 168, 170, 228, 229
nitroglycerin ointment, 2% 167
nitroprusside 179, 189, 201
nitrous oxide 83, 84
norepinephrine 156, 158, 163, 177, 179, 200, 202, 265
norethindrone 462, 463, 469, 472, 473
norethindrone acetate 469, 472
norethynodrel 469, 472
norgestrel 469, 472, 473
normeperidine 72
nortriptyline 44
nortriptyline hydrochloride 43, 47
noscapine 362, 365
novobiocin 497, 511, 513, 517
nylidrin 171, 172
nylidrin hydrochloride 156
nystatin 552, 557, 558, 560

660 Pocket Nurse Guide to Drugs

O

opium tincture 326, 327
orphenadrine 108, 112, 116, 117, 119
ouabain 228, 231, 232, 235, 252, 257
oxacillin 499, 504
oxacillin sodium 496, 498, 501, 502
oxandrolone 489, 490
oxazepam 3, 11, 15
oxidized cellulose 270, 279, 281, 282
oxphencyclimine 307
oxphencyclimine hydrochloride 300, 301, 305
oxphenonium bromide 300, 305
oxtryphilline 342, 350, 353
oxycodone 71, 73, 75, 78
oxymetazoline hydrochloride 358, 360
oxymetholone 489, 490
oxymorphone 73
oxymorphone hydrochloride 71, 76
oxyphenbutazone 493
oxytetracycline hydrochloride 497, 518, 519, 521
oxytocin 402, 406, 411, 478-480

P

pamoate 18
pancreatin 338-340
pancrelipase 338-340
pancuronium 128, 129
pancuronium bromide 122, 130
papaverine 171, 172
papaverine hydrochloride 156, 173
paraaminosalicylic acid (PAS) 258, 497, 544, 547, 548, 550
paragoric 326-328
paraldehyde 91, 93, 100, 101, 102, 103, 106
paramethadione 91, 97
paramethasone 412, 420
parathyroid hormone 438, 448-450
pargyline 179

pemoline 54, 56, 57, 60, 62
penicillamine 390-394
penicillin 394, 498, 499, 505, 511, 515, 519
penicillin G 496-498, 500
penicillin V 496-498, 500, 531
pentaerythritol tetranitrate 156, 164, 167
pentazocine 72, 73, 77
pentazocine hydrochloride 71, 76
pentazocine lactate 71, 76
pentobarbital 3, 5, 7, 10, 193
pentobarbital sodium 70
pentoxifylline 156, 171, 172, 173
perphenazine 24, 25, 30, 37, 316, 321
phenazopyridine 497, 534, 538, 540
phendimetrazine 63, 67
phendimetrazine tartrate 54, 63, 65
phenelzine sulfate 43, 49, 50
phenindione 270, 273
phenmetrazine 63, 67
phenobarbital 91, 92, 94, 101, 102, 193, 247, 258, 268, 311, 314, 389, 464
phenobarbital sodium 93
phenolphthalein 329, 333
phenothiazene 301
phenoxybenzamine 177, 188, 194
phenoxybenzamine hydrochloride 176, 183
phenprocoumon 270, 273
phensuccimide 91, 92, 93, 96
phentermine 54, 63, 65, 67
phentolamine 51, 162, 177, 188, 194
phentolamine hydrochloride 176, 182
phentolamine mesylate 182
phenylbutazone 266, 382, 383, 385, 387, 435, 461, 464, 488, 493
phenylephrine 42, 157, 160, 202, 263
phenylephrine hydrochloride 136, 137, 140, 156, 159, 358, 361

Generic Drug Index 661

phenylpropanolamine 67
phenylpropanolamine
 hydrochloride 54, 63, 65, 358,
 361
phenylthiazines 464
phenytoin 10, 91, 92, 93, 95, 101,
 102, 104, 105, 193, 252, 253,
 254, 258, 262, 264, 266, 268,
 269, 311, 314, 461, 523, 548
phenytoin sodium 93
physostigmine 145
physostigmine salicylate 136, 142
physostigmine sulfate 136, 142
phytonadione 277, 279-284
pilocarpine 141, 147
pilocarpine hydrochloride 142
pilocarpine nitrate 136, 142
pindolol 176, 177, 181, 193
piperacetazine 24, 25, 28, 36
piperacillin sodium 496, 498, 503
piperazine 569, 574, 576-578, 582
plantago seed 329, 333
plasma 236, 237, 239, 247
plasma protein fraction 236, 237,
 239, 249
poliomyelitis 562, 564
polycarbophil 329, 332
polyestradiol 612
polyestradiol phosphate 614
polymyxin B sulfate 496, 532-534
polythiazide 203, 211, 214
posterior pituitary extract 402-404,
 406
potassium 244, 245
potassium chloride solution
 236-238, 241, 243, 244
potassium citrate 398
potassium guaiacolsulfonate 365,
 366
potassium iodide 362-364, 438,
 443, 447
povidone-iodine 569, 572, 576,
 578, 582
pramoxine hydrochloride 148, 151
prazepam 3, 11, 15, 314
prazosin 177, 180, 188, 194
prazosin hydrochloride 176, 183

prednisolone 412, 420
prednisone 412, 421, 611-613,
 615
prilocaine 148, 149
prilocaine hydrochloride 152
primaquine 569, 576, 577, 579,
 582
primaquine phosphate 572
primidone 91, 92, 93, 95, 101,
 102
probenecid 395-398
probucol 285, 287, 290
procainamide 219, 252, 253, 255,
 260, 264, 268
procainamide sustained release 260
procaine 149, 505
procaine penicillin G 496, 498,
 500
procaine hydrochloride 148, 152
procarbazine 597, 601
procarbazine hydrochloride 596,
 599
prochlorperazine 24, 25, 30, 37,
 316, 321
prochlorperazine edisylate 30,
 316, 321
prochlorperazine maleate 30, 316,
 321
procyclidine hydrochloride 108,
 111
progesterone 462, 462
progestin 460, 461, 470, 471, 474,
 475, 477
prolactin 402, 409-411
promazine 25, 28, 36, 317
promazine hydrochloride 316, 321
promethazine hydrochloride 316,
 319, 375, 377, 380
propantheline bromide 300, 301,
 305
proparacaine hydrochloride 148,
 149, 151
propoxyphene 73, 78
propoxyphene hydrochloride 71,
 76
propoxyphene napsylate 71, 76,
 106

662 Pocket Nurse Guide to Drugs

propranolol 160, 176, 177, 193, 233, 252, 253, 255, 260, 262, 265, 267, 269, 289, 311, 314, 443-450
propranolol hydrochloride 182, 438, 443, 446
propylhexedrine 358, 359, 361
propylthiouracil 438, 443, 445, 446
protamine sulfate 276
protirelin 438, 439, 441
protriptyline 43, 44
protriptyline hydrochloride 43, 47
pseudoephedrine 246, 358
pseudoephedrine hydrochloride 358, 361
pseudoephedrine sulfate 358, 361
psyllium 329, 332
psyllium hydrocolloid 329, 332
psyllium hydrophilic muciloid 329, 332
pyrantel pamoate 569, 574-576, 579
pyrazinamide 497, 544, 547, 548
pyridostigmine 122, 125, 126, 129
pyridoxine 394, 548
pyrilamine 377
pyrilamine maleate 375, 380
pyrimethamine 296, 569, 572, 573, 576, 579, 582
pyrvinium pamoate 569, 574, 576, 579, 583

Q

quinacrine 569, 573, 576, 577, 583
quinestrol 454, 457
quinethazone 203, 211, 214
quinidine 10, 132, 196, 219, 252, 253, 254, 255, 260, 264, 267, 268, 269, 311, 534
quinidine gluconate 252, 259
quinidine polygalacturonate 252, 260
quinidine sulfate 252, 259, 260
quinine 247, 311, 534, 569, 576, 579, 584

quinine dihydrochloride 572, 584
quinine sulfate 571, 572

R

rabies 562, 565
racemic amphetamine sulfate 58
radioactive iodine 438, 443-445, 447
ranitidine 310, 311, 313, 315, 423
rauwolfia 176, 183, 196
red cell concentrates 248
rescinnamine 176, 184
reserpine 176, 177, 178, 180, 183, 187, 233
rifampin 268, 461, 497, 544-546, 548-551
Ringer's solution 236, 237, 238, 241
rubella (German Measles) 562-564
Rubeola (Measles) 562, 564

S

salbutamol 342, 343, 349
salicylamide 370, 373
salicylate 207, 219, 247, 399, 435
salicylate salts 383
salsalate 382, 384
saralasin 179, 200
scopalomine 137, 316, 317, 318, 324
scopalomine hydrobromide 136, 137, 139, 316, 318
secobarbital 3, 5, 8
senna 330
senna concentrate 329, 333
senna pod 329
senna, whole leaf 334
sennosides A + B 329, 334
silver sulfadiazine 497, 534, 538, 540
smallpox 562, 565
sodium bicarbonate 310, 311, 398, 583
sodium bicarbonate solution 236-238, 244, 246
sodium chloride 238

Generic Drug Index 663

sodium iodide 438, 443, 444, 447, 448
sodium nitrite 201
sodium nitroprusside 176, 180, 187, 201, 228, 229
sodium phosphate 329, 334, 355
sodium polystyrene sulfonate 245
sodium salicylate 370, 372, 382, 384
sodium thiosalicylate 382, 384
sodium thiosulfate 201, 591
somatotropin 410
sorbitol 245
spectinomycin 497, 511, 513, 516, 517
spironolactone 203, 216, 217, 218
stanozolol 489, 491
streptinomycin 496, 497, 523, 524, 526, 527, 531, 544-546, 548, 550
streptokinase 270, 277, 278, 281
streptozocin 611-613, 615, 617
succinylcholine 122, 128, 129, 131, 132
succinylcholine chloride 131
sucralfate 310, 311, 313, 315
sufentanil 73
sufentanil citrate 71, 76
sulfacetamide 497, 534, 539
sulfacytine 496, 534-536
sulfadiazine 496, 534-536, 538, 569, 573, 579
sulfadoxine 569, 572, 579
sulfamerazine 496, 534, 537, 538
sulfamethazine 497, 534, 538
sulfamethizole 496, 497, 534-536, 538, 540
sulfamethoxazole 496, 497, 534, 535, 537, 538, 569, 573, 579
sulfaphenazole 266
sulfasalazine 496, 534-536
sulfinpyrazone 395-399
sulfisoxazole 496, 497, 534-536, 538, 539
sulfonamide 435
sulfoxone sodium 497, 550, 551
sulindac 382, 383, 385, 388, 389

T

tamoxifen 611, 612, 614, 616
tartrazene 42, 45
taurine 240
temazepam 3, 11, 15
terbutaline 348, 349
terbutaline sulfate 342, 346
terpin hydrate 362, 364-366
testolactone 611, 612, 614
testosterone 459, 484-486
testosterone cypionate 458, 484, 486
testosterone enanthate 458, 484, 486
testosterone propionate 484, 486, 487
tetracaine 148, 149, 152
tetracaine hydrochloride 148, 151
tetracycline 132, 294, 311, 315, 497, 569, 579
tetracycline hydrochloride 497, 518-521
tetrahydrozoline 359
tetrahydrozoline hydrochloride 358, 359, 361
theophylline 54, 66, 68, 69, 70, 203, 224-226, 311, 314, 342, 350, 353, 354
theophylline ethylenediamine 342, 350, 352
theophylline monoethanolamine 342, 350, 352
theophylline sodium glycinate 342, 350, 353
thiabendazole 569, 574-577, 579, 584
thiamylal sodium 83, 86, 88
thiethylperazine maleate 316, 321, 324
thioamides 443-445
thiocyanate 202
thioguanine 596-598
thiopental sodium 83, 86, 88
thioridazine 24, 28, 36
thiothixene 24, 37
thiothixene hydrochloride 25, 32
thioxanthene 301

664 Pocket Nurse Guide to Drugs

thiphenamil hydrochloride 300, 306
thrombin 270, 279, 281
thyroglobulin 438-440, 442
thyroid stimulating hormone (TSH) 402, 409-411, 438, 439, 441-443
thyroid U.S.P. 438-440, 442
thyrotropin-releasing hormone (TRH) 441, 442
thyroxin 287
ticarcillin 504
ticarcillin disodium 496, 498, 503
timolol 141, 145, 177, 193
timolol maleate 136, 143, 176, 182
tobramycin 496, 523, 525, 526, 528
tolazamide 426, 434, 436
tolazine 171, 172
tolazine hydrochloride 156, 173
tolbutamide 289, 426, 434, 436, 523
tolmetin 383, 388, 389
tolmetin sodium 382, 385
tranxene 12
tranylcypromine sulfate 43, 49, 50
travamulsion 236
trazodone 48, 49
triamcinolone 412, 421
triamcinolone acetonide 354, 355
triamterine 203, 216, 217, 218
triazolam 3, 11, 15
trichlofos sodium 3, 17, 18, 20
trichlormethiazide 203, 211, 213
tridihexethyl chloride 300, 305
triethylene thiophosphoramide 586, 587, 588, 590
trifluoperazine 24, 31, 37
triflupromazine 36
triflupromazine hydrochloride 24, 27, 316, 321
trifluridine 562, 563, 566, 567
trihexphenidyl hydrochloride 108, 111
trilium 12

trimeprazine 376
trimeprazine tartrate 375, 380
trimethadione 91, 92, 97, 103
trimethaphan 132, 178, 188, 189
trimethobenzamide 316, 317, 324, 325
trimethobenzamide hydrochloride 316, 323
trimethoprim 496, 497, 534, 535, 537, 541-543, 569, 573, 579
trimipramine 44
trimipramine maleate 43, 47
tripelennamine citrate 375, 380
tripelennamine hydrochloride 375, 380
triprolidine 377
triprolidine hydrochloride 375, 380
tropicamide 136, 137, 139
tubocurarine 122, 128, 129, 131, 132, 207, 211
tyramine 601

U

undecylenic acid 552, 558, 560
urea 136, 144, 203, 222-224
urokinase 270, 277-279, 281

V

valproic acid 91, 92, 100, 103, 107, 266
vancomycin 511, 513, 516, 517
vasopressin 402-404, 406, 408
vasopressin tannate 403-406
vecuronium 122, 129, 131
verapamil 179, 180, 186, 199, 200, 252, 253, 255, 261, 265, 269
vidarabine 562, 563, 566, 567
vinblastine 608
vinblastine sulfate (VB) 607, 608
vincristine 608, 609
vincristine sulfate (VCR) 607, 608
vitamin B12 298, 531
vitamin C 294
vitamin D 438, 448-450
vitamin K 12 84

Generic Drug Index 665

vitamin K 32 84
vitamin supplements 237, 249, 250
VP-16 608

W

warfarin 270, 273, 274, 311, 314
whole blood 236, 237, 239, 241,
247, 248

X

xanax 12
xylometazoline 358
xylometazoline hydrochloride 358,
361

Trade Name Index

A

Abbokinase 278
Acetazolam 143, 220
Acetazolan 98
Achromycin 518
Achromycin IM 518
Acidulin 339
ACTH 422
Acthar 422
ACTH gel 422
Actidil 380
Adapin 46
Adipex 65
Adrenalin Chloride 158, 344, 360
Adriamycin 604
Adroyd 490
Adrucil 598
Advil 386
Aeroseb-Dex 418
Aerosporin 533
Afrin 360
Afrinol Repetabs 360
Aftate 560
Agoral, Plain 334
A-hydrocort 420
Airbron 366
Akineton 110
Akrinol 560
Albamycin 513
Albuminar 239
Albutein 239
Aldactone 217
Aldomet 185
Aldoril 191
Alka-Seltzer 372
Alkeran 588
Allertoc 380
Alphaderm 419
Alphadrol 419

Alpha Redisol 297
ALterna Gel 312
Alupent 346
Aluprin 373
Amcill 502
Amen 463
Americaine 150
A-methapred 420
Amicar 280
Amidate 89
Amikin 525
Amiline 46
Aminosalicylic Acid 547
Aminosyn 239
Amitril 46
Amnestrogen 457
Amoxil 502
Amphojel 312
Amyl Nitrate 166
Amytal 6
Amytal Sodium 93
Anabol 490
Anadrol 490
Anaprox 386
Anaspaz 303
Anavar 490
Ancef 506
Ancobon 554
Ancotil 554
Andesterone 459
Android 487
Android-G 459
Android T 486
Andronaq 486
Anectine 131
Angidil 166
Anhydron 214
Anitrem 111

Trade Name Index 667

Anorex 65
Anspor 506
Antabuse 19, 601
Antepar 578
Antiminth 579
Antispas 306
Anti-tuss 364
Antivert 319
Antrenyl 305
Anturan 396
Anturane 396
A.P.L. Secules 466
Apo-Carbamazepine 99
Apo-Chlordiazepoxide 12
Apo-Diazepam 13, 88
Apo-Fluphenazine 29
Apo-Flurazepam 14
Apo-Haloperidol 32
Apo-Imipramine 47
Apo-Meprobamate 21
Apo-Oxazepam 15
Apo-Perphenazine 30
Apo-Primidone 95
Apo-Trifluoperazine 31
Apresoline 185
Aquamephytoin 277, 282, 280
Aquamox 214
Aquatag 214
Aquatensen 213
Aralen 578
Aramine 159
Arfonad 187
Aristocort 421
Aristocort intralesional 421
Aristospan 421
Arlidin 173
Arthrolate 384
Arthropan 384
Articulose 420
Artrane 111
A.S.A. 372
Ascendin 48
Ascriptin 372
Asmolin (1:400) 343
Aspergum 372
Asthma Meter 344
Atarax 20, 319, 380

Athrombin 273
Ativan 14
Atromid-S 286, 407
Atropine Sulfate 138
Atropisol 138
Augmentin 502
Aventyl 47
Avitene 281
Avlosulfan 551
Azene 12
Azlin 503
Azmacort 355
Azo-Gantanol 538
Azo-Gantrisin 538
Azolid 385
Azulfidine 536

B

Bacarate 65
Bactocill 500
Bactrim 537, 579
Banlin 305
Banthine 305
Basaljel 312
Bayer Aspirin 372
Bayer Children's Aspirin 372
Bayer Timed-Release 384
Beclovant 355
Beconase 417
Beef Lente Ilentin II 428
Beef NPH Ilentin II 427
Beef Regular Ilentin 427
Beef Regular Ilentin II 427
Benadryl 111, 365, 379
Benadryl Cough Syrup 365
Benadryl Hydrochloride 318
Bendylate 379
Benemid 396
Benisone 417
Bentyl 306
Bentylol 306
Benuryl 396
Benzadrine 58
Benzedrex 361
Betadine 578
Betalin 12 297
Betaloc 181

668 Pocket Nurse Guide to Drugs

Betapar 420
Bicillin 500
BiCNU 588
Bilron Pulvules 339
Bisco-Lax 332
Blenoxane 589
Bleph Liquifilm 539
Blocadren 182
Bonine 319
Brethine 346, 347
Bretylol 257
Brevicon 472
Brevital Sodium 88
Bricanyl 346
Brietol Sodium 88
Bristacycline 518
Bronkmeter 345
Bronkosol 345
Bucladin-S 318
Bufferin 372
Bufferin Arthritis Strength 384
Bufopto Atropine 138
Bumex 209
Buminate 239
Buprenex 73, 74
Butal 6
Butazem 6
Butazolidin 385
Butesin Picrate 150
Buticaps 6
Butisol Sodium 6

C

Calan 186, 261
Calcimar 450
Calderol 450
Caldesene 561
Calurin 372
Candex 561
Cantil 304
Capastat Sulfate 547
Capoten 186
Carafate 313
Carbacel 142
Carbocaine 152
Cardiazem 186
Cardilate 166

Cardioquin 260
Cas-Evac 333
Catapres 185
Ceclor 506
Cedilanid-D 257
CeeNU 589
Cefadyl 506
Cefizox 508
Cefobid 507
Celbenin 501
Celestone 417
Celestone phosphate 417
Celestone soluspan 417
Celontin 92, 96
Centrax 15
Cephulac 335
Cerubidine 604
Chel-Iron 292
Chloralvan 20
Chlormene 378
Chloromycetin 522
Chlor-PZ 26
Chlortab 378
Chlor-Trimeton 378
Chlorzide 212
Chocolate Ex-Lax 333
Cholan-DH 339
Choledyl 353
Choloxin 286
Chronulac 335
Cinobac 542
Cin-Quin 259
Ciramine 378
Circlidrin 173
Citanest Hydrochloride 152
Claforan 508
Cleocin HC1 513
Cleocin Pediatric 514
Cleocin Phosphate 514
Clinatine 31
Clinoril 385
Clistin 378
Cloderm 417
Clomid 466
Clonopin 92, 98
Clorprom 26
Cloxapen 501

Trade Name Index 669

Codone 365
Cogentin 110
Colace 335
Colestid 286
Cologel 332
Colonil 327
Coly-Mycin M 533
Coly-Mycin S 533
Comfolax 335
Compazine 30, 321
Control 65
Corgard 181
Coricidin Decongestant Nasal Mist 360
Cort-Dome 419
Cortef 419
Cortef acetate 419
Cortenema 419
Corticotropin 422
Corticotropin gel 422
Cortifoam 420
Cortigel 422
Cortone acetate 417
Cortril 419
Cortril acetate 419
Cortrophin zinc 422
Cortrosyn 422
Cosmegen 604
Cotazym 339
Cotazym-S 339
Coughettes 365
Coumadin 273
Cruex 561
Crysticillin 500
Crystodigin 256
Cuprimine 392
Curretab 463
Cyclaine 150
Cyclanfor 173
Cyclocort 417
Cyclogyl 138
Cyclopar 518
Cyclospasmol 173
Cydel 173
Cylert 60
Cytomel 441
Cytomine 441

Cytosar 598
Cytotoxan 588, 592

D

Dalmane 14
Dantrium 118
Daranide 144
Daraprim 579
Darbid 304
Daricon 305
Darvon 73, 76
Darvon-N 76, 106
Datril 373
Day-Barb 6
DDAVP 406
Deaner 61
Decaderm 418
Decadron 418
Decadron-LA 418
Decadron phosphate 355, 418
Decadron phosphate respihaler 418
Deca-Durabolin 490
Decanoate 29
Decapryn 379
Decaspray 418
Decholin 339
Declomycin 519
Deladumone 458
Delalutin 463
Delatestryl 486
Delaxin 119
Delestrogen 456
Delta-cortef 420
Deltalin 450
Deltasone 421, 615
Demerol 73, 75
Demulen 472
Demulen 1/35 472
Dendrid 566
Depakene 92, 100
Depen 392
Depletile 64
Depo-estradiol cypionate 456
Depogen 456
Depo-Medrol 420
Depo-Provera 463, 615
Depo-Testadiol 458

670 Pocket Nurse Guide to Drugs

Depo-Testosterone 486
Deprex 46
Desenex 561
Desferal 293
Desoxyn 59
Desyrel 48
De-Tone 256
Dex-A-Diet II 65
Dexadrine 59
Dexampex 59
Dexasone-LA 418
Dexatrim 65
Dexone 418
Diabinese 407, 436
Diabeta 436
Diadax 65
Diafen 379
Diamox 92, 98, 143, 220
Diamox Parenteral 144
Diapid 406
Diasone Sodium 551
Dibenzyline 183
Dicarbosil 312
Dicodid 365
Didrex 64
Dienestrol 456
Dietac 65
Dilantin 92, 93, 95, 258
Dilaudid 73, 74
Dilin 352
Dilor 352
Dilosyn 379
Dimetane 378
Diprosone 417
Disalcid 384
Disipal 112
Diuchlor-H 212
Diulo 214
Diurcardin 213
Diurese 213
Diuril 212, 406
Diuril (Sodium) 212
Dobutrex 158
Dolene 76
Dolobid 384
Dolophine 73, 75
Dopar 112

Dopram 69
Dorbane 333
Doriden 20
Dorsacaine 150
Doxycycline hyclate 519
Dramamine 318
Drisdol 450
Drolban 614
D-S-S 335
DTIC-Dome 589
Dulcolax 332
Durabolin 490
Duracillin A.S. 500
Dura-estrin 456
Duralone 420
Duranest 152
Duraquin 259
Duratest 486
Duratestrin 458
Duretic 213
Duricef 506
Duvoid 302
DV 456
Dycholium 339
Dycill 501
Dyclone 150
Dyflex 352
Dymelor 436
Dynapen 501
Dyrenium 217

E

Econopred 421
Ecostatin 560
Ecotrin 372
Ectasul Minus 343
Edecrin 208
Edisylate 30
E.E.S. 512
Efedron Nasal 360
Efedsol-1% 360
Effersyllium 332
Efricel 140
Efudex 598
Elavil 46
Elspar 604
Embolex 272

Trade Name Index 671

Emfabide 352
Emite-Con 322
E-Mycin 512
EMYCT 614
Enanthate 29
Endep 46
Enduron 213
Enovid 5 mg 473
Enovid-E 473
Entron 292
E-Pam 13, 88
Epifrin 143
Epinal 143
Epitrate 143
Eppy 143
Epsom Salt 334
Equanil 21
Ergotrate maleate 480
Erypar 512
Erythrocin Lactobionate IV 512
Erythrocin Stearate 512
Eserine Sulfate 142
Esidrix 212
Eskalith 52
Eskalith-CR 52
Estate 456
Estinyl 457
Estrace 456
Estradurin 461, 614
Estratab 457
Estratest 458
Estrovis 457
Ethrane 84
Ethril 512
Etroxin 440
Euthroid 441
Eucatropine Hydrochloride 134
Evex 457
Exna 212
Ex-Obese 65

F

Fansidar 579
Fastin 65
Feen-A-Mint 333
Feldene 386
Feminone 457

Femogen 457
Fenylhist 379
Feosol 292
Feostat 292
Fergon 292
Fer-In-Sol 292
Ferndex 59
Fero-Gradumet 292
Ferralet Plus 292
Ferranol 292
Ferrolip Plus 292
Ferronord 292
Flagyl 578
Flamazine 538
Flaxedil Triethiodide 130
Fleet Brand 353
Flexeril 119
Flexon 119
Florinef 418
Florinef acetate 418
Florone 418
Floropryl 143
Fluidil 214
Fluonid 419
Fluothane 84
Fluoroplex 598
FML liquifilm 419
Follutein 466
Folvite 297
Forane 84
FreAmine III 240
FUDR 598
Fulvicin 560
Fumerin 292
Fungizone 554, 560
Furadantin 542
Furalan 542
Furamide 578
Furoxone 578

G

Gantonol 536
Gantrisin 536, 539
Garamycin 525
Gelfilm 281
Gelfoam 281
Geocillin 503

672 Pocket Nurse Guide to Drugs

Geopen 503
Geriamic 459
Gesterol L.A. 463
Glaucon 143
Glucotrol 436
Glycotuss 364
Glynazan 353
Glyrol 144
Glysennide 334
Grifulvin 560
Grisactin 560
Gris-Peg 560
Gyne-Lofrimin 560
Gynogen 457

H

Halciderm 419
Halcion 15
Haldol 32, 321
Haldrone 420
Halodrin 459
Halog 419
Halotex 560
Harmonyl 184
Halotestrin 487
Hedulin 273
Hepahydrin 339
Hepathrom 272
Heprinar 272
Herpes Liquifilm 566
Hespan 239
Hexadrol 418
Hexadrol phosphate 418
Hexyphen 111
Hispril 379
Histerone 486
H.M.S. Liquifilm 420
Homatrocel 138
Homatropine Hydrobromide 138
Honvol 456
Hormonin 456
H.P. Acthar Gel 422
Humorosol 142
Humulin N Human NPH 428
Humulin R 427
Hydeltrasol 421
Hydeltra-T.B.A. 421

Hydergine 173
Hydrazol 220
Hydrea 599
Hydrochloride 28, 32, 99, 379
Hydrocortisone acetate 420, 419
Hydrocortisone phosphate 420
Hydrolase 332
Hydromox 214
HydroxDiuril 212
Hygroton 214
Hylorel 184
Hyperstat 187
Hypnomidate 89
Hypoproval-P.A. 463
Hytakerol 450

I

Ilosone 512
Ilotycin 512
Ilotycin Gluceptate IV 512
Ilozymes 339
Imavate 47
Imferon 292
Imodium 327
Impril 47
Inapsine 89, 321
Inderal 182, 260, 289, 446
Indocid 385
Indocin 385
Inhal-Aid 356
Inspir Ease 356
Insulatard NPH 428
Intrabutazone 385
Intralipid 240
Intropin 158
Ionamin 65
Ismelin 184
Ismotic 144
Isobec 6
Iso-Bid 166
Isolait 173
Isophrin 159
Isoptin 186, 261
Isopto Atropine 138
Isopto Carbachol 142
Isopto Carpine 142
Isopto Eserine 142

Trade Name Index 673

Isopto Homatropine 138
Isopto Hyoscine 139
Isordil 166
Isotrate 166
Isuprel Hydrochloride 158, 345
Isuprel Mistometer 345

K

Kantrex 525
Kaopectate 223
Kayexalate 245
Keflex 506
Keflin 506
Kefzol 506
Kelex 292
Kemadrin 111
Kenacort 421
Kenalog 421
Kestrin 457
Ketaject 89
Ketalar 89
Kona Kion 280, 282
Kondremul 334
Ku-Zymes HP 339

L

L.A. Formula 332
Lamprene 551
Lanoxin 256
Largactil 26
Larotid 502
Lasix 208
Lemiserp 183
Lentard 428
Lente Iletin I 428
Lente Purified Pork 429
Leucovorin Calcium 297
Leukeran 588
Levate 46
Levo-Dromoran 73, 74
Levophed 42
Levophed Bitartrate 158
Levothroid 440
Levsin 303
Libritabs 12
Librium 12
Lidex 419

Lidocaine 259
Limit 65
Linocin 514
Lioresal 118
Liop-Hepin 272
Liposyn 240
Liquaemin 273
Liquamar 273
Liquifilm 142
Lithane 52
Lithizine 52
Lithobid 52
Lithonate 52
Lithonate-S 52
Lithotabs 52
Locorten 419
Loestrin 1.5/30 472
Loestrin 1/20 473
Lofene 327
Lomotil 327
Loniten 186
Lo/Ovral 473
Lopin 286
Lopresor 181
Lopressor 181
Loprox 560
Lopurin 396
Lorelco 287
Lorfan 81
Lorodopa 112
Loxipac 34
Loxitane 34
Lozol 214
Ludiomil 48
Lufyllin 352
Lugol's Solution 445, 447
Lumial 7
Luminal 92, 94
Luminal Sodium 93, 94
Lysodren 615

M

Macrodantin 542
Magan 384
Maleate 29, 30
Malogen CYP 486
Mandol 507

674 Pocket Nurse Guide to Drugs

Maolate 118
Marezine 318
Marplan 50
Matulane 599
Maxibolin 490
Maxidex 418
Mazanor 64
Mazepine 99
Measurin 372, 384
Mebaral 92, 94
Meclomen 386
Mediatric 458
Medihaler-Epi 344
Medihaler-Iso 345
Medilium 12
Meditran 21
Medrol 420
Medrol acetate 420
Medrol Enpak 420
Mefoxin 507
Megace 463, 615
Melfiat 65
Mellaril 28
Menest 457
Menrium 458
Mephyton 280
Meprospan 21
Meprospan-400 21
Mercurasol 225
Mer-estrone 457
Mersalyn 225
Mesantion 95
Mestinon 125, 126
Mesylate 293
Metahydrin 213
Metamucil 332
Metandren 487
Metandren linguets 487
Metaprel 346
Methabolic 490
Methampex 59
Methergine 480
Methidate 59
Meticortelone acetate 421
Meticorten 615
Meti-Derm 420
Metopirone 422

Metreton 421
Metryl 578
Metubine 130
Meval 13, 88
Mexate 598
Mezlin 503
Micronase 436
Micronor 463, 473
Microseal Drug Delivery system
  (MDD), 171
Midamor 217
Milk of Magnesia 312, 334
Milontin 92, 93, 96
Milprem 458
Miltown 21
Minipress 183
Minocin 519
Minocin IV 519
Mintezol 579
Miradon 273
Mithracin 604
Mitrolan 332
Mixtard 428, 433
Moban 34
Mobidin 384
Modane 333
Modane Bulk 332
Modecate 29
Moderil 184
Modicon 472
Moditen 29
Mol-Iron 292
Monistat 560
Monocid 507
Motrin 386
Moxam 508
Mucomyst 366
Murocel 143
Mustargen 588
Mutamycin 589
Myambutol 546
Myaxene 131
Mychel 522
Mycifradin 524
Myciguent 524
Mycostatin 561
Mydfrin 140

Trade Name Index 675

Mydriacyl 139
Myleran 588
Myochrisine 392, 393
Myotonachol 302
Mysoline 92, 93, 95
Mytelase 124
Mytrate 143

N

Nafcil 501
Nafrine 361
Nalate 384
Nalfon 386
Nandrolate 490
Nandrolin 490
Naprosyn 386
Naqua 213
Narcan 81
Nardil 50
Nasalcrom 355, 418
Nasalide 355
Naturetin 213
Navane 32
Nebcin 525
NegGram 542
Nembutal 6
Neobiotic 524
Neo-Cultol 335
Neocyten 119
Neoholan 339
Neoloid 333
Neomycin 524
Neo-Polycin 534
Neosar 588
Neosporin 534
Neo-Synephrine 42, 159
Neo-Synephrine Hydrochloride 140, 360
Neo-Synephrine II, Long-Acting 361
Neothylline 352
Neotrizine 538
Neptazine 144, 220
Nesacaine 151
Netromycin 525
Niac 286
Niclocide 578

Nicobid 286
Nicolar 286
Nicomyl 546
Nilstat 561
Nipride 187
Nisentil 73, 74
Nitrex 542
Nitro-Bid 167
Nitrodisc 167
Nitro-Dur 167
Nitroglycerin 166
Nitrol 167
Nitrostat 166
Nizoral 560
Noctec 20
Noe-Barb 6
Noludar 20
Nolvadex 614
Norcuron 131
Nordette 472
Norflex 119
Norinyl 2 mg 472
Norinyl 1 + 50 472
Norinyl 1 + 80 472
Norisodrine Aerotrol 345
Norisodrine Sulfate 345
Norlestrin 1/50 473
Norlestrin 2.5/150 472
Norlutate 463
Norlutin 463
Norpace 260
Norpramin 45, 46
Nor-QD 473
Nortussin 364
Noscatuss 365
Novafed 361
Novocaine 152, 153
Novochlorhydrate 20
Novocolchine 396
Novodipam 13, 88
Novoflupam 14
Novoflurazine 31
Novohydrazine 212
Novolin N Human NPH 428
Novolin L Lente 429
Novolin R Human 427
Novopentobarb 6

676   Pocket Nurse Guide to Drugs

Novopramine 47
Novoridazinek 28
Novosecobarb 8
Novosemide 208
Novothalidone 214
Novotriptyn 46
Novrad 365
NPH Iletin I 428
NPH Insulin 428
NPH Purified Pork 428
Nubain 73, 74
Numorphan 73, 76
Nupercaine 152
Nupercaine hydrochloride 150
Nuprin 386
Nydrazid 546

O

Ocusert Pilo-20 147
Ocusert Pilo-40 147
Ogen 457
Omnipen 502
Oncovin 608
Ophthalmic 539
Ophthane Hydrochloride 151
Optef 419
Optimine 378
Opto-Pentolate 138
Orasone 421
Ora-Testryl 487
Oratrol 144
Oretic 212
Oreton 486
Oreton methyl 487
Organidin 364
Orinase 436
Ormazine 26
Ortho-Novum 2 mg 472
Ortho-Novum 1/50 472
Ortho-Novum 1/80 472
Ortho-Novum 7/7/7 472
Osmitrol 144
Osmoglyn 144
Ostoforte 450
Ovcon-35 472
Ovcon-50 472
Ovitrin Spray 361

Ovral 473
Ovrette 473
O-V Statin 561
Ovulen 472
Oxalid 385
Ox Bile Extracts Enseals 339
Ox-Pam 15
Oxycel 281
Oxylone 419
Oxlopar 519

P

Pagitane Hydrochloride 111
Pamelor 47
Pamine 303
Pancrease 339
Pancreatin 339
Pancreatin Enseals 339
Panectyl 380
Panheprin 272
Panmycin 518
Panophylline Forte 353
Panwarfin 272
Paradione 97
Paradrine 140
Paraflex 119
Parapectolin 327
Parasal Sodium 547
Parisdol 111
Parlodel 466
Parnate 50
PAS Sodium 547
Pathilon 305
Pavulon 130
Paxipam 14
PBZ-SR 380
Peganone 96
Penthrane 84
Pentids 500
Pentocaine Hydrochloride 151,
   152
Pentogen 6
Pentothal 88
Pen-Vee-K 500
Pepto-Bismol 327
Percocet 75, 78
Percodan 75

Trade Name Index 677

Percorten acetate 417
Percorten pivalate 417
Pergonal 466
Periactin 379
Peridol 32
Peritrate 167
Permitil 29
Pertofrane 46
Pethidine HCl 75
Petn Plus 167
Petrogalan plain 335
Pfizerpen 500
Phenazine 30
Phenergan 319, 380
Phenolax 333
Pheno-Square 7
Phospholine Iodide 142
Phosphic-Soda 334
Pilocar 142
Pima 364
Pipanol HCl 111
Pipracil 503
Pitocin 479
Pitressin 406
Pitressin Tannate in oil 405, 406
Pituitrin 406
Placidyl 20, 45
Plaquenil Sulfate 392, 578
Plasbumin 239
Plasmanate 239
Plasma Flex 239
Plasmatein 239
Platinol 589
Plegine 65
PMB 458
Polycillin 502
Polymox 502
Ponderal 64
Pondimin 64
Ponstan 373
Ponstel 373
Pork Lente Iletin II 428
Port NPH Iletin II 428
Pork Regular Iletin II 427
Potassium Iodide 364
Povan 579
Prantal 304

Precef 507
Predcor-TBA
Predulose 421
Premarin 456
Primatene Mist 344
Principen 502
Priscoline 173
Privine Hydrochloride 360
Proaqua 212
Pro-Banthine 305
Probolik 490
Procan 260
Procan-SR 260
Procardia 186
Procyclid 111
Profac-O 463
Progelan 463
Progestilin 463
Proketazine 29
Prolamine 65
Prolixin 29, 321
Proloid 440
Proloprim 542
Promamyl 26
Promapar 26
Pronestyl 260
Pronestyl-SR 260
Propadrine Hydrochloride 361
Propanthel 305
Propine 143
Prostaphlin 501
Prostigmin Bromide 124, 125
Prostigmin Methysulfate 125, 302
Prostin/15M 480
Prostin E2 480
Prostin F2 alpha 480
Protamine, Zinc and Iletin I 429
Protamine, Zinc and Iletin II 429
Protamine Zinc Insulin 429
Protenate 239
Proventil 343
Provera 463
PSP-IV 421
Purified Lente 428
Purified NPH 428
Purinethol 598
Purodigin 256

678 Pocket Nurse Guide to Drugs

P.V. Carpine 142
Pyopen 503
Pyranistan 378
Pyribenzamine 380

Q

Quadetts 538
Quadnite 380
Quarzan 304
Quelicin 131
Questran 286
Quide 28
Quietae 21
Quinaglute Duro-Tabs 259
Quinate 259
Quinidox Extentabs 259
Quinora 259

R

Raudixin 183
Rau-Sed 183
Rauwiloid 184
Rectoid 419
Redisol 297
Regitine Hydrochloride 182
Regitine Mesylate 183
Reglan 323
Regonol 125
Regular Concentrated Ilentin II, purified pork 427
Regular Ilentin I 427
Rela 118
Relaxil 12
Relefact TRH 441
Remsed 319, 380
Renese 213
Renoquid 536
Reserpoid 183
Respihaler 355
Restoril 15
Ridaura 392
Rifadin 546, 551
Rimactane 546, 551
Rimifon 546
Riopan 312
Ritalin 59
Rivotril 98

Robalate 312
Robamol 119
Robaxin 119
Robidone 365
Robidrine 361
Robimycin 512
Robinul 304
Robitussin 364
Rocaltrol 450
Ro-chlorozide 212
Ro-Hist 380
Rohydra 379
Rohypnol 89
Rolabromophen 378
Rolaids 312
Rolavil 46
Rolidrin 173
Romethocarb 119
Romilar CF 365
Rondomycin 519
Roniacol 173
RP-Mycin 512
Rubramin PC 297
Rufen 386
Rynacrom 355

S

Sal Hepatica 334
Salicylamide 373
Saluron 213
Sanorex 64
Sarisol 6
SAS-500 536
Secogen Sodium 8
Seconal 8
Seconal Sodium 8
Sectral 181
Sedadrops 7
Sed-Tensse 303
Semilente Ilentin 427
Semilente Insulin 427
Semilente Purified Pork Prompt Insulin 427
Senokot 333
Senokot Suppositories 333
Septra 537, 579
Seral 8

Trade Name Index 679

Serax 15
Serentil 28, 42
Seromycin 547
Serophene 466
Serpasil 183
Sertan 95
Seventil 28
Silvadene 538
Sinemet 112
Sinequan 46
Sinutab Long-lasting Sinus Spray 361
SK65 76
Sk-Pramine 47
SK-Soxazole 537
Solazine 31
Solfoton 7
Solganal 392, 393
Solu-Cortef 420
Solu-Medrol 420
Solu-Predalone 421
Solurex-LA 418
Soma 118
Sorbide 166
Sorbitrate 166
Spanestrine P 457
Span-Test 486
Sparine 321
Sparini 28
Spenaxin 119
Spenduo 458
Spinhaler 357
SSKI 364
Stadol 73, 74
Staphcillin 501
Statobex 64
Stelazine 31
Stemetil 30
Steribolic 490
Stilbestrol 456
Stilbilium 456
Stiphostrol 456, 614
Stoxil 566
Streptase 278
Streptomycin 524
Sublimaze 74, 89
Sucostrin 131

Sucrets Cough Control Lozenge 365
Sudafed 361
Sulcrate 313
Suldiazo 538
Sulf-10 539
Sulfamyd 539
Sulfamylon 538
Sulfenta 76
Sulfonamide Duplex 537
Sumycin 518
Super Anahist 361
Surfacaine 150
Surfak 335
Surgicel 281
Surital 88
Surmontil 47
Susadrin 167
Sus-Phrine (1:200) 343, 348
Sux-Cert 131
Symmetrel 112, 565
Synalar 419
Synkayvite 290
Synophylate 353
Synthroid 440
Sytobex 297
Syntocinon 479, 481

T

Tacaryl 379
TACE 456
Tagamet 16, 313
Tagamet Hydrochloride 313
Talwin 73
Talwin Lactate 76
Talwin NX 76
Tandearil 385
Tapazole 446
Taractan 31
Tarasan 31
Tavist 378
Teebacin 547
Teebacin Acid 547
Teebaconin 546
Tega-Flex 119
Tegopen 501
Tegretol 92, 93, 99, 407

680 Pocket Nurse Guide to Drugs

Temaril 380
Tenormin 181
Tensilon 124, 126
Tenuate 64
Tepanil 64
Terfluzine 31
Teronac 65
Terramycin 519
Terramycin IM 519
Terramycin IV 519
Teslac 614
Tessalon 366
Testaqua 486
Testate 486
Testoject 486
Testradiol-90/4 458
Testred 487
Tetracyn 518
Tetracyn IM 518
Tetracyn IV 518
Theelin 457
Theofort 353
Theophylline 353
Theo-Syl R 225
Thiodyne 384
Thiolate 385
Thiomerin Sodium 225
Thiotepa 588
Thiosulfil 536
Thiosulfil-A 538
Thorazine 26, 320
Thrombin Topical 281
Th-Sal 385
Thypinone 441
Thyrar 440
Thyrocrine 440
Thyrolar 441
Thyro-Teric 440
Thytropar 441
Ticar 503
Tigan 323
Timoptic 143
Tinactin 561
Tindal Maleate 29
Ting 561
Titralac 313
T-lonate P.A. 486
Tofranil 45, 47

Tofranil-PM 47
Tolectin 385
Tolinase 436
Tolzol 173
Topicort 417
Tora 65
Torecon 321
TRAL 304
Trandate 183
Transdermal Infusion System 170
Transdermal Therapeutic System 170
Transderm-Nitro 167, 171
Transderm-Scop 318, 324
Transderm-V 171
Tranxene 99
Travamulsion 240
Travasol 240
Trecator SC 547
Tremin 111
Trental 173
Trest 306
Trexan 81
Tricilon 421
Triclos 20
Tridesilon 417
Tridione 92, 97
Trihexy 111
Tri-Kort 421
Trilafon 30, 321
Trimpex 542
Tri-Norinyl 472
Triphasil 472
Triple Sulfa 538
Triptil 47
Trobicin 513
Trocinate 306
Tronothane Hydrochloride 151
Troph Amine 240
Tubarine 130
Tums 312
Turbinaire decadron phosphate 418
Tusscapine 365
Tylenol 373
Tylosterone 458
Tylox 75, 78
Tyzine 361

Trade Name Index 681

U

Ulo 366
Ulone 366
Ultracef 506
Ultralente Ilentin I 429
Ultralente Insulin 429
Ultralente Purified Beef 429
Undecyclenic Compound 561
Unde-Jen 561
Unigen 457
Unipen 501
Unisom 379
Uracel 372
Urazide 212
Ureaphil 144
Urecholine 302
Uremide 538
Urevert 144
Uromide 373
Uticort 417

V

Valdrene 379
Valergen 456
Valisone 417
Valium 88, 92, 93, 97, 118, 119
Valmid 20
Valpin 304
Vancenase 417
Vanceril 355
Vancocin 513
Vaponefrin microNEFRIN 344
Vaporole 166
Vasodilan 173
Vasoprine 173
Vasotec 186
Vasoxyl 159
Vatronol Nose Drops 360
V-Cillin K 500
Veetids 500
Veinamide 240
Velban 608
Velbe 608
Velosef 506
Velosulin 427
Ventolin 343

VePesid 608
Vermizine 578
Vermox 578
Verstran 15
Vescal 183
Vesprin 27, 321
Vibramycin 519
Vibramycin IV 519
Viokase 339
Vira-A 566
Viroptic 566
Visken 181
Vistaject 319
Vistaril 20, 319
Vivactil 47
Vontrol 322
Voranil 64

W

Wampocap 286
Westadone 75
Westcort 420
Winstrol 491
Wyamine Sulfate 159
Wycillin 500
Wytensin 185

X

X-Otag 119
Xylocaine 93, 99, 150, 152
Xylocaine hydrochloride 258
Xylocard 99

Y

Yodoxin 578

Z

Zanosar 615
Zantac 313
Zarontin 92, 96
Zaroxolyn 214
Ziloprin 396
Zinacef 507
Zipan 319, 380
Zovirax 565

Index

A

Acebutolol, 176, 177, 181
Acetazolamide, 91, 92, 98, 103, 136, 143, 203, 218, 219, 220
Acetazolamide sodium, 144
Acetaminophen, 78, 370, 371, 372, 374, 399
Acetazolamide sodium, sterile, 136
Acetohexamide, 426, 436
Acetophenazine, 24, 25
Acetophenazine m, 29
Acetylcholine, 108, 122, 128
Acetylcholinesterase inhibitors, for myasthenia gravis, 122, 123-128
  dosage and administration, 124-125
  interactions with anesthetics, 146
  overdose, 126
  reversal of redness by epinephrine, 146
  reversing the irreversible by PAM, 146
Acetylcysteine, 362, 363, 366, 367
Acetylsalicylic acid, 370, 372
Acriscorcin, 552, 558, 559, 560
ACTH, 211, 219
Actinomyces, 535
Acyclovir, 562, 563, 565, 567-568
Addison's disease, 416
Adenohypophyseal hormones, 402, 403, 408-411
  physiologic actions, 410
ADM, 411
Adrenal antagonist, 611, 615

Adrenal gland, drugs affecting, 412-425
Adrenal gland dysfunction, drugs to diagnose, 412, 416, 422
  dosage and administration, 422
Adrenal insufficiency, 413
Adrenal steroids, 412-425
  administration, 417-421
  and smallpox vaccination, 422
  effect on allergy tests, 422
  effect on TB test, 424
Adrenergic beta blockers, 141
Adrenergic bronchodilators, 342-350
  dosage and administration, 343-347
  effects on nervous system, 349
Adrenergics, 136, 143, 301
  hypertensive crisis, 162
  incompatability with other drugs, 161
Adrenocorticotropic hormone (ACTH), 92, 98, 408, 409, 410, 411, 412, 416, 422
Albumin, human, 236, 237, 239, 240, 247-249
Albuterol, 342, 343, 348, 349
Alcohol, 3, 16, 66, 80, 101, 117, 172, 191, 203, 266, 271, 301, 317, 371, 376, 549, 601
Alcoholism, 21-23, 296
Alcoholism, withdrawal, 24-25
Alcohol withdrawal, 11
Aldoril, 191
Aldosterone, 216

684 Pocket Nurse Guide to Drugs

Alkaline phosphatase, 121
Allopurinol, 395, 396, 397, 399,
607-608, 612
Alpha-adrenergic blockers, 188
Alpha-adrenergic receptor
antagonists, 176, 182-183
Alpha- and beta-adrenergic
receptor antagonist, 176, 183
Alphaprodine, 73
Alphaprodine hydrochloride, 71,
74
Alprazolam, 2, 11, 12
Alseroxylon, 176, 184
Aluminum carbonate, 310, 312,
451
Aluminum hydroxide, 310, 312
Aluminum hydroxide gels, 451
Amantadine, 108, 109, 112, 113,
114, 562, 563, 565
Ambenomium, 122, 124, 125
Amcinonide, 412, 417
Amebiasis, 570-571, 577
Amebic dysentery, 519
Amenorrhea, 454, 462, 471
Amikacin, 497, 523, 525, 526, 528
Amiloride, 203, 216, 217, 218
Amino acids, crystalline, 236,
237, 240, 242, 249, 250
Aminocaproic acid, 270, 278, 279,
280, 281, 283
Aminoglycosides, 132, 207, 492,
523-531
and neuromuscular blockade,
530
toxicity and effects on ear,
526-531
dosage and administration,
524
Aminophylline, 194, 342, 350,
351, 352
Aminosalicylate acid, 497, 544,
547
Amitriptyline, 43, 44, 46
Amobarbital, 2, 5, 6, 93
Amoxicillin, 496, 498, 499, 502,
505

Amoxicillin and K clavulanate,
496, 498, 502
Amoxapine, 43, 49
Amphetamines, 54, 56-57, 58, 67,
219, 246
Amphotericin B, 234, 552, 553,
554, 555-556, 558, 559, 560
Ampicillin, 461, 496, 498, 499,
502, 504
Amyl nitrate, 156, 164, 166, 169,
201
Amyotrophic lateral sclerosis, 132
Anabolic steroids, 489-493
dosage and administration,
490-491
Analgesics, 117, 608, 612
Analgesic antipyretics, 382, 387,
390
nonnarcotic, 370-374
Anaphylactic shock, 157, 162
Anaphylaxis, 375
Androgens, 458-459, 484-488,
611-614
anabolic, 484
dosage and administration,
486-487
Anemias, 489
iron deficiency, 291-296
drugs for, dosage and
administration,
292-293
megaloblastic, drugs for,
dosage and administration,
297
megaloblastic macrocytic,
291, 296-298
neutritional treatment of,
291-298
pernicious, 338
Anesthetics,
administration by injection,
151-152
allergic reaction, 149
CNS depressants, 153
CNS stimulants, 149, 153
dental, 83, 86

Index **685**

Anesthetics—cont'd.
general, 83-90
and cough suppression,
85-86
and post-operative pain, 85
in childbirth, 153
inhalation, 83-86
administration, 84
intravenous, 83, 86-90
dosage and administration,
88-89
local, 148-154, 252
obstetrical, 83
surface applications, 150-151
Angina,
and smoking, 164
and weight loss, 165
drugs to treat, 156, 164-171
and hypertension, 165, 168
dosage and administration,
166-167
ointments, 169
oral drugs to treat, 169
sublingual drugs to treat, 168
with dose bandages, 170-171
pectoris, 439
Angiodema, 375
Angiotensin converting enzyme
inhibitors, 189
Anisindione, 270, 273
Anisotropine methyl bromide,
300, 304
Ankylosing spondylitis, 382, 414
Anorexiants, systemic effect, 67
Anovulation, 471
Anoxia, fetal, 478-479
Antacids, 233, 310-315, 387
interference with other drugs,
311, 314
Antialcohol agents, 19-23
Antianxiety agents, 376
Antibiotics, 496-551
and diarrhea, 328
Anticancer drugs, 581-617
Anticholinergic antiemetics, 316,
317, 318

Anticholinergics, 108, 109, 110,
113, 114, 136, 252
to decrease motility, 300, 301,
302-305, 307, 308
to treat ulcers, 310
Anticholinesterase, 132
Anticoagulants, 104, 270-277
oral, 311, 314, 374, 540
overdose, treatment of, 281
dosage and administration,
272-273
drug interactions with, 275
Anticonvulsants, 10, 11, 91-107
dosage and administration,
94-100
Antidepressants, 43-53
anticholinergic effects, 49
second generation, 44, 48-49
administration and dosage,
48
Antidiabetic agents, 426-437
Antidiarrheal drugs, 326-328
Antidiuretic hormone, (ADH),
402, 403, 412-413
Antidopaminergic antiemetics,
316, 317, 320-321, 324
Antiemetics, 78, 84, 87, 116,
316-325, 381, 608, 612
and Reye's Syndrome, 325
CNS depressant, 317
Antiestrogens, 611, 614
Antihistamines, 108, 109, 111,
113, 115, 266, 593-594
for allergic reactions, 375
dosage and administration,
378-380
antiemetics, 316, 317,
318-319
cold remedies, 375
for nausea and vomiting, 375
Antiinflammatory drugs,
nonsteroidal, 370, 382-389, 390
dosage and administration,
384-386
Antihelminthic therapy, 337
Antihypertensive drugs, 176-202

686　Pocket Nurse Guide to Drugs

Antilipemics, 285-290
  dosage and administration, 286-287
  interference with absorption of fat-soluble vitamins, 288
  interference with other drugs, 289
Antipsychotics, 24-42, 376
  and false positive pregnancy tests, 41
  and hypertension, 41-42
  central nervous system depressants, 25
  cholinergic blockade action, 25
  counteraction of, 109
  dosage and administration, 26-34
  endocrine-dopamine blockade, 35
  long-term therapy, 41
  potentiation of analgesics, 42
Antirheumatoid drugs, 390-394
  dosage and administration, 392
Antispasmodics, to decrease motility, 300, 301, 306, 307, 308
Antitussives, 362, 363, 364-366, 375
Antiviral agents, 562-568
Antiviral drugs, 562, 565
  dosage and administration, 565-566
Antiviral vaccines, characteristics and administration, 564-565
Appetite suppression, 55
Arrhythmia, drugs to treat, 252-269
  dosages and administration, 256-261
Arthritis, 387
  drugs to treat, 390-394
Asparaginase, 602, 603, 604, 605
Aspergillus, 553

Aspirin, 78, 198, 275, 370, 371, 374, 382, 383, 384, 387, 388, 399, 416
  and Reye's Syndrome, 371
Asthma, 375, 413
  bronchial or respiratory disease as consideration, 3, 68, 101, 109, 123, 214, 262, 363, 444
  drugs for, 342-357
Atenolol, 176, 177, 181
Atropine, 125, 126, 129, 136, 137, 194, 252, 253, 254, 258, 262, 264, 266, 300, 302, 307, 326, 327, 328
Atracurium, 122, 130
Auranofin, 390, 391, 392
Aurothioglucose, 390, 392
Autoimmune hemolytic anemia, 414
Azatadine maleate, 375, 378
Azathioprine, 399
Azlocillin sodium, 496, 498, 503, 504

B

Bacillis anthracis, 498
Bacitracin, 132, 496, 511, 513, 516, 517, 554
Back pain, 382
Baclofen, 108, 116, 117, 118, 120, 121
Bacteriodes fragilis, 511
Barbiturates, 2, 5-11, 70, 86, 87, 88, 90, 91, 101, 102, 104, 130, 191, 233, 266, 461
  abuse and control, 5
  anticonvulsant, 10
  central nervous system depressant, 5
  dependence and withdrawal, 5
  dosages and administration, 6-8
  intermediate-acting, 6

Index 687

Barbiturates—cont'd.
long-acting, 7, 94
short-acting, 6, 8
overdose and treatment,
10-11
withdrawal, 101
Beclomethasone, 412, 417
Beclomethasone dipropionate,
342, 354, 355, 356
Belladonna, 137, 300, 302-303,
309
Bendroflumethiazide, 203, 211,
213
Benzathine Penicillin G, 496, 498,
500, 505
Benzocaine, 148, 150
Benzodiazepines, 2, 11-17, 83,
86, 88, 91, 92, 97, 105
central nervous system
depressant, 11, 16
dependence and withdrawal,
16-17
dosages and preparations,
12-15
Benzonatate, 362, 366, 367
Benzphetamine, 54, 63, 64, 67
Benzthiazide, 203, 211, 212
Benztropine, 109
Benztropine mesylate, 108, 110
Benzquin amide hydrochlorides,
316, 322, 325
Beta-adrenergic blockers, 188
Beta-adrenergic receptor
antagonists, 156, 164, 176, 181,
192-194
Beta-blockers, 200, 252, 255
overdose, treatment of, 194
Betamethasone, 412, 417
Bethanecol chloride, 300, 301,
302, 307
Bexoxinate hydrochloride, 148,
150
Bile acids, 285
Bile salts, 338, 339, 340
Bilirubin, 121
Biperiden, 108, 110

Bisacodyl, 329, 330, 332, 336
Bishydroxycoumarin, 270, 272-273
Bismuth salts, 326, 327
Bismuth subsalicylate, 326, 327
Bladder, atonic, 301
Blastomyces, 553
Blood, components and
substitutes, 236, 239
Blood, whole, 236, 237, 239, 241,
247-249
Bleomycin, 586, 587, 589, 590,
594
Bone loss, 489
Brompheniramine maleate, 375,
376, 378
Bronchodilators, 342-357
Buclizine hydrochloride, 316, 318
Bumetanide, 203, 206, 208, 209,
210
Bupivacaine, 148
Bowel, hyperactive, 301
Brain edema, 205
Bretylium tosylate, 252, 253, 254,
257, 262, 264, 265
Bretylium,
in hypotension, 265
Bromocriptine mesylate, 465, 466,
468
Bupivacaine, 149, 151
Buprenorphine, 71, 72, 73, 74
Burn therapy,
role of anabolic steroids in,
489
Bursitis, 414
Busulfan, 586, 587, 588, 590, 592
Butabarbital, 2, 5, 6
Butamben picrate, 148, 150
Butyrophenone, 24, 32, 301
Butorphanol, 72, 73, 77
Butorphanol tartrate, 71, 74

C

Caffeine, 68, 69, 311, 314
Caffeine sodium benzoate, 54, 66,
69

688 Pocket Nurse Guide to Drugs

Calciferol, 438, 448, 449, 450
Calcitonin, 438, 448, 449, 450
Calcitriol, 438, 448, 449, 450
Calcium, 247
    in muscular contraction, 117
Calcium carbasprin, 370, 372
Calcium carbonate, 310, 312
Calcium channel blockers, 156,
    164, 189, 198-199, 252, 255
Calcium gluconate, 448
Calcium metabolism, drugs to
    alter, 438, 448-451
        dosage and administration,
            450
Calcium replacements,
    intramuscular, 241
Calcium undecylenate, 552, 558,
    561
Cancer, 78, 454, 455, 462, 484,
    489
    drugs to control in specific
        tissues, 611-617
        dosage and administration,
            614-615
    drugs to treat, 581-617
    drugs that attack DNA,
        586-595
        dosage and administration,
            588-589
    drugs that block DNA
        synthesis, 596-601
        dosage and administration,
            598-599
    drugs that block mitosis,
        607-609
        dosage and administration,
            608
    drugs that block RNA and
        protein synthesis, 602-606
        dosage and administration,
            604
Cancer chemotherapy, and
    diarrhea, 328
Candicidin, 552
Candida, 553, 558
Candidal infection, 461

Capreomycin, 497, 544, 547, 548
Captopril, 176, 179, 180, 186,
    189, 200
Carbachol, 136, 142
Carbamazepine, 91, 93, 99, 103,
    106, 311, 314, 402, 404, 407
Carbenicillin disodium, 496, 498,
    503, 504
Carbenicillin indanyl sodium, 496,
    498, 503, 504
Carbidopa-levadopa, 108, 109,
    112, 113, 116
Carbinoxamine maleate, 375, 377,
    378
Carbonic anhydrase, 211
Carbonic anhydrase inhibitors,
    136, 141, 143-144, 145, 146,
    203, 204, 218-222
        and potassium supplements,
            221
        dosage and administration,
            220
        enhancement of potassium
            excretion, 219
Carboprost tromethamine, 478,
    480, 481
Carboxymethylcellulose, 329, 332
Cardiac or Cardiovascular disease,
    as consideration, 21, 44, 57, 72,
    109, 160, 187, 241, 253, 301,
    306, 311, 330, 348, 358, 376,
    388, 404, 460, 485, 490, 510
Cardiac glycosides, 228-235
        effect on ECG, 234
        pharmacokinetics, 231
        therapeutic strategy, 230
Cardiotonic drugs, 228-235
Carisoprodol, 108, 116, 118
Carphenazine, 24, 25
Carphenazine maleate, 29
Carmustine, 586, 587, 588, 590,
    592
Cascara sagrada, 329, 330, 333
Castor oil, 329, 333, 336
    emulsified, 329, 333, 336
Catecholamines, 265

Cathartics, 329-337
saline, 329, 334, 337
stimulants, 329, 332-334, 336-337
Cefaclor, 496, 506
Cefadroxil monohydrate, 496, 505, 510
Cefamandole nafate, 496, 507, 509, 510
Cefaperazone sodium, 496, 507, 509, 510
Cefazolin sodium, 496, 505, 506, 510
Cefonicid sodium, 496, 507, 509
Ceforanide, 496, 507, 509
Cefotaxime sodium, 496, 508, 509, 510
Cefoxitin sodium, 496, 507, 509, 510
Ceftizoxime sodium, 496, 508, 509, 510
Cefuroxime sodium, 496, 507, 509
Cellulose, oxidized, 270, 279, 281, 282
Cellulose, regenerated oxidized, 270, 279, 281, 282
Central Nervous System, (CNS) depressants, 117
Central Nervous System, (CNS) stimulants, 54-70
abuse, 55
for narcolepsy and hyperkinesis, 54, 56-62
dosage and administration, 58-61
for respiratory stimulation, 54, 66-70
dosage and administration, 69
to suppress appetite, 54, 63-67
dosage and administration, 64-65
Cepalothin sodium, 496, 505, 506
Cephalexin, 496, 505, 506

Cephalosporins, 496-497, 505-510
dosage and administration, 506-508, 510
Cephapirin sodium, 496, 505, 506, 510
Cephradine, 496, 505, 506, 510
Cerebral edema, 414
Cerebral injury, 117
Cerebral palsy, 117
Chlamydia, 519, 521, 535, 541
Chlonazepam, 91
Chlophedianol, 362, 366, 367
Chloral hydrate, 17, 18, 20
Chlorambucil, 586, 588, 590, 591
Chloramphenicol, 266, 497, 521-523
dosage and administration, 522
Chloramphenicol palmitate, 497, 521, 522
Chloramphenicol sodium succinate, 497, 521, 522, 523
Chlorazepate, 2, 11, 12, 91, 93, 103, 314
Chlorazepate dipotassium, 99
Chlordiazepoxide, 2, 11, 12, 311, 314, 458
Chloroprocaine, 148, 149, 151
Chloroquine, 569, 572, 576, 578, 580
Chlorotheophylline, 376
Chlorothiazide, 402, 403, 406
Chlorotrianisene, 454, 456
Chlorphenesin, 108, 116, 118
Chlorpheniramine maleate, 375, 377, 378
Chlorpropamide, 402, 403, 404, 407, 408, 426, 436
Chlorpromazine, 24
counteraction of quanethidine, 41
Chlorpromazine hydrochloride, 316, 317, 320
Chlorprothixene, 25, 31
Chlorothiazide, 203, 211, 212, 214, 215

690   Pocket Nurse Guide to Drugs

Chlorothiazide sodium, 203, 211, 212

Chlorzoxazone, 108, 116, 119, 120

Cholesterol, 164, 194, 285, 290

Cholestyramine, 233

Cholestyramine resin, 285, 286, 287, 288-289

Choline salicylate, 382, 384

Choline theophyllinate, 342, 350, 353

Cholinergic crisis, 123

Cholinesterase inhibitor, 122, 131

Cholinomimetics, 136, 141, 142-143, 145

Chorioretinitus, 414

Chvostek's sign, 247, 448

Ciclopirox olamine, 552, 558, 559, 566

Cimetidine, 16, 193, 267, 268, 310, 311, 313, 314-315

Cinoxacin, 497, 541, 542, 543

Cirrhosis with ascites, 415

Cisplatin, 586, 587, 589, 590, 593

Citrated caffeine, 54, 66, 69

Clemastine, 375, 377, 378

Clindamycin, 132, 496, 511, 513, 516, 517

Clindamycin palmitate, 496, 511, 513

Clindamycin phosphate, 496, 511, 513

Clidinium bromide, 300, 304

Clioguinol, 552, 558, 559, 560

Clocortolone, 412, 417

Clofazimine, 497, 550, 551

Clofibrate, 285, 286, 287, 289, 402, 403, 404, 407

Clomiphene citrate, 465, 466, 467

Clonazepam, 92, 98, 101, 103, 105, 178, 180, 185, 187, 188, 189, 197

Clonidine hydrochloride, 176

Clortermine, 54, 63, 64, 67

Clostridium difficile, 511

Clostridium perfringens, 498

Clostridium tetani, 498

Clotrimazole, 552, 558, 559, 560

Cloxacillin sodium, 496, 498, 499, 501

Coagulation, 270-271, 279, 281

Coagulation testing, 275-277

Cocaine hydrochloride, 148, 150

Coccidioides, 553

Codeine, 362, 363, 364, 370

Codeine phosphate, 71, 73, 74, 326, 327

Codeine sulfate, 71, 74, 326, 327

Colchicine, 395, 396, 397, 398

Colestipol hydrochloride, 285, 286, 287, 288-289

Colistimethane sodium, 497, 532, 533

Colistin methane sulfonate, 497, 532, 533

Colistin sulfate, 497, 532, 533

Colitis, ulcerative, 415

Collagen hemostat, microfibrillar 270, 279, 281, 282

Complex seizures, 93

Congestive heart failure, 219
   drugs to treat, 228-235

Conjunctivitis, allergic, 414

Contraceptives oral, 454, 462, 469-477
   amounts of progestin and estrogen, 472-473
   potential adverse reactions, 474-475

Coombs' test, 197

Copper metabolism, 393

Corneal marginal ulcers, allergic, 414

Cortical focal seizures, 92

Corticosteroids, 211, 219, 393, 593, 594

Corticosteroid therapy, role of anabolic steroids in, 489

Corticotropin, 410

Cortisol, 409, 412, 419-420

Cortisone, 98, 412, 417

Corynebacterium diptherium, 498

Cosyntropin, 412, 416, 422

Index **691**

Cough, drugs to treat, 362-367
 dosage and administration,
 364-366
Coumarin, 266, 272-273, 274,
 277, 289, 523
Coumarin overdose, treatment of,
 277
CPD (citrate-phosphate-dextrose),
 239
CPDA (citrate-phosphate-dextrose-
 adenine), 239
Creatinine phosphokinase, (CPR),
 267, 268
Cretinism, 443
Cromolyn sodium, 342, 354, 355,
 356
Cryptochordism, 468
Cryptococcus, 553
Crystalline, 297
Curare, 122, 130
 Neostigmine antidote for, 128
Cushing's syndrome, 354, 416,
 425, 613
Cyanocobalamin, 291, 297
Cyclandelate, 156, 171, 173, 174
Cyclic AMP, 68, 229, 342, 350
Cyclizine hydrochloride, 316, 318
Cyclizine lactate, 316, 318
Cyclobenzaprine, 108, 116, 119,
 120
Cyclomethycaine sulfate, 148, 150
Cyclooxygenase, 382
Cyclopentolate, 137
Cyclopentolate hydrochloride, 136
Cyclophosphamide, 586, 587,
 588, 590, 592
Cycloplegia, 136-141
 drugs producing, 136
Cyclopropane, 68
Cycloserine, 497, 544, 547, 548
Cyclothiazide, 203, 211, 214
Cycrimine hydrochloride, 108, 110
Cyproheptadine hydrochloride,
 375, 378
Cystic fibrosis, 338
Cytarabine or Ara-C, 596, 597,
 598, 600

D

Dacarbazine, 586, 587, 589, 590,
 593
Dactinomycin, 602, 603, 604, 606
Dantrolene, 108, 116, 117, 118,
 120, 121
Danthron, 329, 333
Dapsone, 497, 550, 551
Daunorubicin, 602, 603, 604, 606
Deanol, 54, 56, 61
Decongestants, 358-361
 dosage and administration,
 360-361
Deferoxamine mesylate, 291, 293,
 294, 295
Dehydrochloric acid, 338, 340
Demecarium, 141
Demecarium bromide, 136, 142
Demeclocycline HCl, 496, 518,
 519
Dental inflammation,
 postoperative, 415
Depolarizing drugs, 122, 131
Depression, 54
Dermatitis, contact, 413
Dermatitis, seborrheic, 413
Deserpidine, 184
Deserpine, 176
Desipramine, 43, 44, 46
Deslanoside, 228, 231, 232, 252,
 253, 257
Desmopressin acetate, 402, 403,
 404, 406
Desonide, 412, 417
Desoximetasone, 412, 417
Desoxycorticosterone, 412, 413,
 417
Dexamethasone, 412, 416, 418
Dexamethasone sodium phosphate,
 342, 354, 355
Dexchlorpheniramine
 hydrochloride, 375, 379
Dextrans, 236, 237, 239, 242,
 249, 278
Dextroamphetamine sulfate, 54,
 56, 59

692 Pocket Nurse Guide to Drugs

Dextromethorphan hydrobromide, 362, 363, 365
Dextrose,
in saline, 241
in water, 236, 237, 238
Dextrose solution, hypertonic, 236, 237, 239, 241, 249, 250
Dextrothyroxine, 285, 286, 287, 290
Diabetes,
as consideration, 40, 50, 56, 105, 145, 147, 192, 211, 215, 216, 221, 284, 290, 330, 348, 350, 351, 358, 391, 442, 488, 545, 559, 617
drugs to treat, 426-437
Diabetes insipidus, 205
drugs to treat, 402-408
Diabetes mellitus, 426
Diabetes, Type I, 426
Diabetes, Type II, 435
Diarrhea, treatment of, 326-328
Diazepam, 2, 11, 13, 83, 86, 87, 88, 91, 92, 93, 97, 98, 102, 103, 105, 108, 116, 117, 118, 119, 120, 266, 311, 314
Diazoxide, 176, 179, 180, 187, 189, 200-201, 266
Dibenzoxazepine, 24, 34
Dibenzyline, 183
Dibucaire, 148, 149, 150, 152
Dichlorphenamide, 136, 144
Dicloxacillin sodium, 496, 498, 499, 501
Dicumarol, 270, 272-273
Dicyclomine hydrochloride, 300, 306
Dienestrol, 454, 456
Diethylpropion, 54, 63, 64, 67
Diethylstilbestrol (DES), 454, 456, 458
Diethylstilbestrol diphosphate, 611, 612, 614
Diflorasone, 412, 418
Diflunisal, 382, 383, 384

Digestants, 338-340
dosage and administration, 339
Digitalis, 145, 160, 194, 196, 207, 211, 219, 228, 231, 233, 234, 235, 247, 253, 254, 264, 265, 290, 442, 448, 531
Digitoxin, 228, 230, 231, 232, 252, 253, 256
Digoxin, 199, 200, 228, 230, 231, 232, 252, 253, 256, 311, 315
Dihydroergotamine, (DHE), 272
Dihydrogenated ergot, alkaloids, 156, 171, 173, 174
Dihydrotachysterol, 438, 448, 449, 450
Dihydroxyaluminum amino-acetate, 310, 312
Dihydroxyaluminum sodium carbonate, 310, 312
Diiodohydroxyquin, 569, 578
Dilaudid, 74
Diloxamide furoate, 569, 571, 578
Diltiazem, 176, 179, 180, 186, 189, 200
Dimenhydrinate, 316, 317, 318, 376, 381
Dimercaprol, 226
Dinoprostone, 478, 480, 481
Dinoprost tromethamine, 478, 480, 481
Diphemanil methylsulfate, 300, 301, 304
Diphenhydramine hydrochloride, 108, 111, 308, 316, 317, 318, 362, 365, 367, 375, 376, 377, 379, 381
Diphenidol hydrochloride, 316, 317, 322, 324, 325
Diphenoxylate hydrochloride, 326, 327, 328
Diphenylpyraline hydrochloride, 375, 379
Diphtheria, 511
Dipivefrin, 136, 143
Direct acting vasodilators, 156

Index 693

Disopyramide phosphate, 252, 253, 255, 260, 265, 268-269
Disulfiram, 19-23, 266, 601
Diuretics, 176, 177, 180, 194, 203-227, 228, 229
    effect on tubular transport, 204
    non-thiazide with thiazide-like action, 214
Dobutamine, 156, 157, 158, 160, 162, 163, 228, 229
Docusate calcium, 329, 335
Docusate sodium, 329, 335
Domperidone, 316, 317, 322
Dopamine, 108, 156, 157, 158, 160, 162, 163, 228, 229, 265
Doxapram, 54, 66, 68, 69, 70
Doxepin, 43, 44, 46
Doxorubicin, 602, 603, 604, 606
Doxycycline, 496, 518, 519, 520, 521
Doxylamine succinate, 375, 376, 379
Dromostanolone propionate, 611-612, 614
Droperidol, 87, 89, 316, 317, 320
Droperidol & Fentanyl, 83, 86
Dwarfism, 409, 489
Dyclonine hydrochloride, 148, 150
Dyphylline, 342, 350, 352
Dysmenorrhea, 469

E

Eaton-Lambert syndrome, 132
Echothiophate, 141
Echothiophate iodide, 136, 142
Eclampsia, 196
Econazole nitrate, 552, 558, 559, 560
Eczema, 375
Edema, 205, 211
Edrophonium, 122, 123, 124, 125, 126, 129
Electrolyte imbalance, 236
Emetine, 569, 571, 578, 580-581

Emphysema, bronchial, 415
Enalapril, 176, 179, 186, 189
Endocrine disorders, 454
Endometrial bleeding, 462
Endorphins, 71
Enflurane, 68, 83, 84
Enteritis, 415
Enuresis, 43
Ephedrine, 228, 229
Ephedrine sulfate, 342, 343, 348, 349, 358, 360
Epilepsy, 117
Epileptic seizures, 91
Epinephrine, 136, 141, 143, 145, 156, 157, 158, 160, 162-163, 194, 342, 343-344, 348, 349, 358, 359, 360, 376, 393, 593, 594
Epinephrine bitartrate, 136, 143
Epinephryl borate, 136, 143
Equilibrium,
    effect of antiemetics on, 316
Ergocalciferol, 438, 448, 449, 450
Erogonovine maleate, 478, 480
Erythema multiforme, 413
Erythrityl tetranitrate, 156, 164, 166
Erythromycins, 219, 496, 511, 512, 515, 516
Erythromycin base, 496, 511, 512, 517
Erythromycin estolate, 496, 511, 512, 517
Erythromycin ethylsuccinate, 496, 511, 512
Erythromycin gluceptate, 496, 511, 512, 515
Erythromycin lactobionate, 496, 511, 512, 515, 517
Erythromycin stearate, 496, 511, 512
Estradiol, 454, 456
Estradiol cypionate, 454, 456, 458
Estradiol valerate, 454, 456

694 Pocket Nurse Guide to Drugs

Estramustine phosphate sodium, 611, 612, 614
Estrogens, 454-461, 469, 611, 614
  administration, 456
  conjugated, 454, 456, 458
  esterified, 454, 457, 458
  in combinations, 458-459
Estrogen deficiency, 454
Estrogenic substance, 454, 457
Estrone, 454, 457, 458
Estropipate, 454, 457
Ethacrynic acid, 203, 206, 207, 208, 210
Ethambutol, 497, 544, 545, 546, 548, 549
Ethchlorvynol, 17, 18, 20, 45
Ethinamate, 18, 20
Ethinyl estradiol, 454, 457, 458, 472, 473
Ethionamide, 497, 544, 547, 548
Ethopropazine, 108, 111
Ethosuximide, 91, 92, 96
Ethotoin, 91, 96
Ethylestrenol, 489, 490
Ethynodiol diacetate, 469, 472
Etidocaine, 148, 149, 152
Etomidate, 83, 86, 87, 89
Etoposide, 607, 608, 610
Eucatropine hydrochloride, 136, 137, 139
Expectorants, 362, 363, 364
Extended insulin zinc suspension, 426, 429

F

Factor VIII, 249
Fat emulsion, 236, 237, 240, 242, 249, 251
FD&C number 5, 45, 198, 245
FD&C yellow number 5, 42, 592
Fecal softeners, 329, 335, 337
Fenamate, 386
Fenfluramine, 54, 63, 64, 66, 67
Fenoprofen, 382, 383, 386, 387, 389
Fentanyl, 71, 73, 74

Fentanyl citrate, 83, 86, 89
Ferrocholinate, 291, 292
Ferroglycine sulfate, 291, 292
Ferrous fumarate, 291, 292
Ferrous gluconate, 291, 292
Ferrous sulfate, 291, 292
Fertility agents, 465-468
  administration, 466
Floxuridine, 596, 597, 598
Flucytosine, 552, 553, 554, 556
Fludrocortisone, 412, 413, 418
Fluid deficit, 236
Fluid excess, 236
Fluids and electrolytes, 236-251
  dosages and administration, 238-240
Flumethasone, 412, 419
Flunisolide, 342, 354, 355, 412, 418
Flunitrazepam, 83, 86, 87, 89
Fluocinolone, 412, 419
Fluocinonide, 412, 419
Fluorometholone, 412, 419
Fluorouracil, or 5-FU, 596, 597, 598, 600
Fluoxymesterone, 459, 484, 485, 487
Fluphenazine, 24, 25, 29, 316, 321
Fluphenazine decanoate, 29
Fluphenazine enanthate, 29
Fluprednisolone, 412, 419
Flurazepam, 2, 11, 14
Folic acid, 102, 105, 266, 291, 296, 297
Follicle-stimulating hormone (FSH), 402, 408, 409, 410, 411, 465
Fungal infections, drugs to treat, 552-561
Fungal infections, systemic, drugs to treat, 552
  dosage and administration, 554-555
Fungal infections, topical, drugs to treat, 552, 557-561
Furazolidone, 569, 573, 578

Index   695

Furosemide, 203, 206, 207, 208, 210

G

Gallamine, 128, 129
Gallamine triethiodine, 122, 130
Gelatin film, absorbable, 270, 279, 281, 282
Gelatin sponge, absorbable, 270, 279, 281
Gemfibrozil, 285, 286, 287, 289
Gentamicin, 497, 523, 524, 525, 526, 528
German measles, 564
G-6-PD deficiency, 577
Giardiasis, 573, 577
Gilles de la Tourette syndrome, drugs to treat, 25
Gitalin, 228, 231
Glaucoma, 205, 219, 221
    as consideration, 16, 44, 45, 57, 109, 117, 132, 137, 160, 193, 205, 262, 308, 376
    drugs to treat, 136, 141-147
    and cataracts, 145
    dosage and administration, 142-144
    emergency treatment of, 141, 145
    test for, 139
Glipizide, 426, 436
Glucagon, 431
Glucocorticoids, 356, 390, 391, 409, 412, 413, 416, 422, 425, 611, 612, 615, 616
    conditions treated with, 413-415
Glucose, 234
Glutanic acid, 338, 339
Glutethimide, 18, 20
Glyburide, 426, 436
Glycerin, 136, 144, 145, 329, 335
    and hyperglycemia, 147
Glycerin suppositories, 329, 333, 336-337
Glycerol guaiacolate, 362, 364

Glycopyrrolate, 300, 304
Glycoside mixtures, 232
Gold sodium thiomalate, 390, 391, 392
Gonorrhea, 498
Gout, 289, 382
    drugs to treat, 395-399
    dosage and administration, 396-397
Gouty arthritis, 414
Grand mal seizures, 5, 19, 92, 101
Graves' disease, 444
Grey syndrome, 523
Griseofulvin, 552, 558, 559, 560
Growth hormone (GH), 402, 408, 410, 411
Growth stimulation, 489
Guanabenz, 176, 178, 180, 185, 188, 189, 197
Guanadrel, 176, 178, 180, 184, 195
Guanethidine, 176, 178, 180, 187, 188, 195-196
Guanethidine sulfate, 184
Guanifenesin, 362, 363, 364

H

Halazepam, 2, 11, 14
Halcinonide, 412, 419
Haloperidol, 25, 32, 316, 321
Haloprogin, 552, 558, 559, 560
Halothane, 68, 84, 86
Hay fever, 375
Heart failure, congestive, 415
Helminth (worm) infestations, drugs to treat, 574-575
Hemoglobin, 291
Hemophilia, 249
Hemostatic Agents, 270, 279-284
    dosage and administration, 280-281
Heparin, 270, 271, 275, 276
Heparin overdose, treatment of, 276
Hepatitis B, 562, 563
Hetastarch, 236, 237, 239, 242, 249

696 Pocket Nurse Guide to Drugs

Hexafluorenium, 122, 128, 131
Hexocyclium methylsulfate, 300, 304
Hexylcaine hydrochloride, 148, 150
Hiccups, drugs to treat, 24
Histamine, 375
Histoplasma, 553
Hives, 375
Hodgkin's disease, 586-587, 597
Homatropine, 137
Homatropine hydrobromide, 136, 138
Homatropine methylbromide, 300, 303
Hookworms, 575, 577
H_2 receptor antagonists, 310, 313, 314-315
Human chorionic gonadotropin (HCG), 465, 466, 467, 468
Hydantoins, 91, 95, 102
and oral hygiene, 104-105
Hydralazine, 176, 179, 180, 185, 188, 189, 197-198
Hydrochloric acid, 338, 339, 340
Hydrochlorothiazide, 191, 203, 211, 212
Hydrocodone bitartrate, 362, 363, 365
Hydrocortisone, 412, 419-420
Hydroflumethiazide, 203, 211, 213
Hydromorphone hydrochloride, 71, 73, 74
Hydroxyamphetamine hydrobromide, 136, 137, 140
Hydroxychloroquine, 569, 572, 576, 578, 580
Hydroxychloroquine salts, 390, 391, 392, 393
Hydroxycobalamin, 291, 297
Hydroxymagnesium aluminate, 310
Hydroxyprogesterone, 462, 463
Hydroxystilbamidine isethionate, 552, 553, 554
Hydroxyurea, 596, 597, 599, 601

Hydroxyzine hydrochloride, 18, 20-21, 316, 319, 375, 379
Hydroxyzine pamoate, 18, 20-21, 316, 319, 375, 379
Hyperkalemia, treatment of, 245
Hyperkinesis, 54, 55, 56, 57
Hyperkinetic retardation, drugs to treat, 25
Hyperlipidemia, 251
treatment of, 285-290
Hypertension, 205
drugs for,
causing hypotension, 190
combined with diuretics, 191
drugs to treat,
dosage and administration, 181-186
therapeutic strategy, 180
drug types, 177-179
Hypertensive emergencies, 180
Hypertensive emergency drugs, 176, 187, 189
Hyperthyroidism, drugs to treat, 438, 443-448
dosage and administration, 446-447
Hypervolemia, 237
Hypnotics, 376
Hypoglycemic agents, oral, 426, 434-437
dosage and administration, 436
Hypoglycemics, oral, 540
Hypothrombinemia, 281
Hypothyroidism, drugs to treat, 438-443
dosage and administration, 440-441
Hypothyroid treatment, effects on other glands, 439
Hypovolemic shock, 237
Hypoxanthine, 395
Hyposcyamine hydrobromide, 300, 303
Hyposcyamine sulfate, 300, 303

Index 697

I

Ibuprofen, 382, 383, 386, 389
Idoxuridine, 562, 563, 566, 567
Imipramine, 44
Imipramine hydrochloride, 43, 47
Imipramine pamoate, 43, 47
Immunosuppressive drugs, 390
Impotence, treatment of, 484
Indandiones, 273, 274, 277
Indandione overdose, treatment of, 277
Indapamide, 203, 211, 214
Indole, derivative of parachlorobenzoic acid, 382, 385
Indomethacin, 193, 382, 383, 385, 388
Infantile spasms, 92
Influenza, 562, 564
Innovar, 85
Insulin, 250, 398, 426-434
    allergic reaction to, 430
    mixing of two kinds, 431
Insulin preparations, administration and properties, 427-429
Insulin zinc suspension, 426, 428
    prompt 426, 427
Intermittent Positive Pressure Breathing (IPPB), 86
Interstitial cell-stimulating hormone (ICSH), 402, 408, 410
Intestine, atonic, 301
Intralipid, 236, 240
Intraocular pressure, 205
Iodinated glycerol, 362, 363, 364
Iodine, 444, 445
Iodochlorhydroxyquin, 552, 558, 560
Iodoquinol, 569, 571, 578, 581
Iritis and iridocytosis, 414
Iron overdose, treatment of, 296
Iron toxicity, antidote, 291, 293
Iron-dextran, 291, 292, 295
Isocarboxazid, 43, 49, 50

Isoetharine hydrochloride, 342, 345, 348, 349
Isoetharine mesylate, 342, 345, 348, 349
Isoflurane, 83, 84
Isoflurophate, 136, 141, 143
Isoniazid, 266, 424, 497, 544, 545, 546, 548-549
Isophane insulin suspension (NPH), 426, 428
Isopropamide iodide, 300, 304
Isoproterenol, 157, 160, 162-163, 194, 342, 345, 349
Isoproterenol hydrochloride, 156, 158
Isoproterenol sulfate, 342, 345, 349
Isosorbide, 136, 144, 145
Isosorbide dinitrate, 156, 164, 166, 228, 229
Isoxsuprine, 156, 172, 173, 174

J

Jacksonian seizures, 92

K

Kanamycin, 224, 497, 523, 524, 525, 526, 527
Karaya gum, 329, 332
Keratitis, 414
Ketamine, 83, 86, 87, 89
Ketoconazole, 552, 553, 554, 557
Ketone tests, false positives, 107
Klebsiella, 541

L

Labetalol, 178, 188, 195
Labetalol hydrochloride, 176, 183
Labor, stimulation of, 478
Lactulose, 329, 331, 335, 337
Larva migrans, cutaneous, 575
Laxatives, 329-337
    bulk forming, 329, 332, 336
    and cathartics, dosage and administration, 332-335
Lee-White test, 275

698 Pocket Nurse Guide to Drugs

Legionnaire's disease, 511
Leprosy, drugs to treat, 497, 550-551
Leucovorin, 601
Leucovorin calcium, 291, 296, 297, 298
Leukemia, 414
Levallorphan hydrochloride, 82
Levallorphan tartrate, 71, 80, 81
Levarterenol, 42, 157, 160, 162, 194, 196, 263
Levodopa, 108, 109, 112, 113, 115, 116
    and MAO inhibitors, 115
Levonorgestrol, 469, 472
Levopropoxyphene napsylate, 362, 365, 367
Levorphanol tartrate, 71, 73, 74
Levothyroxine sodium (T_4), 438, 439, 440, 442
LH, 465, 469
Lidocaine, 91, 93, 99, 103, 148, 149, 150, 152, 246, 252, 253, 254, 258, 259, 262-263, 264, 266-267
    effect on CPK levels, 267
Lincomycin, 132, 496, 511, 513, 515, 517
Liothyronine sodium, (T_3), 438, 439, 441, 442
Liotrix, 438, 439, 441, 442
Lipid pneumonia, 337
Liposyn, 236, 240
Lithium, 43, 51-53, 247
    and diabetes insipidus, 53
    and polyuria, 52-53
    treatment of mania, 52
Lithium carbonate, 43, 51, 52, 443
Lithium citrate, 43, 51, 52
Liver disease, as consideration, 3, 21, 40, 101, 222, 241, 287, 326, 340, 371, 545
Lomustine, 586, 587, 589, 590, 592
Loop diuretics, 203, 204, 206-211
Loperamide, 326, 327, 328
Lorazepam, 2, 11, 14

Loxapine, 24, 25, 266
Loxapine succinate, 34
Lubricants, 329, 334, 337
Lung, rheumatoid, 390
Luteinizing hormone (LH), 402, 408, 409, 410, 411
Luteotropic hormone (LTH), 402, 409, 410
Lymphoma, 414
Lypressin, 402, 403, 404, 406

M

Mafenide acetate, 497, 534, 538, 540-541
Magaldrate, 310, 312
Magnesium carbonate, 310, 312
Magnesium citrate, 329, 334, 337
Magnesium hydroxide, 310, 312, 329, 334
Magnesium oxide, 310, 312
Magnesium phosphate, 310, 312
Magnesium salicylate, 382, 384
Magnesium sulfate, 132, 329, 334
Magnesium sulfate solution, 236, 237, 238, 241, 246
Magnesium trisilicate, 310, 312
Malaria, 570-571, 580
Mannitol, 136, 144, 145, 203, 222-224, 593
    and kanamycin, 224
MAO Inhibitors, 49-51, 77, 160, 196, 301, 358
    dosage and administration, 50
    for treatment of phobias, 50
Maprotiline, 43, 48
Mazindol, 54, 63, 64, 67
Mebendazole, 569, 574, 575, 576, 578, 581
Mecamylamine, 178, 246
Mechlorethamine, 586, 587, 588, 591
Meclizine hydrochloride, 316, 319
Meclofenamate sodium monohydrate, 382, 383, 386
Medroxyprogesterone, 462, 463, 611, 612, 613, 615
Medrysone, 412, 420

Index 699

Mefenamic acid, 370, 371, 372
Megestrol, 462, 463, 611, 612, 613, 615
Melphalan, 586, 588, 590, 591
Menadiol sodium diphosphate, 270, 279, 280, 281, 283
Menadione, 270, 279, 280, 284
Menadione sodium busulfite, 270, 279, 280, 281, 282
Meningitis, 521
Menotropins, 465, 466, 467, 468
Menstrual cramps, 382
Mepenzolate bromide, 300, 304
Meperidine, 71, 72, 73, 75, 77, 80, 328
Mephentermine, 157, 159, 160, 161
Mephentermine sulfate, 156
Mephenytoin, 91, 95
Mephobarbital, 91, 93, 94
Mepivacaine, 148, 149, 152
Meprobamate, 18, 19, 21, 458
Mercaptomerin sodium, 203, 224, 225
Mercaptopurine, 399, 596, 597, 598
Mersalyl with theophylline, 203, 224, 225, 226
Mesoridazine, 25, 42
Mesoridazine besylate, 24, 28
Mestranol, 472, 473
Metaproterenol sulfate, 342, 346, 348, 349
Metaraminol, 157, 160, 161, 162, 164, 196
Metaraminol bitartrate, 156, 159
Methacycline HCl, 496, 518, 519
Methadone, 71, 73, 75, 82
Methamphetamine, 54, 56, 59, 458
Methandriol, 489, 490
Methandrostenolone, 489
Methantheline bromide, 300, 305
Methazolamide, 136, 144, 203, 218, 220
Methdilazine hydrochloride, 375, 376, 379

Methicillin sodium, 496, 498, 499, 501, 504
Methimazole, 438, 443, 446
Methisazone, 562, 563, 567
Methixene hydrochloride, 300, 306
Methocarbamol, 108, 116, 117, 119
Methohexital, 86, 87, 88
Methotrexate, 296, 540, 596-597, 598, 601
Methoxamine, 156, 157, 159, 160, 162
Methoxyflurane, 83, 84
Methscopolamine bromide, 300, 303
Methsuximide, 91, 92, 96
Methycyclothiazide, 213
Methyldopa, 176, 178, 180, 185, 187, 189, 191, 197
Methylergonovine maleate, 478, 480
Methylphenidate, 54, 56-57, 59, 62
Methylprednisolone, 412, 420
Methyltestosterone, 458, 484, 485, 487
Methyprylon, 17, 18, 20
Metoclopramide, 300, 301, 302, 307, 308, 316, 317, 323, 594
Metocurine, 122, 128, 129
Metocurine iodide, 130
Metolazone, 203, 211, 214
Metoprolol, 176, 177, 181, 193
Metronidazole, 569, 571, 573, 576, 578, 581-582
Metyrapone, 412, 416, 422
Metyrosine, 179
Mezlocillin sodium, 496, 498, 503, 504
Miconazole, 552, 558, 559, 560
Miconazole nitrate, 552, 553, 555, 557
Microseal Drug Delivery System (MDD), 171
Migraine, 193, 470
Milontin, 96

700   Pocket Nurse Guide to Drugs

Mineral oil, 329, 334, 335, 337
Mineralocorticoids, 412, 413, 416, 422
Minimum alveolar concentration (MAC), 84
Minocycline HCl, 496, 518, 519, 520, 521
Minoxidil, 176, 179, 180, 186, 189, 198
Miotic drugs, and blurred vision, 146
Mithramycin, 602-603, 604, 606
Mitomycin, 586, 587, 589, 590, 595
Mitotane, 611, 612, 613, 615, 616
Molidone, 24, 25
Monoamine Oxidase (MA) inhibitors, 43
Monosodium phosphate, 329, 334
Morphine, 71, 72, 73, 75
Motion sickness, 375
Mountain sickness, 205
Moxalactam disodium, 496, 508, 509, 510
Mucolytic drugs, 362, 363, 366
Muscle relaxants,
    and CNS depressants, 117
    centrally acting, 108
    dosage and administration, 118-119
Muscle spasms, 108, 116, 117
    drugs to treat, 118-119
Multiple sclerosis, 117
Mumps, 562, 564
Myasthenia gravis, 122-128, 530
    diagnosis of, 130
Myasthenic crisis, 123
Myasthenic vs. cholinergic crisis, differentiation of, 124, 126, 127
Mycobacteria, 544-545
Mycoplasmic diseases, 511
Mycosis fungoides, 413
Mydriasis, 136-141
    producing drugs, 136-141
    and cycloplegia producing drugs, dosage and administration, 138-140

Myoglobin, 291
Mysoline, 93
Myoclonic seizures, 92, 100

N

Nadolol, 176, 177, 180
Nafcillin sodium, 496, 498, 499, 501, 504
Nalbuphine, 71, 73, 75, 77
Nalidixic acid, 497, 541, 542, 543
    and false urine test results, 543
Naloxone, 81-82
Naloxone hydrochloride, 71, 80, 81
Naltrexone, 71, 80, 81, 82
Nandrolone decanoate, 489, 490
Nandrolone phenpropionate, 489, 490
Naphazoline hydrochloride, 358, 359, 360
Naproxen, 382, 383, 386, 389
Naproxen sodium, 382, 383, 386, 389
Narcolepsy, 54, 55, 57
Narcotic analgesics, 71-80, 301, 317, 381
    abuse, 77
    and antagonists, 71-82
    and CNS depressants, 80
    and cough suppression, 79
    and respiratory depression, 79
    dosage and administration, 74-76
    endorphin-like, 71
    in treatment of pain, 73
    tolerance and dependency, 72
Narcotic antagonists, 71, 80-82
    and respiratory depression, 82
    dosage and administration, 81
Narcotic dependency, 77
Narcotic overdose, 72
Nausea and vomiting, drugs to control, 24-25
Neisseria gonorrhoea, 498
Neisseria meningitis, 498

Index 701

Neomycin, 496, 497, 523, 524, 527, 534
Neostigmine, 122, 123, 126, 127, 129
    antidote for Curare, 128
    and atropine, 127
Neostigmine bromide, 122, 124-125
Neostigmine methylsulfate, 122, 125, 300, 301, 302, 307, 308, 309
    muscarinic side effects, 125
Nephrotic edema, 414
Netilmicin, 497, 523, 525, 526, 528
Neurohypophyseal hormones, 402-408
    dosage and administration, for diabetes insipidus, 406-407
Neuromuscular blocking drugs, 122, 128-133
    and antibiotics, 132
    dosage and administration, 130-131
    effect on breathing, 128-129, 132
    not to be used as anesthetics, 129, 132
    prolonging the effects of, 132
    reversal of effects, 129
Niacin, 285, 286, 287, 289-290
    increasing effects of anti-hypertensives, 289
Niclosamide, 569, 575, 576, 578
Nicotinic acid, 285, 286, 289
Nicotinyl alcohol, 156, 172, 173, 174
Nifedipine, 176, 179, 186, 189, 199-200
Nitrofurantoin, 497, 541, 542, 543
Nitrogen mustard, 586
Nitroglycerin, 156, 164, 166, 168, 228, 229
Nitroglycerin ointment, 167
Nitroprusside, 179, 189
Nitroprusside overdose, treatment of, 201

Nitrous oxide, 83, 84, 85
Nocardia, 535, 541
Nondepolarizing drugs, 122, 130-131
Norepinephrine, 265
    drugs interfering with storage or release, 176, 183-184, 188
Norethindrone, 462, 463, 469, 472, 473
Norethindrone acetate, 469, 472-473
Norethynodrel, 469, 473
Norgestrel, 469, 473
Normeperidine, 72
Nortriptyline, 43, 44, 47
Noscapaine, 362, 365
Novobiocin, 496, 511, 513, 517
Nylidrin, 156, 171, 172, 173, 174
Nystatin, 552, 558, 559, 561

O

Obesity, 54, 63, 439, 460
Opioids, 72
    antidiarrheal, 326-328
Opium tincture, 326, 327, 328
Optic neuritis, 414
Opto-Tropinal, 138
Organomercurials, 203, 224-227
    and mercury poisoning, 226
    dosage and administration, 225
Organophosphorus pesticides, 132
Orphenadrine, 108, 112, 116, 117, 119
Osmotic agents, 136, 141, 144, 146
Osmotic diuretics, 203, 204, 222-224
Osteoarthritis, 382
Osteoporosis, 489
Ototoxic drugs, 381
Ouabain, 228, 231, 232, 235, 252, 253, 257
Oxacillin sodium, 496, 498, 499, 501-502, 504

702 **Pocket Nurse Guide to Drugs**

Oxandrolone, 489, 490
Oxazepam, 2, 11, 15
Oxazolidinediones, 91, 97
Oxicam, 386
Oxtriphylline, 342, 350, 353
Oxycodone, 71, 73, 75, 78
Oxymetazoline hydrochloride, 358, 360
Oxymetholone, 489, 490
Oxymorphone, 71, 73, 76
Oxyphenbutazone, 382, 383, 385, 387, 493
Oxyphencyclimine hydrochloride, 300, 301, 305, 307
Oxyphenonium bromide, 300, 305
Oxyphenbutazone, 488, 493
Oxytetracycline HCl, 496, 518, 519, 521
Oxytocic drugs, 478-481
    dosage and administration, 479-480
Oxytocin, 402, 403, 478, 479, 480-481

P

Paget's disease, 449
Pain, 73, 77-78, 85
PAM, 146
Pancreatectomy, 338
Pancreatic antagonist, 611, 615
Pancreatic cancer, 338
Pancreatin, 338, 339, 340
Pancreatitis, 77, 338
Pancrelipase, 338, 339, 340
Pancuronium, 122, 128, 129
Pancuronium bromide, 130
Panhypopituitarism, 409
Papaverine, 156, 171, 172, 173, 174
Para-aminosulicylic acid (PAS), 497, 544, 545, 547, 548, 550
Parachlorobenzoic acid, 382, 385
Paracoccidioides, 553
Paraldehyde, 91, 100, 101, 102, 103, 106
    reaction with plastic, 106
    rectal, 93

Paralytic ileus, 113
Paramethadione, 91, 97
Paramethasone, 412, 420
Parasites, drugs for, 569-584
    side effects, 578-579
Parathyroid, drugs affecting, 438-451
Parathyroid hormone, 438, 448, 449, 450, 451
Paregoric, 326, 327, 328
Parkinsonism, drugs to control, 108-116
    dosage and administration, 110-112
Parkinson's disease, 465, 468, 530, 563
Partial thromboplastin time (PTT), 275, 276
Pellagra, 290
Pelvic endometriosis, 454
Pemoline, 54, 56, 57, 60, 62
Pemphigus, 413
Penicillamine, 390, 391, 392, 393, 394
Penicillin G, 496, 497, 500
Penicillin V, 496, 497, 498, 500, 531
Penicillins, 496, 497-505
    antipseudomonas, 496, 498, 503
    biosynthesized, 496, 497, 500
    broad spectrum, 496, 498, 502
    cross-sensitivity with penicillamine, 394
    dosage and administration, 500-503
    Penicillinase-resistant, 496, 498, 499, 501-502
    repository, 496, 498, 500
    substitutes, 496, 511-518
        dosage and administration, 512-514
Pentaerythritol tetranitrate, 156, 164, 167
Pentazocine, 72, 73, 77

Index   703

Pentazocine hydrochloride, 71, 76
Pentazocine lactate, 71, 76
Pentobarbital, 2, 5, 6
Pentoxifylline, 156, 171, 172, 173, 174
Peptic ulcer, 301
Perphenazine, 24, 25, 30, 316, 321
Petit mal seizures, 92
Phendimetrazine, 67
Phendimetrazine tartrate, 54, 63, 65
Phenelzine sulfate, 43, 49, 50
Phenindione, 270, 273
Phenmetrazine, 67
Phenobarbital, 2, 5, 7, 91, 92, 94, 101, 102, 190, 247, 311, 314, 389
Phenobarbital sodium, 93
Phenolphthalein, 329, 333
Phenothiazene, 301
Phenothiazines, 24-42
    aliphatic, 24, 26-28
Phenoxybenzamine, 177, 188, 194
Phenoxybenzamine hydrochloride, 176, 183
Phenprocoumon, 270, 273
Phensuximide, 91, 92, 93, 96
Phentermine, 54, 63, 65, 67
Phentolamine, 162, 177, 188, 194
Phentolamine hydrochloride, 176, 182
Phentolamine mesylate, 176, 182
Phenylbutazone, 266, 382, 383, 385, 387, 435, 461, 488
Phenylephrine, 42, 157, 160, 196, 263
Phenylephrine hydrochloride, 136, 137, 140, 156, 159, 358, 360-361
Phenyloxybutazone, 493
Phenylpropanolamine, 67
Phenylpropanolamine hydrochloride, 54, 63, 65, 358, 361
Phenylpropionic acid derivatives, 382, 386

Phenytoin, 91, 92, 93, 95, 101, 102, 104, 193, 252, 253, 254, 258, 262, 264, 266, 269, 311, 314, 461, 523, 548
    cardiac effects, 105
Pheochromocytoma, 180, 182, 196
Physostigmine, 145
Physostigmine salicylate, 136, 142
Physostigmine sulfate, 136, 142
Phytonadione, 270, 279, 280, 281, 282, 283, 284
Pilocarpine, 141
    sustained release, 147
Pilocarpine nitrate, 136, 142
Pindolol, 176, 177, 181, 193
Pinworms, 574, 577
Piperacetazine, 24, 25, 28
Piperacillin sodium, 496, 498, 503
Piperazine, 24, 29-31, 569, 574, 576, 577, 578, 582
Piperidine, 24, 28
Piroxicam, 382, 383, 386, 389
Pituitary glands, drugs affecting, 402-411
Plantago seed, 329, 332
Plasma, 236, 237, 239, 247-249
    protein fraction, 236, 237, 239, 247-249
Pneumocytosis, 573
Pneumonia, 511
Poliomyelitis, 562, 564
Polycarbophil, 329, 332
Polyestradiol phosphate, 611, 612, 614
Polymyxins, 132, 497, 532-534
Polymyxin B sulfate, 497, 532, 533, 534
Polystyrene sulfonate, 245
Polythiazide, 203, 211, 213
Pork roundworms, 575
Porphyria, drugs to treat, 24
Posterior pituitary extract, 402, 403, 404, 406
Post-menopausal symptoms, 454
Potassium chloride solution, 236, 237, 238, 241, 243-245

704 Pocket Nurse Guide to Drugs

Potassium citrate, 398
Potassium iodide, 362, 363, 364, 443, 444, 447
Potassium-sparing diuretics, 203, 204, 216-218
Povidone iodine, 569, 572, 576, 578, 582
Pralidoxime (PAM), 146
Pramoxine hydrochloride, 148, 151
Prazepam, 2, 11
Prazosin, 176, 177, 180, 183, 188, 194-195
Prednisolone, 412, 420
Prednisone, 412, 420, 611, 612, 613, 615
Pregnancy, labor, and lactation, as consideration, 4, 16, 40, 44, 49, 63, 71, 101, 103, 160, 175, 180, 193, 196, 198, 215, 216, 246, 269, 271, 282, 285, 296, 301, 311, 312, 330, 348, 351, 376, 383, 391, 416, 435, 444, 455, 462, 464, 465, 469, 484, 490, 515, 520, 523, 530, 541, 553, 576, 597-603, 608, 612
Prilocaine, 148, 149, 152
Primaquine, 569, 572, 576, 577, 579, 582
Primidone, 91, 93, 95, 101, 102
Probenecid, 395, 396, 397, 398-399
Probucol, 285, 287, 290
Procainamide, 219, 252, 253, 255, 260, 263, 264, 268
  in hypotension, 263
Procaine, 149, 152
Procaine Penicillin G, 496, 498, 500, 505
Procarbazine hydrochloride, 596, 597, 599, 601
Prochlorperazine, 24, 25, 30, 316, 321
Prochlorperazine edisylate, 30, 316, 321
Prochlorperazine maleate, 316, 321

Procyclidine hydrochloride, 108, 111
Progesterone, 462, 463
Progestins, 455, 462-464, 469, 611, 615, 616
Proketazine Maleate, 29
Prolactin, 402, 409, 410, 411, 465
Promazine, 25
Promazine hydrochloride, 316, 317, 321
Promethazine hydrochloride, 316, 319, 375, 377, 380
Propantheline bromide, 300, 305
Proparacaine, 148, 149, 151
Propoxyphene, 73, 78
Propoxyphene hydrochloride, 71, 76
Propoxyphene napsylate, 71, 76, 106
Propylhexedrine, 358, 359, 361
Propylthiouracil, 438, 443, 445, 446
Prostaglandins, 382
Protamine sulfate, 276
Protamine zinc insulin suspension, 426, 429
Protirelin, thyrotropin releasing hormone, 438, 439, 441
Proteus, 541
Prothombin time (PT), 277, 284
Protriptyline, 44
Protriptyline hydrochloride, 43, 47
Propranolol, 160, 176, 177, 182, 193, 233, 252, 253, 255, 260-261, 265, 267, 269, 311, 314
Propranolol hydrochloride, 438, 443, 444, 445, 446
Pseudomonas aeruginosa, 499, 525, 532, 535
Pseudoephedrine, 246
Pseudoephedrine hydrochloride, 358, 361
Pseudoephedrine sulfate, 358, 361
Psoriasis, 413, 601
Psoriatic arthritis, 414
Psychomotor seizures, 93

Index 705

Psyllium hydrocolloid, 329, 332
Psyllium hydrophilic mucilloid, 329, 332
Pulmonary edema, 205
Pulmonary fibrosis, 415
Pupil, dilated, 136-141
Purpura, 375
Pyramethamine, 296
Pyrantel pamoate, 569, 574, 575, 576, 579
Pyrazinamide, 497, 544, 547, 548
Pyridine hydrochloride, 115
Pyridostigmine, 122, 125, 126, 129
Pyridostigmine bromide, 122, 125
Pyridoxine, 394, 548
Pyrilamine maleate, 375, 377, 380
Pyrimethamine, 569, 572, 573, 576, 579, 582-583
Pyrrole, derivative of parachlorbenzoic acid, 382, 385
Pyrvinium pamoate, 569, 574, 576, 579, 582-583

Q

Quinacrine, 569, 573, 576, 577, 583-584
Quinestrol, 454, 457
Quinethazone, 203, 211, 214
Quinidine, 132, 196, 219, 311
    and hypotension, 268
Quinidine gluconate, 252, 253, 254, 259, 263, 264, 267-268
Quinidine polygalacturonate, 252, 253, 254, 260, 263, 264, 267-268
Quinidine sulfate, 252, 253, 254, 259, 263, 264, 267-268
Quinine, 246, 311, 569, 571, 572, 576, 579, 584

R

Rabies, 562, 563, 565
Radioactive iodine, 438, 443, 444, 445, 447

Ranitidine, 310, 311, 313, 315
Rauwolfia, 176, 183, 196
Relaxants, skeletal muscle, 116-121
Renal disease, as consideration, 3, 16, 21, 129, 241, 287, 311, 317, 371, 383, 388, 391, 395, 490, 510, 545
Rescinnamine, 176, 184
Reserpine, 176, 178, 180, 183, 187, 188, 196-197, 233
Respiratory stimulation, 54, 55
Reye's syndrome, 325, 371
Rheumatoid arthritis, 382, 414
    drugs to treat, 390-394
Rhinitis, 375
Rickettsiae, 521
Rifampin, 461, 497, 544, 545, 546, 548, 549-550, 551
Ringer's solution, 163, 210, 236, 237, 238, 448
    lactated, 236, 237, 238, 247, 282
Rubramin PC, 297

S

Salbutamol, 342, 343, 349
Salicylamide, 370, 372
Salicylates, 207, 219, 247, 370-374, 382, 384, 399, 435
Saline, hypertonic, 236, 237, 238
Saline, hypotonic, 238
Saline, isotonic, 236, 238
Salsalate, 382, 384
Saralasin, 179, 200
Sarcoidosis, 415
Schizophrenia, drugs to treat, 33
Scopolamine, 137, 316, 318
Scopolamine hydrobromide, 136, 139, 316, 318
Secobarbital, 2, 5
Sedative-hypnotics, 80
Sedative-hypnotics and Anti-anxiety agents,
    dependence and tolerance, 3
    dosages and preparations, 20-21

706   **Pocket Nurse Guide to Drugs**

Sedatives, 191, 376
Seizures, 50, 103
  drugs to treat, 92
Senna concentrate, 329, 330, 333
Senna pod, 329, 330
Senna, whole leaf, 329, 330, 334
Sennosides A & B, 329, 334
Serratia, 541
Serum sickness, 413
SGOT, 121
Shigella, 535
Shock, 157
Silver sulfadiazine, 497, 534, 538, 540-541
Sleeping medications, 301, 317
Smallpox, 562, 565
Smallpox vaccination, 422
Sodium bicarbonate, 398
Sodium bicarbonate overdose, treatment of, 246
Sodium bicarbonate solution, 236, 237, 238, 246-247
Sodium iodide, 438, 443, 444, 447
Sodium nitrite, 201
Sodium nitroprusside, 176, 180, 187, 188, 201, 228, 229
Sodium phosphate, 329, 334
  with sodium biphosphate, 329, 334
Sodium salicylate, 370, 372, 382, 384
Sodium thiosalicylate, 382, 384-385
Sodium thiosulfate, 201, 591
Somatropin, 410
Sorbitol, 245
Spasms, 108, 116
Spasticity, 108, 116
Spasticity, drugs to treat, 118
Spectinomycin, 496, 511, 513, 516, 517
Spinal cord injury, 117
Spirochetes, 519
Spironolactone, 203, 216, 217, 218
Sprue, 415

Stanozolol, 489, 491
Staphydococcus aureas, 498, 511
Status epilepticus, 11, 93, 94, 100, 101, 102
Steroids, 207, 234
Stevens-Johnson syndrome, 540
STH, 410
Streptococcus pneumonia, 498
Streptokinase, 270, 277, 278-279, 281
Streptokinase, effects of streptococcal infection on, 279
Streptomycin, 497, 523, 524, 527, 531, 544, 545, 546, 548, 550
Streptozocin, 611, 612, 613, 615, 617
Stroke, 117
Succinimides, 91, 96, 102, 105
  and oral hygiene, 105
Succinylcholine, 122, 128, 129, 131, 132
Succinylcholine chloride, 131
Sucralfate, 310, 311, 313, 315
  interfering with other drugs, 315
Sufenatil, 73
Sufentanil citrate, 71, 73, 76
Sulfacetamide, 497, 534, 539
Sulfacytine, 497, 534, 535, 536
Sulfadiazine, 497, 534, 535, 536, 569, 573, 579
Sulfadoxine and pyrimethamine, 569, 579
Sulfamerazine and sulfadiazine, 497, 534, 537-538
Sulfamerazine, sulfadiazine, and sulfomethazine, 497, 534, 537-538
Sulfamethizole, 497, 534, 535, 536
Sulfamethizole and phenazopyridine, 497, 534, 537-538, 540
Sulfamethoxazole, 497, 534, 535, 536
Sulfamethoxazole and phenazopyridine, 497, 534, 538

Index 707

Sulfamethoxazole and Trimethoprim, 497, 534, 535, 537, 569, 573, 579
Sulfaphenazole, 266
Sulfasalazine, 492, 534, 535, 536
Sulfinpyrazone, 395, 396-397, 398-399
Sulfinpyrazone, potentiation of hypoglecemic agents by, 398
Sulfisoxazole, 497, 534, 535, 536-537, 539
Sulfisoxazole and phenazopyridine, 497, 534, 538
Sulfonamides, 435, 497, 535-541
Sulfonylureas, 435
Sulfoxone sodium, 497, 551
Sulindac, 382, 383, 385, 388-389
Sulindac, effects on liver function tests, 388
Sympathetic nervous system depressants, 177
Sympathetic nervous system inhibitors, 176, 184, 189
Sympathomimetics, 233
  for hypotension and shock, 156-164
    dosage and administration, 158-159
Syphilis, 498
Systemic lupus erythematosus, 413
Sytobex, 297

T

Tamoxifen, 611, 612-613, 614, 616
Tapeworms, 575, 583
Tartrazine, 42, 45, 198, 245, 592
Temazepam, 2, 11, 15
Temporal lobe seizures, 93
Tenosynovitis, 414
Terbutaline sulfate, 342, 346-347, 348, 349
Terpin hydrate, 362, 364
Testolactone, 611-612, 614
Testosterone, 459, 484, 486

Testosterone cypionate, 458, 484, 486
Testosterone enanthate, 458, 484, 486
Testosterone propionate, 484, 486
Tetanus, drugs to treat, 24
Tetany, 247
Tetracaine, 148, 149, 152
Tetracaine hydrochloride, 148, 151
Tetracyclines, 132, 311, 315, 496, 518-521, 569-579
    dosage and administration, 518-519
Tetrahydrozaline hydrochloride, 358, 359, 361, 496, 518
Theophylline, 54, 66, 68, 69, 311, 314, 342, 350, 353
Theophylline ethylenediamine, 342, 350, 352
Theophylline monoethanolamine, 342, 350, 353
Theophylline sodium glycinate, 342, 350, 353
Thiabendazole, 569, 574, 575, 577, 579, 584
Thiamylal sodium, 83, 86, 88
Thiazide, 230
    and related diuretics, 203, 204, 211-216
    diuretics effect on parathyroid test, 215
Thiethylperazine maleate, 316, 321, 324
Thioamides, 443, 444
Thiocyanate, 202
Thioguanine, 596, 597, 598
Thiopental sodium, 83, 86, 88
Thioridazine, 24, 28
Thiordazine hydrochloride, 28
Thiothixene, 24, 25
Thiothixene hydrochloride, 32
Thioxanthenes, 24, 31-32, 301
Thiphenamil hydrochloride, 300, 306
Threadworms, 575
Thrombin, 270, 279, 281, 282

708 Pocket Nurse Guide to Drugs

Thrombocytopenia, 414
Thrombolytics, 270, 277-279
  dosage and administration, 278
Thyroglobulin, 438, 439, 440, 442
Thyroid, drugs affecting, 438-451
Thyroid-stimulating hormone (TSH), 402, 409, 410, 411, 438, 439, 441, 442, 443
Thyroid storm, 193
Thyroid U.S.P., 438, 439, 440, 442
Thyrotoxicosis, 193
Thyrotropin, 410
Ticarcillin disodium, 496, 498, 503, 504
Timolol, 141, 145, 146, 177, 193
Timolol maleate, 136, 143, 176, 182
Tobramycin, 497, 523, 525, 526, 528
Tolazamide, 426, 436
Tolazoline, 171, 172
Tolazoline hydrochloride, 156, 173, 174
Tolbutamide, 289, 423, 426, 436
Tolmetin, effects on liver function test, 388
Tolmetin sodium, 382, 383, 385-386, 388-389
Tolnaftate, 552, 558, 561
Tone, drugs affecting, 300-309
Tonic-clonic seizures, 92
Total Parenteral Nutrition (TPN), 249-250
Toxoplasmosis, 573, 580, 582
Tranquilizers, 78, 80, 301, 317
Transaminase, 199
Transdermal Infusion System (TIS), 170
Transdermal Therapeutic System (TTS), 170
Tranylcypromine sulfate, 49, 50
Travamulsion, 236, 240
Trazodone, 43, 48, 49
Trendelenburg position, 174

Treponema pallidum, 498
Triamcinolone, 412, 420
Triamcinolone acetonide, 342, 354, 355
Triamterene, 203, 216, 217, 218
Triazolam, 2, 11, 15
Trichlormethiazide, 203, 211, 213
Trichomoniasis, 572-573, 577
Triclofos sodium, 17, 18, 20
Tricyclic antidepressants, 43, 160, 219, 301, 358, 404
  anticholinergic effects, 44
  dosage and administration, 46-47
  toxicity, 44
Tridihexethyl chloride, 300, 305
Triethylenepthiophosphoramide, 586, 587, 588, 590
Trifluoperazine, 24, 25, 31
Triflupromazine, 24
Triflupromazine hydrochloride, 316, 321
Trifluridine, 562, 563, 566, 567
Trihexyphenidyl hydrochloride, 108, 111
Trimeprazine tartrate, 375, 376, 380
Trimethadione, 91, 92, 97, 103
Trimethaphan, 132, 178, 188, 189
Trimethaphan camsylate, 176, 180, 187, 202
Trimethobenzamide hydrochloride, 316, 317, 323, 325
Trimethoprim, 497, 541, 542, 543
Trimipramine, 44
Trimipramine maleate, 43, 47
Tripelennamine citrate, 375, 380
Tripelennamine hydrochloride, 375, 380
Triprolidine hydrochloride, 375, 377, 380
Tropicamide, 136, 137, 139
Trousseau's sign, 247, 448
Tuberculosis, drugs to treat, 497, 544-550
  dosage and administration, 546-547

Index 709

Tuberculosis, pulmonary, 415
Tubocurarine, 122, 128, 129, 132, 207, 211
Tubocurarine chloride, 130
Turbo-inhaler, 357
Typhoid fever, 521

U

Ulcers, drugs to treat, 310-315
    dosage and administration, 312-313
Ulcer crater coating, 310, 313, 315
Undecylenic acid, 552, 558, 561
Urea, 136, 144, 145, 203, 222-224
Urinary tract infections, drugs for, 497, 541-544
    dosage and administration, 542
Urokinase, 270, 278-279, 281
Urticaria, 375, 415

V

Vaccines, 562
Valproate, 266
Valproic acid, 91, 92, 100, 103, 107
    and false-positive ketone tests, 107
Vancomycin, 496, 511, 513, 516, 517
Vasculitis, 390
Vasodilators, 176, 179, 185, 189, 228, 229
    angiotensin converting enzyme inhibitor, 176, 186
    calcium channel blockers, 176, 186
    for peripheral vascular disease, 156,
    and hypotension, 174-175
        dosage and administration, 173
Vasopressin, 402, 403, 404, 406, 408

Vasopressin tannate, 402, 403, 404, 405, 406
Vasopressors, 194
Vecuronium, 122, 129, 131
Verapamil, 176, 179, 180, 186, 199, 252, 253, 254, 261, 265, 269
Vidarabine, 562, 563, 566, 567
Vinblastine sulfate, or VLB, 607, 608, 610
Vincristine sulfate, or VCR, 607, 608, 609
Virilization, 485
Vitamin B_6, 115
Vitamin B_{12}, 291, 296, 297, 531
Vitamin C, increasing absorption of iron, 294
Vitamin D, 438, 448, 449, 450, 451
Vitamin K_1, 270, 277, 279, 280, 282, 283, 284
Vitamin K_3, 270, 279, 280, 284
Vitamin K deficiency, 281

W

Warfarin, 270, 273, 274, 311, 314
Whipworms, 574
Wilms' tumor, 607
Wilson's disease, 393-394

X

Xanthines, 342, 350-354, 395
    dosage and administration, 352-353
Xylometazoline hydrochloride, 358, 359, 361

Y

Yellow fever, 562, 565

Z

Zollinger-Ellison syndrome, 310